D0887212

Stakeholder Health
Insights from New Systems of Health

Editors: Teresa F. Cutts and James R. Cochrane

Developed with Support from the Robert Wood Johnson Foundation

Stakeholder Health, c/o FaithHealth Division, Wake Forest Medical Baptist Center, Medical Center Blvd., Winston-Salem, NC 27157

ISBN: 978-0-692-70728-9

Editors: Teresa F. Cutts and James R. Cochrane
Cover Picture: Community Members, North Carolina Event, 2016
Suggested Citation: Cutts, T. & Cochrane, J.R., Editors (2016). *Stakeholder Health: Insights from New Systems of Health.* USA: Stakeholder Health Press.

Graphic Designer: Kelli Smith

Printed in the United States of America

This book is printed on archival-quality paper that meets requirements of the American National Standard for Information Sciences, Permanence of Paper, Printed Library Materials, ANSI Z39.48-1984.

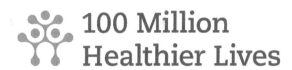 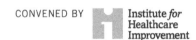

CONVENED BY 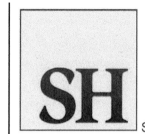 Institute *for* Healthcare Improvement

Stakeholder Health

March 31, 2016

Dear Colleagues:

I am delighted to write a letter of introduction and commendation for this second Stakeholder Health offering to our field: Insights from New Systems of Health.

As Lead Transformative Adviser and former Vice President of Patient Centered Medical Home Development at Cambridge Health Alliance and Executive Lead,100 Million Healthier Lives at the Institute for Healthcare Improvement, I am constantly involved in the gritty, illuminating and challenging work of trying to improve health, well-being and equity in our country and across the globe. I am honored to be a part of the Stakeholder Health movement and to have the members of Stakeholder Health as partners in the 100 Million Healthier Lives movement.

As stewards in this shared movement together, we recognize that to truly improve health, we need to embrace that health is created by the mental, physical, social and spiritual dimensions of our lives interacting together in a beautiful and complex whole–and that it is created in the context of community. In addition, we believe it is not possible to move the needle on health outcomes for the population without a dedicated focus on health equity. In a country where two children growing up two miles apart can expect a 25 year difference in life expectancy, this is both a practical and a moral imperative. We cannot improve our health rankings in the world without improving the well-being of those who aren't thriving; by unleashing the trapped and untapped potential of our most vulnerable and marginalized residents, we have the potential to create wholeness in our communities and in our country. In a shrinking world where the developing world and the developed world coexist in our own hearts, in our communities and around the globe, it is a deep recognition of our interconnectedness as a human family that offers us the opportunity to create the beloved community envisioned by Dr. Martin Luther King Jr.

Stakeholder Health's movement has been dedicated to creating this wholeness in our communities since its inception. Stakeholder Health's members are unabashedly focused on care for the poor and marginalized and are not afraid to embrace their faith and/or missional heritage and responsibilities for caring for all. They constantly focus on pushing the language and traditional views of the field on health and health care far beyond the comfort zone of most health systems. As other health systems begin the journey to population health, this narrative, along with the real world examples of what it means to walk on this journey to whole person, whole community health and well-being, is critically needed.

This book offers a rich and detailed review of some of the best and most promising work being done to build health system and community partnerships. From a new platform for how to re-invent the electronic medical or health record to reflect the person's journey of health (vs. a billing or service delivery capture) to disruptive leadership practices to adapt to our chaotic times to how trauma-informed care to building resiliency and mental health prevention efforts can be implemented both within and across health systems and the broader community, I found the book to be chockful of illuminating examples that help create a path for health systems on the journey. It serves as both a fantastic resource guide and a thoughtful and delightfully written "textbook" for community health improvement that appeals to a broad audience: those working clinically, operationally and administratively inside health systems, in faith and other communities, as well as in public health and other clinical settings.

In short, I highly recommend this book to all readers who care deeply about growing health, well-being, equity, justice and interconnectedness in our broader world. I hope that it serves as a useful resource guide for you, whatever your role in health and health care is, whatever your specific aims or passions are. It has deeply enriched our path in 100 Million Healthier Lives; we look forward to growing into the lessons learned and invite you to contribute to the next stage of the path.

Together,

Somava Saha Stout, MD MS
Executive Lead, 100 Million Healthier Lives
Institute for Healthcare Improvement

Table of Contents

Acknowledgments

Stakeholder Health is deeply indebted to the Robert Wood Johnson Foundation, for funding this book and its future dissemination. We particularly wish to thank our program officer, Amy Slonim and her team, for their graciousness and help in getting this book to print. Eileen Barsi deserves special praise for her critical copy editing efforts on the whole book. Lastly, we wish to thank our Stakeholder Health sponsoring organizations, 44 contributing authors and all the members of Stakeholder Health with whom we have co-created and learned since 2011.

Introduction

Teresa Cutts, Gerald Winslow, Gary Gunderson,
Kirsten Peachey and Marice Ashe

Welcome to the second generation of learning from Stakeholder Health! Stakeholder Health is a voluntary movement of people working within health care systems who see an opportunity to address the underlying causes of poor health in our communities. We are committed to **open source learning** and **a shared mission which we initially** articulated in an 80-page monograph, presented to senior leadership at the Dept. of Health and Human Services in April 2013. In it, we outlined a framework for the health outcomes of the broader population, including its most vulnerable citizens, by strategically shifting existing resources and partnering with diverse stakeholders. We believe in:

> **Addressing the social complexity of the most challenging patients** by engaging them **at the "neighborhood" level,** working **with large-scale community partnerships,** and **proactively using existing resources** such as charity care or community health assets.

(For more details on our over 50 health system and other partners and scope/scale of our work, see Appendix 1: Stakeholder Health: Our Story.)

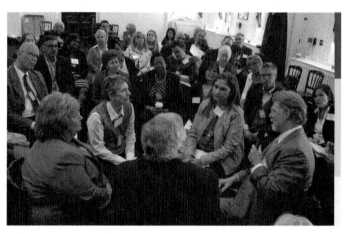

White House Partners in Health Meeting, April 2015, Washington, DC.

This second book is intended to serve as a guidebook for those of us working inside health systems. We wrote it to raise awareness of the power of the "social determinants of health" as predictors of health outcomes, and to foster aspirations for how health systems can better address these determinants (the focus of Chapter Two). However, while we continue to use the expression "social determinants of health" in this learning document, we also wonder if this language best serves our vision. By calling the many external factors that impact health, "determinants" do we foster an attitude of inevitability? The settled conviction of the members of Stakeholder Health is that social variables that often have devastating effects on health, can be and should be understood, addressed, and ameliorated. One of the signature characteristics of the movement represented by Stakeholder Health is a willingness to challenge conventional language and the conceptual frameworks that hinder rather than facilitate the health of whole communities. Stakeholder Health focuses on introducing new language intentionally; we want to expand and challenge the consciousness of health system audiences, governing bodies, public health and community practitioners and even faith communities, to see that they are all part of a broader system of health.

Stakeholder Health seeks to push the edge of innovation, always moving beyond "what is" current, standard practice and thinking in health systems and public health. We intend to be change agents. Many of our systems are faith-based (whether in name or tradition) and all are "mission-driven." We are committed to caring for the poor, marginalized and vulnerable: "the least of these." Therefore, in this

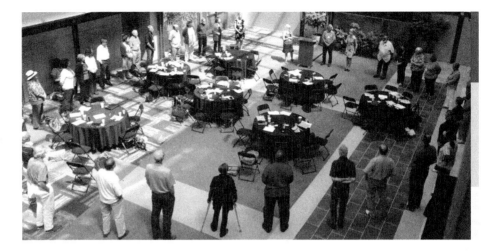

Chawumba Gathering, July 2014, Winston Salem, NC

book, you will find great detail about many promising practices that often receive cursory mention in other publications. We boldly claim the moral ground of social justice and a desire to achieve equity in the health of our nation's diverse communities.

In all these dimensions, Stakeholder Health and this book reflect a dynamic world of learning and practicing in healthcare and other realms. Forty-four contributors, often with very different voices, crafted the following chapters. As you read, you will encounter different and, at times, divergent voices, often from those operating on the margins of their named guilds and disciplines. Through a rich array of different lenses these authors have brought new clarity to the issues and topics addressed here. For example, while most chapters focus inside the boundaries of the U.S. health systems, Chapter Six, on community health asset mapping, brings in voices from our colleagues in Africa who trained many Stakeholder Health partners in their foundational process that was endorsed by the World Health Organization. So, too, you will note that Chapter Ten pushes explicitly to the outer edges of global health, broadly defined, to signal again that we are already beyond U.S. boundaries and limits in our learning about changing how health is fostered and healthcare is delivered.

Overall, our chapters seek to address these critical questions:

1) How should we think differently about and help improve social conditions in which our most vulnerable neighbors live?

2) How do we move toward establishing essential healthcare as a basic human right?

3) How do we help achieve health and other types of equity in our communities?

4) How do we use our positional authority and work in health systems to engage hearts and spirits of our local communities, as well as of our own employees?

5) How do we creatively and sustainably move health outcomes and the delivery of healthcare upstream in an environment with constrained resources?

The original Stakeholder Health monograph went about as far as one could in addressing these questions before the Affordable Care Act was firmly in place. As workers and leaders in the institutions most affected by that legislation, we were quite aware of the highly negotiated—most would say "compromised"—nature of those thousands of pages of small print. Many in the field did not even think it would survive review by the Supreme Court. But once it did and as enrollments proceeded on a remarkable scale, we now focus on the terrain on which the Affordable Care Act must not only take root, but flourish. Of course, the terrain differs quite radically depending on whether one lives in a "Medicaid expansion state" or a state pushing far into the land of creative "waivers," so our tactics must be varied and nuanced to be relevant to local conditions. We wrote this book to outline a vision of what is possible now, here, and with the institutions and array of assets at hand with which we can weave a new future for all people across our oft divided nation.

Therefore, we offer you a treasure trove of both practice and vision for innovative ideas and work from our very own health systems and other partners. Chapter Two sets the stage for the integrative thread of social determinants of health, laying a foundation for what follows. Chapter Three is on leadership, offering a blueprint of unique ways of both thinking and doing that are required in these dynamic times in the healthcare landscape. Chapter Four offers a comprehensive overview of relational information technology; it follows a person's journey of health, rather than suggesting an IT system devoted to supporting billing or service delivery alone. Chapter Five delves into a variety of community health navigation programs and systems, with a very deep dive into the work and everyday lives of community health workers.

Chapter Six gives a granular review of community asset mapping models, the theory driving why such mapping is important, as well as implications for work with health systems and building communities with a focus on achieving health, equity and justice. Chapter Seven offers new community-based and community-driven resiliency models to help with the "healing of our land," reviewing why integrated behavioral health, both inside and outside of health systems, is essential. Chapter Eight expands beyond "return on investment" or even "social return on investment" to not only highlight even more robust and integrated financial accounting systems that enhance community health, but also illuminate the financial impact of community-based work within our health systems.

Chapter Nine brings an overview of philanthropic practices to help build a more systemic and integrated practice to funding and building community health improvement. Chapter Ten looks forward to the global health implications of our work and sets the stage for how the boundaries of Stakeholder Health expand beyond U.S. borders. Lastly, and perhaps most importantly, Chapter Eleven reminds us of our mission, purpose and power as health systems, invoking the heart of healthy communities.

This book is not likely to be our last, for the edge of our learning will continue to be revisited as we pass other key landmarks on the path to what science and faith can imagine. Even as we look to the future, we are compelled to be deeply accountable for what is possible now and here. Thus, the collaborative learning captured in these chapters is meant to be both immediately applicable to our current practice and turn on a bright light to guide our future vision. Our deepest hope is that this book will spur more authentic dialogue and productive action to promote mercy, grace and justice in our very chaotic and, often, unjust world.

Thanks in advance for reading with us. We hope you enjoy the journey and, if you aren't already part of our work, will become part of the kinship of Stakeholder Health.

FULL AUTHORSHIP LISTING

Teresa Cutts, PhD, Asst. Research Professor, Wake Forest School of Medicine, Div. of Public Health Science, Dept. of Social Sciences and Health Policy, Winston Salem, NC

Gerald Winslow, PhD, Vice President of Mission and Culture, Loma Linda University Health, Loma Linda, CA

Gary R. Gunderson, MDiv, DMin, DTh (Hon), Vice President of FaithHealth, Wake Forest Baptist Medical Center, Professor, Faith and Health of the Public, Wake Divinity School and Wake Forest School of Medicine, Winston Salem, NC

Kirsten Peachey, MDiv, MSW, DMin, Director, Congregational Health Partnerships and Co-Director, The Center for Faith and Community Health Transformation, Advocate Health Care, Chicago, IL

Marice Ashe, JD, MPH, Founder and CEO, ChangeLab Solutions, Oakland, CA

For more information about this chapter, please contact **Teresa Cutts** at e-mail, cutts02@gmail.com or phone, (901) 643-8104.

CHAPTER 2

A Systems Thinking Approach to the Social Determinants of Health

Marice Ashe with Dora Barilla, Eileen Barsi and Stephanie Cihon

In our last monograph, Stakeholder Health (SH) described the "social determinants of health" in terms of providing "integrated care for socially complex people in socially complex neighborhoods" (Health Systems Learning Group, 2013). This acknowledged that the factors that have the greatest impact on health are not medical interventions or individual lifestyle choices, but instead arise from the environments in which we live, work and play. It also introduced the Social Ecological Model to focus attention on the environments (or the "places") that provide the socioeconomic, cultural and environmental conditions in which community health either thrives or fails.

Here we further explore the social determinants of health through the lens of systems thinking. Systems thinking is defined as a practice that takes a comprehensive approach to complex events or phenomena seemingly caused by a myriad of isolated, independent, and usually unpredictable factors or forces (Senge, 2006). It shifts the "mind from seeing parts to seeing wholes, from seeing people as helpless reactors to seeing them as active participants in shaping their reality, from reacting to the present to creating the future" (Senge, 2006, p. 69). So the essence of systems thinking lies in a shift of thinking to see interrelationships rather than linear cause-effect chains, and longer-term processes of change rather than simply snapshots in time.

Systems thinking reflects four fundamental characteristics (Peterson, 2010):

- *Dynamism*: Multiple specific phenomena evolve in relation to each other. Rather than seeing only isolated events (e.g., asthma, graduation, and employment rates), systems thinkers see the patterns of relationship (e.g., how unemployment is connected to higher school absences due to uncontrolled childhood asthma). When these patterns of relationship are projected over time, the historic data can be used to make predictions for the future.

- *Complexity*: Besides numerous stakeholders being involved in a living system, its full complexity lies in its ever-evolving and partially non-predictable adaptation to new circumstances and its patterns of resilience that are self-preserving, self-organizing and goal-seeking in expressing its integrity or wholeness (Meadows, 2008). The challenge to the systems thinker, while embracing the unpredictable, is to find mutuality despite the diverse, divergent or siloed interests of those involved, as these key characteristics of a system emerge.

- *Interdependency*: Seemingly isolated phenomena actually are intimately connected and influence each other over time.

- *Hard to communicate*: Words are often inadequate for explaining dynamic problems driven by the interdependency of multiple players with diverse interests.

Systems thinkers look for patterns of interaction among complex phenomena in order to better understand, analyze and articulate the current effectiveness of a system, and to diagnose how the system can be improved over time (see also Chapter 10 in this document for further discussion on complexity and "complex living systems").

Systems Thinking and Population Health

Every effective hospital administrator knows that a well-run hospital has multiple service lines, existing within even larger complex systems, that must interact efficiently to achieve the best outcomes for both patients and employees. In fact, a single glitch in the system—a laboratory test that is late or provides inaccurate results—can have ripple effects across the whole care-delivery apparatus. The most successful administrators ensure that attention is given to even the relatively small problems (such as under-staffed laboratory services), in service of the interdependent functions and smooth functioning throughout the entire hospital.

Likewise, a person's health is rooted in those broader complex systems, too. It is now widely accepted that the environment has the greatest impact on health outcomes across populations. We will refer to the following case study related to childhood asthma throughout this chapter. Asthma is an

CASE STUDY: CHILDHOOD ASTHMA
(ChangeLab Solutions, 2014)

Think of a child who is repeatedly hospitalized with uncontrolled asthma. Despite the best that medicine can offer, if the child lives in substandard housing with mold climbing walls and bed posts or with roaches or other vermin spreading asthma triggers, medical interventions alone will not prevent the continuous recurrence of disease. In fact, building code standards, tenants' legal rights, and the availability of healthy and affordable housing have a direct impact the child's health. To effectively address the asthma, these non-medical issues must become a central focus of attention. We could depict this relationship with a simple diagram:

POOR HOUSING ⇢ ASTHMA

Yet, we also know the impact of asthma on school attendance, which is directly related to educational achievement. In 2008, asthma accounted for approximately 14.4 million lost school days nationwide (American Lung Association, 2012). A study of over 9,000 students in a predominantly African American urban school district in St. Louis, Missouri found that students with any degree of asthma experienced, on average, 30 percent more absent days than those without asthma. Students with moderate to severe asthma experienced, on average, 4.3 times the number of absences of non-asthmatic children (Moonie, Sterling, Figgs, & Castro, 2006). In a study conducted in an inner-city school in Los Angeles, students with asthma missed, on average, two more days of school than children without asthma (Bonilla, Kehl, Kwong, Morphew, Kachru & Jones, 2005). Students who attended schools with the highest concentrations of low-income students were more likely to miss school because of asthma than those at schools with higher income students (Meng, Babey, & Wolstein, 2012).
We can now extend the diagram like this:

POOR HOUSING ⇢ ASTHMA ⇢ SCHOOL ABSENTEEISM

Further, we also know that chronic absenteeism leads to lower educational attainment (Thies, 1999), and this, in turn, has significant impacts on future employability, social capital, and psychological resiliency (Levine, 2003). We can expand our simple diagram to reflect multiple feedback loops and pathways, showing how poverty creates a systemic reality of increasingly poor health with a negative feedback loop (housing):

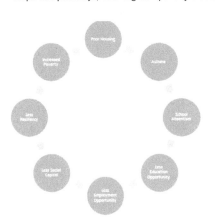

Of course, going even further, within the family, when a child is absent from school due to illness, a parent or guardian must be available to care for the child. Do the parents' jobs offer sick leave benefits? If not, must one of the parents take unpaid time away from work? Will his or her job be at risk if too many unpaid days are taken? Again, without basic prevention, the ripple effects of having a single child suffer from asthma have profound impacts on all aspects of family stability and economic achievement.

But even that is not all. There is a strong link between child poverty and other chronic health conditions beyond asthma:

- Children from families in poverty are more likely to be obese than their non-poor peers of the same age, of the same gender, and within the same geographic region (Centers for Disease Control and Prevention, 2015b; Singh, Siapush, & Kogan, 2010).

- Children from families in poverty are more likely to be identified as having developmental delays than their non-poor peers of the same age, of the same gender, and within the same geographic region (Brooks-Gunn & Duncan, 1997; Child Trends DataBank, 2013).

- Children from families in poverty are more likely to be identified as having learning disabilities than their non-poor peers of the same age, of the same gender, and within the same geographic region (Brooks-Gunn & Duncan, 1997).

increasingly common disease, found in all income groups but significantly more common in children living in poverty. It provides a rich landscape to illustrate the Triple Aim of improved experience of care, reducing per capita cost of care, and improving the health of populations (Bisognano & Kenney, 2014), and to point to SH's addition of a fourth ("quadruple") aim of equity.

What are the Social Determinants of Health?

The World Health Organization states that the "social determinants of health" reflect the conditions in which people are born, grow, live, work and age (World Health Organization, 2015). Healthy People 2020 highlights the importance of addressing the social determinants of health as one of the overarching national population health goals of the current decade (Secretary's Advisory Committee on National Health Promotion and Disease Prevention, 2010). The CDC gives deeper meaning to this definition when it calls upon health leaders to advance health equity by addressing the social determinants of health (Marmot, 2007; Williams, Costa, Odunlami, & Mohammed, 2008).

As the asthma case study above illustrates, the most basic conditions of everyday life—like the structural quality of the family home, or whether the parents have jobs with leave benefits to care for their sick children—have overwhelming influence on health outcomes, not just on asthma but on all other preventable chronic health conditions as well. We know that having access to quality food, recreation, housing, transportation, public safety, education and jobs are associated with how long we will live (Robert Wood Johnson Foundation, 2015). These aspects of family and neighborhood living conditions—beyond a person's genetic inheritance and even beyond their poverty levels—have lasting consequences for health (Jutte, Miller, & Erickson, 2015). When these basic aspects of civic life fail, a person is exposed to "toxic stress" which influences gene expression and brain development with direct and indirect negative consequences for health (Jutte et al., 2015). In fact, fully one-fourth of the differences in health in mid- to late-life can be attributed to neighborhood differences during young adulthood (Jutte et al., 2015). (See Life Expectancy Table below.)

Because the social determinants of health have such a profound impact on health outcomes, we now say that a person's zip code is far more important than their genetic code in determining health outcomes (Jutte et al., 2015; Lavizzo-Mourey, 2012). We can measure this clearly through demographic data: the most impoverished neighborhoods in our nation, comprised predominantly of persons of color, have a life expectancy 15 to 25 years less than higher income and predominantly white neighborhoods.

Life Expectancy at Birth by Zip Code[*]

City	Higher Income and Predominantly White Neighborhoods	Lower Income and Predominantly Persons of Color Neighborhoods	Years of Difference
Cleveland, OH (Norris & Howard, 2015)	88	64	24
Kansas City, KS	83	69	14
Lincoln, NE (Andersen, 2015)	90's	60's	25-30
Minneapolis/St. Paul, MN	83+	75	8+
New Orleans, LA	80	55	25
San Joaquin Valley, CA	87	75	12
Washington, DC	84	77	7

*The data from this table is taken from the Robert Wood Johnson Foundation. (2015a). City Maps. Retrieved December 5, 2015, from www.rwjf.org/en/library/articles-and-news/2015/09/city-maps.htm

Excerpt from Williams, D., (2012) "Miles to Go before We Sleep: Racial Inequities in Health" Journal of Health and Social Behavior, Sage. 53(3) 279, 285.

Research suggests that three key factors may each contribute to the residual effect of race after socioeconomic status (SES) is controlled (Williams & Mohammed, 2009).

- First, indicators of SES are not equivalent across race. Compared with whites, blacks and Hispanics have lower earnings at comparable levels of education, less wealth at every level of income, and less purchasing power because of higher costs of goods and services in their communities (Williams & Collins, 1995).

- Second, health is affected not only by one's current SES but by exposure to social and economic adversity over the life course. Racial ethnic minority populations are more likely than whites to have experienced low SES in childhood and elevated levels of early life psychosocial and economic diversity that can affect health in adulthood (Colen, 2011). In national data, early life SES helps explain the black-white gap in mortality for men (Warner & Hayward, 2006). Another recent study linked early life adversity to multiple markers of inflammation for adult African Americans but not for whites (Slopen et al., 2010), suggesting a link to allostatic load. Allostatic load, or the cumulative biological burden exacted on the body through daily adaption to stress, particularly unremitting physical and emotional stress, is considered to be a risk factor for several diseases, including cardiovascular disease, diabetes, obesity, depression and cognitive impairment, as well as both inflammatory and autoimmune disorders (Djuric et al, 2008).

- Third, a growing body of evidence documents that racism is a critical missing piece of the puzzle in understanding the patterning of racial disparities in health. Institutional racism and personal experiences of discrimination are added pathogenic factors that can affect the health of minority group members in multiple ways (Williams & Mohammed, 2009). Discrimination can lead to reduced access to desirable goods and services, internalized racism (acceptance of society's negative characterization) can adversely affect health, by eroding the individual's sense of value (Jones, 2000), racism can trigger increased exposure to traditional stressors (e.g., unemployment), and experiences of discrimination are psychosocial stressors. For example, perceived discrimination/racism has been shown to play a role in unhealthy behaviors such cigarette smoking, alcohol/substance use, improper nutrition, and refusal to seek medical services (Lee, Ayers, & Kronenfeld, 2009; Peek et al, 2011).

Arguably, the most consequential effects of racism on health are due to residential segregation by race, a mechanism of institutional racism (Williams & Collins, 1995). Segregation can restrict socioeconomic attainment and lead to group differences in SES and health. It also creates pathogenic neighborhood conditions, with minorities living in markedly more health-damaging environments than whites and facing higher levels of acute and chronic stressors. Although the majority of poor persons in the United States are white, poor white families are not concentrated in contexts of economic and social disadvantage with an absence of an infrastructure that promotes opportunity in the ways that poor blacks, Latinos, and Native Americans are. The neighborhoods where minority children live have lower incomes, education, and home ownership rates and higher rates of poverty and unemployment compared with those where white children reside. In 100 of America's largest metropolitan areas, 75 percent of all African American children and 69 percent of all Latino children are growing up in more negative residential environments than are the worst-off white children (Acevedo-Garcia, Osypuk, McArdle, & Williams, 2008).

These extraordinary differentials in life expectancy are due primarily to an overburden of preventable chronic diseases in low income communities of color that can be addressed best by taking a systems approach to health outcomes. Through systems thinking, we know that we have to look for the fundamental causes of the problems we are trying to solve. This means that we must find the interrelationships between the structural issues that affect health issues such as the quality of housing and education in a community; access to job training and economic opportunity; exposure to interpersonal or community-level violence; and the realities of historic, institutional and internalized racism. (See the sidebar, Racism and the Social Determinants of Health.)

County Health Rankings *(County Health Rankings & Roadmaps, 2015a)*

Research conducted by the Population Health Institute at the University of Wisconsin demonstrates that clinical medical care accounts for just 20% of health outcomes while health behaviors, socioeconomic factors and the physical environment account for the remaining 80% of health outcomes (County Health Rankings & Roadmaps, 2015a).

The seemingly distinct measurements on the chart are deceptive as there are tremendous interactions between health factors. Compare two families:

One is a middle class family that lives in a home free of hazards, in a neighborhood that has parks safe for children to play in. They are likely to spend weekends shuttling between youth sporting events, and whether or not they always eat healthfully, they will at least be able to afford plenty of healthy foods. When family members get sick, they likely have access to quality medical care. This family has ready access to all that is needed to live a healthy life.

The other family lives near or below the poverty line. This family is far more likely to live in a neighborhood with an over-proliferation of stores that sell liquor but few fruits or vegetables. This alone affects the family diet (a Health Behavior factor) and safety (Social and Economic factors) as an increased density of liquor stores is correlated with increased community and interpersonal violence (Ashe, Jernigan, Kline, & Galaz, 2003). This family is likely to have limited access to medical care (a Clinical Care factor) and may even have to choose between seeing a doctor or buying medication and paying rent or buying food (Social and Economic factors). The children in this family most likely do not belong to sports teams and may have to play inside their home to keep safe (Social and Economic, and Physical Environment factors).

The health behavior of the family living in or near poverty is likely to be far different than the middle class family with access to all that is needed for a healthful life. In short, poor health disproportionately burdens people who live in places that limit opportunities to live long and well (County Health Rankings & Roadmaps, 2015b).

Yet, when we look at how we spend our health care dollars, we see that just 3-4% of our national health budget is dedicated to disease prevention; the rest is dedicated to medical care delivery (Alley, Asomugha, Conway, & Sanghavi, 2015; Centers for Disease Control and Prevention, 1992; Forsberg & Fichtenberg, 2012; McGinnis, Williams-Russo, & Knickman, 2002). This unbalanced distribution of the national health budget is illustrated by the fact that the nation's largest single investment in prevention, the Prevention and Public Health Fund,

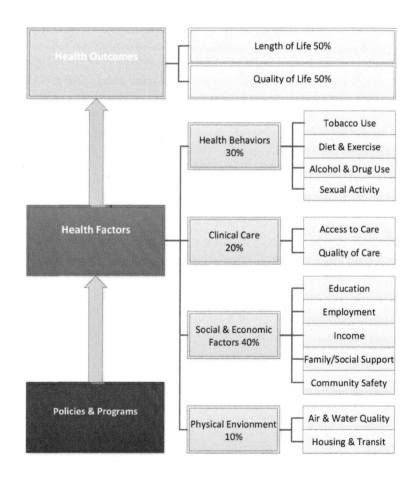

provides $14.5 billion over the next 10 years (Trust for America's Health, n.d.), while the total health care spending for 2014 alone was $3 trillion (Centers for Medicare and Medicaid Services, 2015a). In short, as things stand today, we are challenged to address the 80% of the causative factors for preventable disease with a fraction of the national budget on health. This is an impossible ratio that is bound to lead to failure unless something is done that is dramatically different than the status quo.

The Triple Aim (Bisognano & Kenney, 2012) continues to be the gold standard for the transformation of our health system, linking improved experience of care, reducing per capita cost of care, and improving the health of populations. In our first monograph, SH advocated an even more expansive view: that health equity, strongly linked to social determinants, should be added as a "Quadruple Aim" to insure justice in healthcare and other venues (Health Systems Learning Group, 2013, p. 12). However, despite these calls to action, few health systems are incorporating the relevant tools and processes to address the social determinants of health in their systems of care. Without addressing and integrating the social determinants, the Triple Aim, and certainly not our more expansive Quadruple Aim, will not be realized.

What Can We Do to Address the Social Determinants of Health?

While access to health care for individuals is necessary to close gaps in life expectancy, it is hardly sufficient. Rather, we must work at the systems level by taking a comprehensive approach to complex events or phenomena affecting a person's or a community's life even though these events seem to be caused by a myriad of isolated, independent, and often unpredictable factors or forces (Senge, 2006). Population health means doing business differently: it will require at least an integration of both public health and traditional health care settings. We will need to begin to integrate both clinical and community prevention. The new level of thinking for the emerging health system will require aligning partnerships that are built for health, not just the treatment of symptoms associated with disease. This will require addressing the social determinants with strategic partners not traditionally aligned with the health system. We can no longer think of hospitals, labs, physician offices and clinics as the health system, but include housing, education, and public health. For example, our colleagues at ProMedica have done years of work around improving health outcomes via food security initiatives (see sidebar).

The 5-tiered Health Impact Pyramid developed by CDC director Thomas Frieden (2010) illustrates the various types of interventions that contribute to improving population health. It takes a decidedly systems theory view of what will work, and provides a framework for how to address any number of public health challenges—from preventing chronic diseases, to decreasing HIV/AIDS transmission or teen pregnancy rates, to increasing immunization rates. It demonstrates that the greatest achievements in population health will be secured by implementing interventions at the base levels of the pyramid.

BOTTOM TIER – *Socioeconomic Factors*
The lowest tier represents changes in socioeconomic factors (e.g., poverty reduction, quality educational systems, healthy and affordable housing, etc.). These changes have the greatest potential impact on health outcomes because they affect fundamental conditions in life and simultaneously reach broad segments of society with population-scale policies. Because we know that socioeconomic factors impact up to 40% of the differential in life expectancy, these changes—complex though they may be—provide an overwhelmingly positive impact on health outcomes (Frieden, 2010).

Relevance for asthma prevention
As discussed above, asthma is significantly affected by:

• Poverty: greater likelihood of living in substandard housing, may not have health insurance or be able to afford medication.

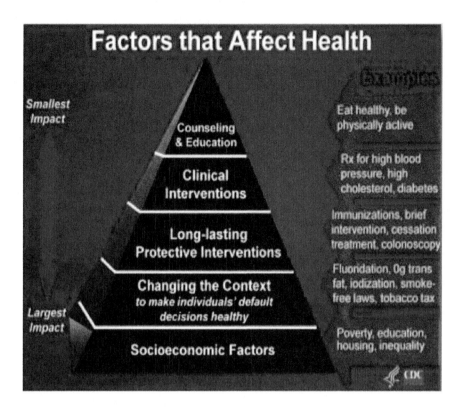

- Homelessness: Shelters are often filled with asthma triggers, and the stress of displacement alone exacerbates asthma.
- Education: Poor education is a risk for health illiteracy not only for the asthmatic child, but also parents.

2ND TIER – *Changing the Context to Make Individual's Default Decisions Healthier*

This tier includes interventions that change the environmental context to make healthy options the standard regardless of education, income, or social services. Examples include access to fluoridated water, elimination of lead and asbestos exposures, improvements in road and vehicle design, iodized salt, removal of trans-fats from foods, policies that encourage use of active transportation (walking, bicycling, public transit, stair use), clean indoor air laws, taxing or differential prices on tobacco, alcohol, and unhealthy foods and beverages (Frieden, 2010). In each instance, the individual does not need to think about choosing a healthy option—it is the norm. Regardless of education, income, or other societal factors, all persons benefit from such interventions.

Relevance for asthma prevention
- If an asthmatic child lives in a home with known asthma triggers such as mold, mildew, roaches, or second hand smoke, there is little hope of preventing illness even if she has perfect adherence to treatment regimes. If that child moves to a home that meets habitability standards free from asthma triggers including secondhand smoke, the likelihood of her health improving increases dramatically.

3RD TIER – *Long-Lasting Protective Interventions*

This tier includes one-time or infrequent protective interventions that do not require ongoing clinical care. Examples of such interventions include immunizations, colonoscopies and smoking cessation programs. Because these interventions operate by reaching people as individuals rather than through a broader base policy strategy, they typically have less impact on population health outcomes than the bottom two tiers of the pyramid (Frieden, 2010).

Relevance for asthma prevention

- Most healthy housing projects fit here as they use a family-by-family or apartment-by-apartment approach to addressing a health concern. For example, it is common that a child with lead poisoning also has asthma, as both health problems are caused by poorly maintained houses. Maintaining housing quality by remediating lead poisoning or asthma triggers for each family with a lead poisoned or asthmatic child provides long-lasting protections, but without the universal approach of creating default conditions or opportunities as in the lowest tiers.

4TH TIER – *Clinical Interventions*

This tier includes direct medical care in a hospital or clinical setting, including home health visits. Evidence-based clinical care reduces disability and increases life expectancy for recipients and we know that it has a 20% impact on overall health outcomes. Nonetheless, in some communities, clinical interventions are often unavailable to low-income residents, especially in states that have not adopted Medicaid expansion under the Affordable Care Act. Further, clinical services can be limited in their effectiveness by a patient's socioeconomic status such as his/her inability to afford medicine; non-adherence to a medication regime due to a lack of education and health literacy; clinic organization, such as single provider vs. rotating providers and physician's expectation of patients' capacity to use the newest technique for control of conditions (Lutfe & Freese, 2005; Phelan & Link, 2005); or the fact that the patient does not have access to healthy and affordable foods, safe places to play, or healthy housing, which are necessary to prevent disease (Frieden, 2010).

Relevance for asthma prevention

- Even patients with all the amenities of middle class life can have asthma. All patients need screening, health education, and medication. Sometimes even the otherwise healthy and wealthy asthmatic patient needs hospitalization.

TOP TIER – *Counseling and Educational Interventions*

This tier includes health education provided during clinical encounters (e.g., nutrition education or smoking cessation classes) or during participation in community-based program (e.g., health fairs, cooking classes at WIC sites, exercise classes, etc.). From a population health perspective, these are often the least effective types of intervention largely because they reach just one person or a small group of persons at a time (Whitlock, Orleans, Pender, & Allan, 2002). Further, they often fail to address the socioeconomic contexts in which healthy choices are or are not default options. They may also fail to communicate effectively across cultural, worldview and discourse gaps that affect how participants behave and act, their so-called "healthworlds" (Germond & Cochrane, 2010), discussed in more detail in Chapter 10. These critiques aside, when applied consistently and repeatedly, counseling and educational interventions can have meaningful impact on the individuals served. For example, behavioral counseling to have safe sex, along with access to clinical interventions such as clean needles and condoms, has reduced HIV risk among the broader population (Frieden, 2010).

Relevance for asthma prevention

- Patients with asthma can significantly reduce their health problems by knowing asthma triggers and learning how to manage symptoms early with the proper use of inhalers and other medicines.

Excerpts from Norris & Howard (2015) "Can Hospitals Heal America's Communities?", p. 1, 2, 8.

Healthcare's role in creating healthy communities through increasing access to quality care, research, and grant-making is being complemented by a higher impact approach: hospitals and integrated health systems are increasingly stepping outside of their walls to address the social, economic, and environmental conditions that contribute to poor health outcomes, shortened lives, and higher costs in the first place.

They are doing so for several reasons: by addressing these social determinants of health through their business and non-clinical practices (for example, through purchasing, hiring, and investments), hospitals and health systems can produce increased measurably beneficial impacts on population and community health. By adopting this "anchor mission," they can also prevent unnecessary demand on the healthcare system. This in turn can contribute to lower costs and make care more affordable for all, especially those truly in need. Simply put, this approach can improve a health system's quality and cost effectiveness while simultaneously significantly benefiting society.

With hospitals and health systems representing more than $780 billion in total annual expenditures, $340 billion in purchasing of goods and services, and more than $500 billion in investment portfolios, this approach expands the set of resources and tools institutions have at their disposal to carry out their mission. It shifts the discussion of community benefit from the margins of an institution's operations to overall accountability, where all resources can be leveraged to benefit the communities in which institutions are located.

Physicians, healthcare administrators, and hospital trustees face an important and historic leadership opportunity that our country and our communities desperately need. Hospitals and health systems throughout the country are beginning to build on their charitable efforts, beyond traditional corporate social responsibility, to adopt elements of an anchor mission in their business models and operations.

Can hospitals and health systems heal America's communities?

For integrated health systems such as Kaiser Permanente, that means intentionally aligning and activating all of the resources of the institution—including sourcing and procurement, workforce pipeline development, training, investment capital, education programs, research, community health initiatives, environmental stewardship, and clinical prevention—to produce total health: a state of complete physical, mental and social well-being for all people.

Social Determinants of Health as Systems Theory for Population Health Improvement

As we reflect on both the County Health Rankings and Frieden's Health Impact Pyramid, it is clear that hugely complex systems must be addressed if we are to have a positive impact on population health. The benefit of using an open systems approach to guide our work is that it demonstrates how positive or virtuous feedback loops can be created so that even small changes in one discreet element of a complex system can have multiple ripple effects on the other elements. In practice, systems thinkers strive to know just the right actions to take or facilitate in order to grow—or "snowball"—positive change throughout an entire system no matter how complex. If we can learn to see the whole of a situation, we also can learn to identify levers of change that are available to create the outcomes we want to achieve. Our partners at Kaiser Permanente have exemplified this approach (see side-bar on the Hospital as Systems Change Leaders).

Addressing the Fundamental Causes of Poor Health and Inequity

We said at the beginning of this chapter that systems thinking shifts the "mind from seeing parts to seeing wholes" (Senge, 2006, p.69). The newly emerging concept of "Health in All Policies" helps us understand how to address the social determinants of health so that our efforts are likely to be the most effective in creating positive ripple effects throughout entire systems. In brief, Health in All Policies is a systems approach to improving the health of a community by incorporating health, equity and sustainability considerations into decision-making across sectors and policy areas (Rudolph et al., 2013). The work of Health Care without Harm and the Democracy Collaborative in relation to changing hospital policies on waste management, procurement, hiring and capital projects offer great examples of how these positive effects can be leveraged across health systems (see http://democracycollaborative.org and https://noharm.org).

The asthma case study above demonstrates the need for a Health in All Policies approach. A growing understanding of the social determinants of health has led to a call for public policy that shapes our social, physical, and economic environments in ways that are more conducive to health (Wilkinson & Marmot, 2003). The Health in All Policies approach takes us far outside of traditional hospital systems, and even outside of public health agencies. The policies that determine whether a person has access to healthy food (ChangeLab Solutions, 2012), clean water (Denzin, 2008), clean air (United States Environmental Protection Agency, 2015), safe places for play and physical activity (National Recreation and Park Association, n.d.), affordable, quality housing (ChangeLab Solutions, 2015), jobs (Partnership for Working Families, n.d.), and schools (Centers for Disease Control and Prevention, 2015c; Cowan, Hubsmith, & Ping, 2011), are typically developed and implemented by agencies other than health departments, including planning, transportation, social services, education, economic development, fire, police, sanitation, and public works (ChangeLab Solutions & Bay Area Regional Health Inequities Initiative, 2010). Community Development Finance Institutions can play an important intermediary role, too (Jutte et al., 2015). To achieve a vision for healthier communities, we need such an approach, one in which every part of government, as well as non-governmental sectors like business, faith, and community based organizations play an active role. That is the idea behind Health in All Policies.

To achieve Health in All Policies, hospitals and all the other leading sectors in civic life must adopt a new approach to decision-making. The new approach requires the various stakeholders, including a community and its assets, to understand how policies and actions affect health. They need to recognize that they are part of an interrelated system and that every part of the system has a direct impact on the community's health outcomes. The stakeholders need to learn to share information and organizational goals and to collaborate to coordinate their efforts.

Effective Health in All Policies initiatives are developed by and for a particular community, and there is no "one size fits all" approach. An initiative's overarching focus must resonate with everyone involved, including public agencies, community leaders and residents. These efforts can be framed around health, wellness, equity, sustainability, or some other core value as defined by a community. While there is variation in local Health in All Policies initiatives, they usually share the same fundamental principles, with an inherent goal of building and nurturing trust among all stakeholders:

• Create an ongoing collaborative forum to help stakeholders and sectors to work together to improve public health;

• Advance specific projects, programs, laws, and policies that enhance public health while furthering stakeholders' core missions; and

• Embed health-promoting practices in the organizational practices of all stakeholders.

We also said at the beginning of this chapter that systems thinking shifts the "mind from seeing people as helpless reactors to seeing them as active participants in shaping their reality, from reacting to the present to creating the future" (Senge, 2006, p. 69). We know through systems thinking that if we take short cuts—such as failing to identify or address fundamental causes of problems, or failing to engage with community and neighborhood leaders—our actions could jeopardize the ultimate success of the social changes being attempted (Senge, 2006).

Failure to Address Fundamental Causes: Oftentimes, short-term "solutions" are used to correct a problem with seemingly positive immediate results. But if action is taken without regard to how a short-term solution affects the entire system, only isolated results will be attained and more fundamental long-term corrective measures will be missed. Systems thinking urges stakeholders to focus on fundamental solutions rather than simply addressing short-term symptoms.

Failure to Release the Existing Energy and Assets of the Community: So often the most powerful stakeholders such as hospitals and government agencies—emboldened by the best of intentions and employing deep expertise from their areas of specialty—try to solve complex problems without engaging with and winning the trust of members of the community most affected by systemic problems. We all know that working with community groups can be unpredictable, volatile and contentious. Historic inequities are felt in real time, anger can surface and trust may be low. Sometimes we don't know which community leaders to trust, and consensus on how best to move forward can seem elusive. Yet, if the very hard work of deep community engagement is glossed over or ignored, those most affected by health inequities battle to deal with problems themselves. Instead of fully engaging and utilizing their own existing community assets and intelligence, community members may remain passive "recipients" of well-intentioned programs or efforts led by so-called "professionals," and the system will never achieve real change.

Recommendations: So, What is a Hospital Leader to DO?

You wouldn't be alone if you have read this chapter and feel burdened with undue expectations and insufficient resources. Most hospital administrators willingly accept the responsibility of aligning all the functions of integrated hospital systems, but have more difficulty dealing with domains beyond the hospital system itself for which they are not directly responsible. For instance, most leaders are not likely to commit to alleviating poverty or solving problems related to historic or systemic racism (which are beyond the control of the health sector alone). Yet, it is abundantly clear that unless and until the socioeconomic and structural issues at the base of the Health Impact Pyramid are addressed, the human and economic costs related to preventable diseases will also not be addressed. Achieving the Triple Aim of improved experience of care, reducing per capita cost of care, and improving the health of populations, not to mention paying attention to SH's "Quadruple Aim" that includes equity, requires engaging in the hard work of changing the systems driving preventable diseases and avoidable costs.

The good news: You are not alone when you seek to find ways to go beyond the limits of traditional institutional boundaries and responsibilities. Many resources are available to help get the job done and innovations are underway that help. The most effective interventions to drive population health improvement—those at the bottom of the Health Impact Pyramid—cannot be achieved by the health sector alone. They require new kinds of partnership with people and organizations in communities (see Chapter 6 on "Transformative Partnerships," HSLG, 2013) in collaboration with multiple government agencies and non-governmental sectors outside of the health sectors' immediate areas of influence or expertise. Evidence for this integration of issues across traditional siloes is found throughout academic literature and increasingly through successes in the field.

At ProMedica, a mission-based, nonprofit, locally owned health care system serving northwest Ohio and southeast Michigan, hunger has been chief among many social determinants of health being addressed in recent years. Driven by a mission to improve the health and well-being of the communities we serve, we began to look at hunger after becoming increasingly aware of its link to obesity and other health concerns across the age spectrum.

Partnerships have been key to our success beginning with a food reclamation program developed in 2013. ProMedica hired two part-time employees to work in the kitchen of the newly opened Hollywood Casino Toledo. These employees reclaim the prepared but unserved, food in the Casino kitchen and package it for distribution to local shelters and communal feeding sites by Toledo Seagate Foodbank. Since inception, the program has expanded to other community locations including several of ProMedica's own hospitals and has provided more than 250,000 pounds of food.

In addition to important community partnerships such as the one with the casino and the food bank, ProMedica understands the importance of directly addressing food insecurity in our patient population. To that end, ProMedica has adopted the Hunger Vital Sign, two-question screen validated by Children's Health Watch. Upon hospital admission, patients are asked the two questions, and those patients with a positive screen are seen by a member of the care team who further assesses the situation. If a need is confirmed, the patient is provided a day's worth of food upon discharge from the hospital, as well as information and assistance about community resources available to them, and how to access those resources.

To take this screening one step further, in April 2015 ProMedica began screening patients in primary care offices and opened its first Food Pharmacy. Patients who screen positive for food insecurity are provided a referral to the food pharmacy where they receive several days of healthy food for themselves and their family. Food choices are based upon the patient's nutrition related diagnosis, if one is present. For example, diabetic patients choose from low sugar options, hypertensive patients choose from low sodium options and patients choose additional protein choices. The referral enables the patient to visit the food pharmacy once per month for up to six months before needing a new referral if they are still in need. Patients at the food pharmacy are also given the opportunity to meet with a registered dietitian to learn more about healthy eating and managing their diagnosis.

Recognizing the importance of eliminating barriers to accessing nutritious, affordable food, in December 2015 ProMedica opened a grocery market in a food desert in Toledo. With seed money from a generous donor, ProMedica designed a 5,000 square-foot market in a four-story building that was previously abandoned. The Market is unique because it employs neighborhood residents in a job training program where each employee will learn all aspects of the market during their 12-month training period. They will also participate in financial literacy programs and other wrap around services to assist them in becoming and remaining self-sufficient. At the end of their 12-month training period they will be better prepared for job opportunities elsewhere in the ProMedica system or with community business partners. By spring 2016, we will complete the second floor build out that will include a teaching kitchen and other classroom space where a variety of programs can be offered to fill gaps that exist in the community.

- **Hospitals Can Support Public Policies that Enhance Community Health**
  Public policy is your best friend. Think about it. Public policy largely determines what happens base level of the Health Impact Pyramid: housing affordability; the quality of local school systems; whether there is access to healthy foods, safe places to walk and play, or smoke-free environments. Every state in the nation can develop public policies based on a Health in All Policies model that ensure the default conditions in which people live are healthy. Most local governments can augment the baseline state rules to tailor public policies so they are even more reflective of local health needs and priorities, too. Hospitals are in a key position to ensure that the public policies in the communities they serve work *for* rather than *against* population health. While this is not necessarily an easy task, it remains a crucial role that is within leaders' competency, running a key social institution.

The good news is that the ChangeLab Solutions website offers a large library of free resources designed exactly to support the policy changes needed to address the social determinants of health. Supported by major philanthropies and many government agencies, ChangeLab Solutions offers model laws and policies plus a wide range of supporting materials to ensure everyday health for all—whether that's providing access to healthy food and beverages, creating safe opportunities for physical activity, or ensuring the freedom to enjoy smokefree air and clean water. The model policy solutions are a great starting place to find what is needed to create a just, vital and thriving community (see www.changelabsolutions.org).

Likewise, the "What Works for Health" section of the County Health Rankings website also highlights explicit multi-sector policy, programs and systems changes, all reviewed and curated for level of evidence supporting the recommendations (see www.countyhealthrankings.org/roadmaps/what-works-for-health).

- **Hospitals can Creatively Leverage Partnerships**
  Partnerships are everywhere and leadership opportunities abound. As anchor institutions driving large portions of local economic activity, hospitals enjoy significant economic and political clout, and have a diverse array of strong allies that can be mobilized to ensure that healthy public policies are the norm. As emphasized in our discussion about Health in All Policies and the excerpts from "Can Hospitals Heal America's Communities?," non-traditional and innovative partnerships across government agencies and multiple sectors of civic life are the new norm to achieve population health. Hospitals are able to exert wonderfully creative leadership in the multiple sectors of civic life—business, economic development, education, faith and more—that can ensure the health message is heard and acted upon by decision-makers (Norris & Howard, 2015).

- **Hospitals Can Engage Local Residents**
  One of the most potent partner groups that hospitals can engage are local residents, who are deeply invested in the health and well-being of their neighborhoods, agencies and citizens. As described in Chapter 6 on community asset mapping, hospital leadership who take the time to truly know and understand the local residents served by a hospital and respond to what information or needs are shared, can enrich community health needs assessment, provide useful data for strategic planning, as well as help health systems do a better job serving patients and families. Such partnerships can yield both improved community health outcomes in the long-run and improved margins in caring for vulnerable populations in the short-term.

- **Hospitals Can Implement Best Practice Models**
  Scientific research is rich and best practices are abundant. An enormous array of readily available resources are at your fingertips—especially related to the 4th tier of the pyramid in changing the context so that default conditions lead to health rather than disease:

  o **National Prevention Strategy** (U.S. Surgeon General, n.d.): This guides our nation to the most effective and achievable means for improving health and well-being. The Strategy prioritizes prevention by integrating recommendations and actions across multiple settings to improve health and save lives. It provides a strong foundation for all prevention efforts and provides evidenced-based recommendations that are most likely to reduce the burden of the leading causes of preventable death and major illness:

- Tobacco Free Living
- Preventing Drug Abuse and Excessive Alcohol Use
- Healthy Eating
- Active Living
- Injury and Violence Free Living
- Reproductive and Sexual Health
- Mental and Emotional Well-Being

o **CDC Community Guide to Preventive Services** (The Community Guide, 2015) and **Community Health Improvement Navigato**r (Centers for Disease Control and Prevention, 2015a): The Guide to Community Preventive Services is a free resource to help you choose programs and policies to improve health and prevent disease in your community. Systematic reviews are used to answer these questions:
  - Which program and policy interventions have been proven effective?
  - Are there effective interventions that are right for my community?
  - What might effective interventions cost; what is the likely return on investment?

The CDC Community Health Improvement Navigator (CHI Navigator) is a website (described in greater detail in Chapter 6) for people who lead or participate in CHI work within hospitals and health systems, public health agencies, and other community organizations. It is a one-stop-shop that offers community stakeholders expert-vetted tools and resources for:
  - Depicting visually the who, what, where, and how of improving community health
  - Making the case for collaborative approaches to community health improvement
  - Establishing and maintaining effective collaborations
  - Finding interventions that have the greatest impact on health and well-being for all.

- **Hospitals can Play a Role in Payment Systems Reforms**
  Payment system reforms are underway. It goes without saying that the financial incentives driving health care delivery today are overwhelmingly dynamic. Hospitals are experimenting on their own to better manage the care of Dual Eligibles to reach the Triple Aim; rethinking the use of their IRS community benefit obligations to address the social determinants of health (Trinity Health, 2015); creating new care delivery models that incorporate trusted community residents as core personnel in a community-based care model; and addressing the social determinants of health through their procurement, workforce development, and other core operations and expenditures (Norris & Howard, 2015). Hospitals can step up to be part of such pilots, particularly, the work being supported by the federal government, too:

o **HHS State Innovation Models (SIMs) Initiative** (Centers for Medicare and Medicaid Services, 2015b): provides financial and technical support to states for the development and testing of state-led, multi-payer health care payment and service delivery models that will improve health system performance, increase quality of care, and decrease costs for Medicare, Medicaid and Children's Health Insurance Program (CHIP) beneficiaries—and for all residents of participating states.

Conclusion

Systems theory offers useful insight into the dynamic and complex changes underway in America's hospitals. We are challenged to find the patterns within the complex phenomenon so that we can address the fundamental conditions—the social determinants of health—that lead to preventable disease, unnecessary costs, and the drain on the economic vibrancy of our nation. This chapter aimed to provide a deeper understanding of these social determinants of health and to offer a series of strategies that will allow hospitals to begin to incorporate the power of a systems approach as they address the many challenges they face.

REFERENCES

Acevedo-Garcia, D., Osypuk, T. L., McArdle, N., & Williams, D. R. (2008). Toward a policy-relevant analysis of geographic and racial/ethnic disparities in child health. *Health Affairs,* 27(2), 321–333. http://doi.org/10.1377/hlthaff.27.2.321

Alley, D. E., Asomugha, C. N., Conway, P. H., & Sanghavi, D. M. (2015). Accountable Health Communities—Addressing Social Needs through Medicare and Medicaid. *New England Journal of Medicine,* 374(1), 1–4. http://doi.org/10.1056/NEJMp1002530

American Lung Association. (2012). *Trends in Asthma Morbidity and Mortality. American Lung Association.* Retrieved from http://www.lung.org/assets/documents/research/asthma-trend-report.pdf

Andersen, E. (2015, June 13). Place Matters: Lincoln maps highlight health disparities across neighborhoods, zip codes. *Lincoln Journal Star.* Retrieved from http://journalstar.com/lifestyles/family/place-matters-lincoln-maps-highlight-health-disparities-across-neighborhoods-zip/article_1be90244-8533-5ad2-9e8b-2b632899cd5d.html

Ashe, M., Jernigan, D., Kline, R., & Galaz, R. (2003). Land use planning and the control of alcohol, tobacco, firearms, and fast food restaurants. *American Journal of Public Health,* 93(9), 1404–8. Retrieved from http://www.pubmedcentral.nih.gov/articlerender.fcgi?artid=1447982&tool=pmcentrez&rendertype=abstract

Bisognano, M. & Kenney, C. (2012). *Pursuing the Triple Aim: Seven Innovators Show the Way to Better Care, Better Health, and Lower Costs.* San Francisco: Jossey-Bass Publishers.

Bonilla, S., Kehl, S., Kwong, K. Y., Morphew, T., Kachru, R., & Jones, C. A. (2005). School absenteeism in children with asthma in a Los Angeles inner city school. *The Journal of Pediatrics,* 147(6), 802–806.

Brooks-Gunn, J., & Duncan, G. J. (1997). The effects of poverty on children. *The Future of Children/Center for the Future of Children, the David and Lucile Packard Foundation,* 7(2), 55–71. http://doi.org/10.4314/ai.v32i1.22297

Centers for Disease Control and Prevention. (1992). Effectiveness in Disease and Injury Prevention Estimated National Spending on Prevention—United States, 1988. *MMWR. Morbidity and Mortality Weekly Report,* 41(29), 529–531. Retrieved from http://www.cdc.gov/mmwr/preview/mmwrhtml/00017286.htm

Centers for Disease Control and Prevention. (2015a). CDC Community Health Improvement Navigator. Retrieved December 4, 2015, from http://www.cdc.gov/chinav/index.html

Centers for Disease Control and Prevention. (2015b). Childhood obesity facts. Retrieved January 5, 2016, from http://www.cdc.gov/obesity/data/childhood.html

Centers for Disease Control and Prevention. (2015c). Local School Wellness Policy. Retrieved December 4, 2015, from http://www.cdc.gov/healthyschools/npao/wellness.htm

Centers for Disease Control and Prevention. (2015d). National Health Interview Survey. Retrieved December 5, 2015, from http://www.cdc.gov/nchs/nhis/quest_data_related_1997_forward.htm#2012_NHIS

Centers for Medicare and Medicaid Services. (2015a). National Health Expenditure Data Historical. Retrieved December 20, 2015, from https://www.cms.gov/research-statistics-data-and-systems/statistics-trends-and-reports/nationalhealthexpenddata/nationalhealthaccountshistorical.html

Centers for Medicare and Medicaid Services. (2015b). State Innovation Models Initiative: General Information. Retrieved December 5, 2015, from https://innovation.cms.gov/initiatives/State-Innovations/index.html

ChangeLab Solutions. (2012). *Green for Greens: Finding Public Funding for Healthy Food.* Oakland, CA. Retrieved from http://www.changelabsolutions.org/publications/green-for-greens

ChangeLab Solutions. (2014). *Not Making the Grade.* Retrieved from http://www.changelabsolutions.org/publications/state-school-financing

ChangeLab Solutions. (2015). *Preserving, Protecting, and Expanding Affordable Housing: A Policy Toolkit for Public Health.* Oakland, CA. Retrieved from http://changelabsolutions.org/publications/affordable_housing_toolkit

ChangeLab Solutions, & Bay Area Regional Health Inequities Initiative. (2010). *Partners for public health: working with local state, and federal agencies to create healthier communities.* Oakland, CA. Retrieved from http://changelabsolutions.org/publications/partners-public-health

Child Trends DataBank. (2013). *Screening and Risk for Developmental Delay.* Retrieved from http://www.childtrends.org/wp-content/uploads/2013/07/111_Developmental-Risk-and-Screening.pdf

Colen, C. G. (2011). Addressing racial disparities in health using life course perspectives. *Du Bois Review: Social Science Research on Race,* 8(01), 79–94. http://doi.org/10.1017/S1742058X11000075

County Health Rankings & Roadmaps. (2015a). Our approach. Retrieved December 4, 2015, from http://www.countyhealthrankings.org/our-approach

County Health Rankings & Roadmaps. (2015b). State Health Gaps. Retrieved December 4, 2015, from http://www.countyhealthrankings.org/health-gaps

Cowan, D., Hubsmith, D., & Ping, R. (2011). *Safe Routes to School Local Policy Guide.* Oakland, CA: Safe Routes to School National Partnership. Retrieved from http://saferoutespartnership.org/resourcecenter/publications/local-policy-guide

Denzin, B. (2008). *Local Water Policy Innovation A Roadmap for Community Based Stormwater Solutions.* American Rivers; Midwest Environmental Advocates. Retrieved from http://www.americanrivers.org/assets/pdfs/reports-and-publications/Local_Water_Policy_Innovation_Stormwater_Oct_20080613.pdf

Djuric, Z., Bird, C., Furumoto-Dawson, A., Rauscher, G., Ruffin, M., Stowe, R. Tucker, K. & Masi, C. (2008). Biomarkers of psychological stress in health disparities research. *Open Biomark Journal*, January 1: 7-19.

Forsberg, V., & Fichtenberg, C. (2012). *The Prevention and Public Health Fund: A critical investment in our nation's physical and fiscal health.* Washington D.C.: American Public Health Association. Retrieved from https://www.apha.org/~/media/files/pdf/topics/aca/apha_prevfundbrief_june2012.ashx)

Frieden, T. R. (2010). A Framework for Public Health Action: The Health Impact Pyramid. *American Journal of Public Health,* 100(4), 590–595. http://doi.org/10.2105/AJPH.2009.185652

Germond, P., & Cochrane, J. R. (2010). Healthworlds: conceptualizing landscapes of health and healing. *Sociology*, 44(2), 307-324.

Health Systems Learning Group (HSLG). (2013). *Strategic Investment in Shared Outcomes: Transformative Partnerships between Health Systems and Communities.* Washington, D.C. Retrieved from http://stakeholderhealth.org/wp-content/uploads/2013/09/HSLG-V11.pdf

Jones C.P. (2000). Levels of racism: a theoretic framework and a gardener's tale. *American Journal of Public Health. 90(8):1212-1215.*

Jutte, D. P., Miller, J. L., & Erickson, D. J. (2015). Neighborhood Adversity, Child Health, and the Role for Community Development. *Pediatrics*, 135(Supplement), S48–S57. http://doi.org/10.1542/peds.2014-3549F

Lavizzo-Mourey, R. (2012). Why health, poverty, and community development are inseparable. edited by. N. Andrews & D. Erickson (Eds.), *Investing in What Works for America's Communities: Essays on People, Place & Purpose,* (pp. 215–225). Retrieved from http://www.whatworksforamerica.org/ideas/why-health-poverty-and-community-development-are-inseparable/#.Vmc3NPPTn4Z

Lee, C., Ayers, S. & Kronenfeld, J. (2009). The association between perceived provider discrimination, health care utilization, and health care status in racial and ethnic minorities. *Ethnicity & Disease*, 19(3): 330-337.

Levine, S. (2003). Psychological and social aspects of resilience: a synthesis of risks and resources. *Dialogues in Clinical Neuroscience,* 5(3), 273–280.

Lutfey, K., Freese, J. (2005). Toward some fundamentals of fundamental causality: Socioeconomic status and health in the routine clinic visit for diabetes. *American Journal of Sociology*, 110, 1326-1337.

Marmot, M. (2007). Achieving health equity: from root causes to fair outcomes: Commission on Social Determinants of Health, Interim statement. *The Lancet,* 370(9593), 1153–1163. Retrieved from http://apps.who.int/iris/handle/10665/69670

Meadows, D. H. (2008). *Thinking in systems: a primer* (D. Wright, Ed.). White River Junction, Vermont: Chelsea Green Publishing.

McGinnis, J. M., Williams-Russo, P., & Knickman, J. R. (2002). The Case For More Active Policy Attention To Health Promotion. *Health Affairs,* 21(2), 78–93. http://doi.org/10.1377/hlthaff.21.2.78

Meng, Y., Babey, S., & Wolstein, J. (2012). Asthma-related school absenteeism and school concentration of low-income students in California. *Preventing Chronic Disease,* 9(2), 1–8. http://doi.org/10.5888/pcd9.110312

Moonie, S. A., Sterling, D. A., Figgs, L., & Castro, M. (2006). Asthma status and severity affects missed school days. *Journal of School Health,* 76(1), 18–24. http://doi.org/10.1111/j.1746-1561.2006.00062.x

National Recreation and Park Association. (n.d.). *Safe Routes to Parks: Improving Access to Parks through Walkability.* Ashburn, VA. Retrieved from http://www.nrpa.org/uploadedFiles/nrpa.org/Publications_and_Research/Research/Papers/Park-Access-Report.pdf

Norris, T., & Howard, T. (2015). *Can Hospitals Heal America's Communities? "All in for Mission" is the Emerging Model for Impact.* Democracy Collaborative. Retrieved from http://democracycollaborative.org/content/can-hospitals-heal-americas-communities-0

Partnership for Working Families. (n.d.). Policy & Tools: Living Wage. Retrieved December 4, 2015, from http://www.forworkingfamilies.org/resources/policy-tools-living-wage

Peek, M., Wagner, J., Tang, H. & Baker, D. (2011). Self-reported racial discrimination in health care and diabetes outcomes. *Medical Care*, 49: 618-625.

Peterson, S. (2010). Systems Thinking for Anyone: Practices to Consider. In J. Richmond, L. Stuntz, K. Richmond, & J. Egner (Eds.), *Tracing Connections: Voices of Systems Thinkers* (pp. 30–51). isee systems, inc. and Creative Learning Exchange.

Phelan, J.C. & Link, B.G. (2005). Controlling Disease and Creating Disparities: A Fundamental Cause Perspective. *J Gerontol B Psychol Soc Sci* (2005) 60 (Special Issue 2): S27-S33doi:10.1093/geronb/60.Special_Issue_2.S27)

Robert Wood Johnson Foundation. (2015). Does where you live affect how long you live? Retrieved December 17, 2015, from http://www.rwjf.org/en/library/features/health-where-you-live.html

Rudolph, L., Ben-Moshe, K., Dillon, L., & Caplan, J. (2013). Health in all Policies: A Guide for State and Local Governments. Washington, DC and Oakland, CA: American Public Health Association and Public Health Institute.

Secretary's Advisory Committee on National Health Promotion and Disease Prevention. (2010). Healthy People 2020 : An Opportunity to Address Societal Determinants of Health in the U.S. Retrieved from http://www.healthypeople.gov/sites/default/files/SocietalDeterminantsHealth.pdf

Senge, P. M. (2006). *The fifth discipline: The art and practice of the learning organization.* Doudbleday.

Singh, G. K., Siapush, M., & Kogan, M. D. (2010). Rising social inequalities in US Childhood Obesity, 2003-2007. *Annals of Epidemiology, 20*(1), 40–52. http://doi.org/10.1016/j.annepidem.2009.09.008

Slopen, N., Lewis, T. T., Gruenewald, T. L., Mujahid, M. S., Ryff, C. D., Albert, M. A., & Williams, D. R. (2010). Early life adversity and inflammation in African Americans and whites in the midlife in the United States survey. *Psychosomatic Medicine, 72*(7), 694–701. http://doi.org/10.1097/PSY.0b013e3181e9c16f

The Community Guide. (2015). The Guide to Community Preventive Services. Retrieved December 4, 2015, from http://www.thecommunityguide.org/index.html

Thies, K. M. (1999). Identifying the educational implications of chronic illness in school children. *The Journal of School Health, 69*(10), 392–397. http://doi.org/10.1111/j.1746-1561.1999.tb06354.x

Trinity Health. (2015). News releases: Trinity Health to Invest in Partnerships that Address Root Causes of Poor Health. Retrieved December 7, 2015, from http://www.trinity-health.org/body.cfm?id=196&action=detail&ref=80.

Trust for America's Health. (n.d.). The Prevention and Public Health Fund: Preventing Chronic Disease and Reducing Long-Term Health Costs. Retrieved December 20, 2015, from http://healthyamericans.org/health-issues/wp-content/uploads/2015/02/Prevention-Fund-Backgrounder.pdf

U.S. Office of Disease Prevention and Health Promotion, & Healthy People 2020. (2015). Social Determinants of Health. Retrieved December 8, 2015, from http://www.healthypeople.gov/2020/topics-objectives/topic/social-determinants-health

U.S. Surgeon General. (n.d.). National Prevention Strategy. Retrieved December 4, 2015, from http://www.surgeongeneral.gov/priorities/prevention/strategy/index.html

United States Environmental Protection Agency. (2015). State and Local Climate Energy Program. Retrieved December 4, 2015, from http://www3.epa.gov/statelocalclimate/local/topics/transportation.html

Warner, D. F., & Hayward, M. D. (2006). Early-life origins of the race gap in men's mortality. *Journal of Health and Social Behavior, 47*(3), 209–226. http://doi.org/10.1177/002214650604700302

Whitlock, E. P., Orleans, C. T., Pender, N., & Allan, J. (2002). Evaluating primary care behavioral counseling interventions. An evidence-based approach. *American Journal of Preventive Medicine, 22*(4), 267–284. http://doi.org/10.1016/S0749-3797(02)00415-4

Wilkinson, R., & Marmot, M. (Eds.). (2003). *Social determinants of health: the solid Facts. World Health Organization Europe* (2nd ed.). World Health Organization. http://doi.org/10.1016/j.jana.2012.03.001

Williams, D. R., & Collins, C. (1995). US socioeconomic and racial differences in health: patterns and explanations. *Annual Review of Sociology, 21*, 349–386. http://doi.org/10.1146/annurev.soc.21.1.349

Williams, D. R., Costa, M. V, Odunlami, A. O., & Mohammed, S. A. (2008). Moving Upstream: how interventions that adress social determinants of health and reduce disparities. *Journal of Public Health Management and Practice, 14*, 8–17. http://doi.org/10.1097/01.PHH.0000338382.36695.42.Moving

Williams, D. R., & Mohammed, S. A. (2009). Discrimination and racial disparities in health: evidence and needed research. *Journal of Behavioral Medicine, 32*(1), 20–47. http://doi.org/10.1007/s10865-008-9185-0

World Health Organization (WHO). (2015). Social determinants of health. Retrieved December 4, 2015, from http://www.who.int/social_determinants/sdh_definition/en/

ACKNOWLEDGMENTS

We gratefully acknowledge and thank the following **ChangeLab Solutions** staff for their contributions to this article:

Christine Fry, MPP, Vice President for Organizational Learning, ChangeLab Solutions

Rebecca Johnson, MPH, Senior Policy Analyst, ChangeLab Solutions

Manel Kappagoda, JD, MPH, Senior Staff Attorney

Jill Tellioglu, LLM, Legal Fellow

Heather Wooten, MCP; Vice President for Programs

FULL AUTHORSHIP LISTING

Marice Ashe, JD, MPH, Founder and CEO, ChangeLab Solutions, Oakland, CA

Dora Barilla, DrPH, President, HC2 Strategies and Executive Leader, Providence Health and Services, Tacoma, WA

Eileen Barsi, GC, Population Health Management and Community Benefit Consultant and Formerly with Dignity Health, San Francisco, CA

Stephanie Cihon, BA, Associate Vice President, Community Relations, Advocacy and Grants, of ProMedica, Toledo, OH

For more information about this chapter, contact **Marice Ashe** at e-mail, mashe@changelabsolutions.org or phone, (510) 302-3380.

CHAPTER 3

Accountable Lives:
Leading Complex Health Structures

Gary Gunderson with Teresa Cutts, Steve Scoggin, Jerry Winslow,
Caroline Battles and Thomas Strauss

The Stakeholder Health (SH) learning community focuses on how we can be deeply accountable for the possibilities latent in the communities and systems for which we provide care. Our focus is on the lives of leaders playing their (our) roles in large institutions, adapting to the profoundly changed present climate of opportunities and challenges. For the most part, Stakeholder Health believes the new climate has great advantages for the future of health and health care. To maximize the possibilities before us, we believe leadership must be intentionally adaptive, not resistant.

This chapter sharpens the focus on being accountable for *our lives as leaders*. This does not require a new paradigm that would split accountability into private and public spheres. The unity is found in a focus on the character of leaders and how that is expressed in the fullness of our lives. Questions of personal character resonate with the same triad that marked the original monograph's recommendation for community: a) a move toward social complexity in *our lives*, b) in sustained partnership, and c) using our own assets.

The embrace of complexity and partnership at social scale set off a learning storm that continues to be manifested in the rest of this collaborative document. This has great implications for our leadership roles within the organizations called health systems, which are as socially complex as the communities we are trying to engage. The priority on partnership also marks a necessary leadership shift as our institutions, like community, are best understood as webs of stakeholders. The third shift, toward a focus on the assets we already possess, is the linking one. Though daunted by the obvious challenges of equity, transparency and trust in such highly structured and hierarchical systems, we know we must find our way with the assets, resources and intelligence to be found among us, our stakeholders and our partners. This is good news, not bad, as it helps us see what is already happening within the health care ecosystem that we can support and strengthen.

The point of the chapter is to frame the work of positional leaders within healthcare organizations in the light of the conceptual framework of Stakeholder Health, understanding the opportunities to align partners in healthcare, public health, and community to achieve optimal health for the whole.

A well-lived leader's life follows the vein of possibility like a miner who seeks precious metal or gemstones. Sometimes it's not that hard—the vein is exposed, waiting for someone to notice that we should point the shovel here, not there. And sometimes, when the policy environment changes radically, as if from mining to farming, the path forward may seem more challenging to find. In institutions accustomed to difficult work, it would be quite unusual to hear from leaders: "We can find money in the less dramatic healthcare arts of prevention; we can work in the sunlight of community, and spend less time in the artificial light of the ER, and do so with partners who share our life's desire for healing."

Our institutions were founded before health, healthcare and public health were differentiated fields speaking different languages. In a sense, we are now called back to the more integrated mission for which we were originally founded. The shift in healthcare, as if from mining to farming, has two distinctive implications for executive leadership.

First is the challenge of *managing the shifting power dynamics* among and between existing stakeholders in the full range of systems that make for health in a particular community. The new possibilities and requirements of population health change the balance of opportunity and power among our very highly privileged institutions. Technology, connectivity, science, transparency and logic all unleash potential gains for the whole community, and they may also strengthen the roles of those formerly viewed as "lower" in the hierarchy. Physicians, who are used to being on an unchallenged pinnacle, find themselves on teams with other needed expertise. We will always need and appreciate highly specialized surgeons, for example, but success in an integrated model of health also rests on the intelligence of many more mid-level providers and an entire ecology of community health workers. The new financial value and improved health outcomes will come from integrating the intelligences of the latter into organizations built around the former.

The new balance will be a more profound change than we have yet experienced. The new roles do not simply *assist* the old roles; if successful, they will make it possible to have *fewer* inpatient beds and operating rooms and fewer operators. If it were purely a matter of power, nothing would change. But we are experiencing another climate shift driven by science and technology that will melt our institutions as surely as Greenland is shedding ice.

We—leadership—are often the *most* powerful and privileged people in the institution, so in the process of securing the possibilities of this era we may be experiencing the loss of some of our power. We will still need smart people at the center, but the value of the intelligence nearer the edges grows in every way. The organization with the smartest, leading-edge people is more likely to be most adapted to the community and the financial advantages found there.

Second, these new possibilities, found in the new models of health, have *practical implications for where we as leaders spend our time*—more among the broad range of stakeholders and less at our desks or with "internal" constituencies. We will spend much less time deciding, more in listening, blending, finding common alignment. This includes listening to those who were paid little attention in the past— and with those who have been (and in some ways still are) competitors. Less time spent convening in the penthouse suite, more on others' streets.

The work of leadership looks filled with freedom and resources to those on the outside, but healthcare organizations are among the most tightly regulated of all. They are accountable to a welter of federal, state, county and city regulations, and then doubly bound by multiple levels of credentialed guilds. Every guild's professional organization is awash with presentations about transformational change even as they work to continue the patter of old privileges. The lived reality is that much of this compliance to law and guild tethers the organization tightly to past science and policy, while it moves into the future with caution and in anything but an even or predictable manner. Some say the first job of the President of the country is defense; so too, with the senior leadership of a hospital. It is simply not possible for any executive at any level to be non-compliant with any of the law or regulatory strictures or ever to be seen to take any of them lightly, forcing much leadership energy and time on defense. This makes severe and often perverse demands on time and cash that have nothing to do with either medical or management science and the health of the public.

This is not an entirely new reality for health leaders, who have always had to navigate the swift and shifting currents of science, technology and public policy. There are times when those flooding currents cut entirely new channels. We seem to be in one of those times.

As leaders we embody the changes we seek. The associated stresses, tensions, ambiguities, perversities and confusions inherent in leadership live inside our bodies, too. Healthcare leaders are among a highly privileged elite, and they spend the vast majority of their waking hours among other highly privileged people. For some years in Memphis, Methodist Le Bonheur Healthcare ran a small program called "Life of Leaders" which wove into a "Mayo-like" (exemplary executive physical) model of health assessment an array of life assessments built on the Leading Causes of Life (Gunderson with Pray, 2009). The experience was initially aimed at clergy who can go years with hardly ever a chance for a safe, frank dialogue about their *own* life, its changes and challenges. The process was then offered to highly placed executives and it revealed that they also lived vulnerably in the open, being constantly seen as the answer to everyone else's problems and hopes.

Healthcare leaders embody a mediating role. They lead structures relevant to every single human in their service areas whom they will often need at the most profound and vulnerable moments in their life journey. The work of leader is typically wide open to view, even when they are not doing anything official, such as walking across the parking lot or getting a cup of coffee. This embodiment is the heart of their challenge: "the body keeps the score." Even a slight rebalancing of whose company they keep may have huge effects in what they know and what their system sees them as knowing.

Hospitals are often compared (with no small irony) to military organizations, especially in terms of the strict authority of hierarchy and command. Armies, of course, are not what they used to be and have had to learn to adjust quite radically to new forms of adversaries. They, too, have undergone fundamental change in shifting their attention to the social factors that currently also shape health over time instead of focusing primarily on one event at a time. "Winning" now demands an empowered, highly adaptive fighting force guided by intelligence as much about psychodynamics as weaponry. How much more true for a healing force? Retired General Stan McChrystal embodies the changes he experienced as a combat leader, now applying those insights to healthcare and other transforming fields (McChrystal, Collins, Silverman & Fussell, 2015). His team focuses on helping organizations develop qualities of robustness and resilience so as to adapt to emergent challenges and opportunities.

The Stakeholder Health logic similarly opens up challenges and, more importantly, opportunities for leadership, by working to bring into active self-conscious alignment the multiple stakeholder and partners whose vital strengths are the sinews of the strength and vitality of the entire health system itself. Whereas the hospital system alone has tended to be the focus of its leaders, this radical re-centering of relationships will, in the future, define the daily walk and work of those who sit in key positions of influence within the highly complex webs of changing relationships among all stakeholders. This will become obvious at the point of care inside the clinical spaces with a shift to teams of mutually empowered professionals not just passively waiting for the direction of the physician. Now the term "clinical space" will include anywhere clinically relevant, and the choices made there, the counsel given, and the activities and interventions undertaken will cross over the whole spectrum affecting health through time. This includes new entrants in the provision of healthcare such as Wal-Mart, CVS, and Rite-Aid. It also includes homeless shelters, places of worship and play, and hairdressers. Financial value is created by lowering the acuity and expense of the care, which totally flips where the money is made from the center to the edge of the system. Few in the hospital world have actually grasped this yet, though there are already outstanding examples, such as Kaiser Permanente's steps toward "total health."

Tectonic tensions are building inside the rigid hospital system we have, between the old world and the inevitable movement toward the new. Changes include those needed in what are often called "corporate support services", including those at the very core—facilities, purchasing, finance, HR and Governance. All of these services now need to be accountable for creating a dynamic web of effects that bring alive the generative relationships within the whole system, with the reasonable expectation that this will positively affect the health of the whole population served. Other chapters in this volume focus on implications for where hospitals put the hundreds of millions of reserve funds they are required to have on hand. Those funds must be considered as multi-relevant assets. Why not place a few percent of them in safe community development partnerships to strengthen the housing trends in the poorest neighborhoods?

Similarly, suppliers, now judged primarily in terms of price, are also crucial variables in the functioning of the whole system: Who we buy from and how their discrete services serve the purposes of a larger system matter. Suppliers, especially of relational and information technology, must be viewed through a more complex lens that sharpens their role in the flow of trust-building information among the partners relevant to aligning our efforts. It is hard enough to list all the factors relevant to the new reality. How is any human supposed to lead it? "Others, besides us, such as corporations like Whole Foods, have already begun to use the principles we promote here (see sidebar below).

LEADERSHIP PRINCIPLES IN ACTION: STAKEHOLDER HEALTH ALIGNMENT WITH NEW CORPORATE MODELS

The authors of both *Firms of Endearment* (*FoE*; see Sisodia, Wolfe & Sheth 2014) and *Conscious Capitalism* (Mackey & Sisodia, 2014) offer many examples, though specific to the corporate or for profit business world, that highlight the structures noted in this piece on leadership. Below are examples and tenets from these new models that fit the leadership principles that Stakeholder Health proposes be put into action within a healthcare setting.

The first distinctive implications for senior leadership involves managing the changed positional and power dynamics among and between existing stakeholders that make for health in a particular place. The authors of *FoE* cite examples of how they are working more closely with local suppliers of produce, cheeses and locally and humanely grown poultry and meat to offer workforce and economic development locally, decrease the carbon footprint and build local goodwill. This changes the landscape of the environment, business relations and stakeholder relationships, for the betterment of the whole.

Secondly, Stakeholder Health notes that such new relationships shape where leaders spend their time—"inside out": outside the walls of offices and more in the "field" listening, blending, finding common alignment and synergies. John Mackey of Whole Foods (Mackey and Sisodia, 2014) shares the story of getting his leaders and employees outside of the confines of the workplace by having them visit places where their products are created and micro-grants have offered local opportunities. He admits that it is hard to put a standard ROI on the impact of these sabbaticals, but all see that for his employees the visits have expanded their work and world, with phenomenal impact on philanthropy, worker productivity, and worker retention.

Likewise, the authors of *Conscious Capitalism* (Mackey & Sisodia, 2014) resonate with the idea that leaders embody the changes they seek, often take a mediating role, and live in the fishbowl of transparency. This openness can be a potential double-edged sword. To be a leader in these times is to have all of your past and potential dirty laundry scrutinized by all, often in inappropriate ways and contexts. John Mackey shares the pain he experienced when being investigated for potential fraud for posts he had made innocently prior to a proposed merger with Wild Oats, as well as the public vilification of his character and motives. On the positive side, leaders can model exactly what they are trying to embody in their institution. John Mackey's letter to his various stakeholders, taking $1 a year for pay from 1997 onward, is a positive example of how "walking the walk and talking the talk" can be powerful.

Our leadership views the need for adaptive, creative, conscious leadership, adjusting to ever-shifting times and work. Our military metaphor, often noted to be too aggressive, nonetheless points to what is needed to transverse the ever changing landscape of payment changes in healthcare and economic downturns in businesses.

The flip of funding flow in our proactive mercy model is also illustrated by this model from Whole Foods (see sidebar) of how so many diverse stakeholders are funded and/or supported or negotiated within the integrated whole, with fairness and equity.

Interestingly, this "flow" also mirrors our advocacy of leadership that works from Inside Out (focusing first on those outside of our hospital walls), Right Side Up (flipping the power dynamics and lifting those stakeholders usually at the bottom of the power pyramid up to the tip), and Out of Control (relishing and adapting to the surprises and changes that will inevitably occur in the market in terms of revenue cycles, particularly "down" quarters in those cycles).

Whole Foods Stakeholder Model

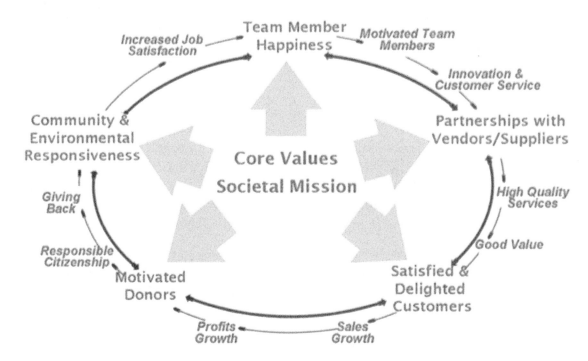

A leaders' role in facilitating the change within our organizations is the mirror of the SH approach to long-term transformation of communities (Health System Learning Group monograph, 2013). The same trilogy of tactical competencies comes to the front:

a. *Move toward social complexity*, in this case, the complex lives, broadly defined, of all the stakeholders. And move toward that complexity as we find it in the places, networks, roles and power relationships in which we find ourselves.

b. *Move in partnerships* nurtured for the scale and duration of the problem—and opportunity (as far as we can imagine into the future).

c. *Invest resources proactively*. The money we need is the money we are already spending on less generative purposes. Be a first mover with the fuel found amid the partnerships already in place.

Stakeholder Health leaders realize their own institutions are so utterly part of the community that the line between inside and outside is dissolving. The business of the hospital is no longer accomplished within its own walls by its employees performing discrete interventions for patients. The wall between within and without disappears as the success of the healing relationship depends on a more complex set of actors spread over a sustained period of time.

One of the things that goes away is the sharp distinction in the roles of the complex lives of the stakeholders. Employees are patients and are at the same time members and often leaders of key partner institutions, influential in the informal and formal networks that encompass the life of the community and members of insurance pools, patrons of stores. Their families spread even farther into the interstices of community, as do those who work for our suppliers. It is easier to remain apart, ignorant of this complexity; easier to think in terms of this and that, inside and outside, us and them. Thinking and acting that way isolates the leaders of what is often the largest institutional identity in the social system—the hospital—in a bubble of our own making without lessening the lived inter-penetration of all the facets of the lives of those in the system.

The institution being led is not apart from the community system in which it functions, finds its life and seeks to fulfill its purpose. This creates anxiety for those who need predictability and control. Yet it is also good news for those able to turn toward the complexity and enter new forms of collaboration with purpose and mission.

Many of the hopeful innovations shared elsewhere in this document are driven by encouraging and releasing the power of the capacities of people in the system who would have previously been contained within a limited prescriptive service role. The icon of this at Wake Forest is the highly effective witness of the Supporters of Health, released from their former role as housekeepers to play a creative role in our toughest communities. In fact, almost every role in the hospital is filled by someone with capacity beyond their conventional job description. High-end doctors can volunteer out of their faith identity. Security officers have been trained as counselors for enhanced roles as *first mental health* responders. People all over the system can be released to play community leadership roles on boards of all kinds of health-relevant organizations. Nurses can be trained as spiritual caregivers. Chaplains can be integrated into transitional care teams in nursing homes, and visiting pastors can be raised up as community healers.

Such cross-functional empowerment opportunities are endless and powerful if aligned with a common vision of cooperation to create a healthier community. This is a goal that resonates with the healthcare systems we help to lead because it fits their avowed missions while also contributing to their financial viability. The opportunity lies in the complex lives of the stakeholders because that complexity is what makes it possible to connect with integrity beyond the simple role definitions that have kept us isolated in our conventional silos. The leadership challenge involved in managing complex roles is no simpler or harder than the challenges handled successfully in earlier times. It is worth the trouble to find those hidden skills and capacities. In a time of shrinking reimbursements and reversed incentives, we must look within ourselves to find what we need. Our counsel is that there is plenty, once we look.

Our challenge as leaders is that complexity cannot be managed as if it were "over there," pertaining to someone or something other than our own lives, our own prerogatives, our own institutions. The complex system of community is not apart from the complex system of our own organization. There is a highly permeable boundary between what is really one system. Our employees, patients, suppliers, Boards and every other person involved cross back and forth constantly.

As leaders we too often think apart from the whole. This has practical implications for the daily work of management. We may understand this via three shifts in the relationship among the patients, families and communities—and the employees, staff and medics who share those roles from time to time. Each of the shifts changes what the leader pays attention to themselves and to what the leader asks their organization to attend.

INSIDE OUT

The first shift is *inside out*—the original exemplar being the 604 partners of the Congregational Health Network of Memphis. The leadership move is to make one's *self* and then one's *organization* connectable with the agents of health that surround the hospital as the ocean surrounds a whale. A community filled with consumers of services is now filled with agents of health who are working in partnership with an array of people, coalitions and organizations that provide services woven in community and by community.

The population in this view is not an entity to be managed, but the thing doing the managing. Those "outside" are not passive consumers. They are agents of their own health through a rich ecology of roles, networks and relationships. The leader of the hospital can make those visible and hold every "internal" system accountable for its connective capacity to the assets "outside." What makes this less daunting than it seems is that all those inside live even more of their lives outside. Once they are freed to speak out of both sites of intelligence, it turns out there is an enormous reservoir of experience and practical knowledge about where and how to connect, and about which hospital policies impede or prohibit the weaving.

Some of these are almost too obvious to see. For example, Wake Forest has long provided free parking to visiting clergy who only had to register to get a badge that worked the exit gate. It was a positive shock when looking for a way to engage the hundreds of community faith groups to realize that more than 1,600 pastors were already registered! How can we strengthen the role they are already in with the patients? Complexity like this is not a problem but a profound opportunity. At Wake Forest another 14,000 people called employees play complex and powerful roles of many kinds in their families (often patients) and communities (where these patients live) that could be systematically honored and strengthened. A leader can set off a cascade of opportunities by making it okay to connect.

In a time of fear, we are all being asked "if you see something, say something." How much more should we be doing this about positive things that could affect the lives of our institutions, communities and, of course, patients? That will not be possible in any organization until its leaders shift what "accountability" means to balance compliance with the old defensive rules with the new behaviors of connectivity so vital to success in complex human populations.

RIGHT-SIDE UP

The second shift of mind is more challenging, but follows from the first. It is the flip toward paying attention to the "bottom" of organizations, the reverse of the old ways. This right-side up attentiveness focuses on creating space and roles for the power and intelligence of those who populate the base of the organization. This is not choosing the new against the old, the janitor against the surgeon, but rather, a blending of all the intelligences available in service of a common goal of health at population scale. Organizations have long carefully tended to the needs and preferences of those of us who live at their "top," but leaders need to pay a balancing dose of attention to those whose roles have been under-valued and strengths left unattended. We need to turn our time and attention upside down in order to get right-side up.

Because leaders lead by modeling what is most important to them, this raises high the need for modeling humility, which may seem like weakness to some but is in fact an essential art and a vital key to the adaptive learning that the future calls for. Good leaders never miss an opportunity to tell about how a successful innovative practice began with the humble recognition of a learning moment. Leaders who once were proud mostly of their *teaching* institutions, now must model the value of a *teachable* institution.

Other chapters lay out an array of tools and techniques, especially those mapping assets, for paying attention to voices and lives in difficult parts of the community. It is somewhat easier, yet more awkward, to bring that kind of curiosity to one's own colleagues and fellow employees. We do not know of any health system that has systematically mapped the webs of influence of its employees in the community they are trying to "serve" (which is the same one the vast majority of the employees live in). Like community assets mapping, the search would be rewarded by an inconvenience of opportunity. The most significant attention should be focused where historically the lowest interest has been shown— among the lowest wage roles. Many of those individuals spend considerable time with patients and thus have a great deal of relevant clinical intelligence. They often have laser clarity about institutional life too and an often-bitter grasp of the relationship between the non-profit corporation and the vulnerable neighborhoods in which they—and many patients—pass their lives.

Stakeholder Health believes that population health schemes will work where our current patient care techniques work. But for those estranged from, stigmatized by or fearful of the present patterns of care and exclusion, population health will fail. We can wait to pay heavily in finance and retrospective data analytics for that failure to happen. Or we could read our communities with new eyes by asking upside-down questions to read the future right-side up.

This right-side-up-ness is not cheap, for it requires the leader to invest in trust with their time and through their behavior. One can't ask and then not act. The lowest wage workers have been recipients of leaders' previous priorities since their first day of work. They've been watching and noticing what matters and may well be wary of giving their trust too quickly to the sound of a new day. Current leaders—or the smarter ones who will replace us—need the intelligence of the whole organization about the places where the biggest opportunities and threats of community scale live. *(See again the sidebar above on Leadership Principles in Action: Alignment with New Corporate Models).*

Stephen Covey, in his Learning at the Speed of Trust *manual (2009, pg. 1) notes that:*

"The ability to establish, extend, and restore trust with all stakeholders-customers, business partners, investors and co-workers-is the key leadership competency of the new global economy."

WEBS OF TRUST

The last shift—toward webs of trust—is even more far-reaching for those of us leaders taught to equate high reliability with high compliance. The new equation is that high reliability equals high adaptive capacity multiplied by speed of trust divided by high compliance.

$$\text{HIGH RELIABILITY} = \frac{\text{HIGH ADAPTIVE CAPACITY X SPEED OF TRUST}}{\text{HIGH COMPLIANCE}}$$

Compliance with established best practices, laws and customs is like an anchor that is essential in organizations dealing daily with thousands of variations and wild things that happen to humans along our path in life. But, in practice, compliance functions to hold us from a premature embrace of the *next* best practice. Ask the poor and they will tell you that deviation from best practice is not random; the short cuts are biased against them and anyone else who presents an inconvenient difference. Compliance is meant to protect the most vulnerable. But it does not favor the possibilities *beyond* the current best practice. The current "best" has fostered systems compliant with the social and economic patterns of privilege that have created very predictable patterns of risk, disease and injury far below what either science or faith deem the minimum acceptable. The current best is not even decent, much less optimal. In this time of change, it is critical that healthcare leaders hold the line protecting patients while pushing that line farther toward mercy and justice, which science, and now policy, make possible.

Trust can accelerate strategy and execution while distrust can and does decelerate those processes. Trust works like waves that create a ripple effect beginning with self trust extending to interpersonal trust that can lead to organizational and community trust (Covey, 2009). Notice that this is an inside-out process that begins with the leader's personal credibility and his or her capacity to extend trust to others. "Trust Taxes" are those decisions and behaviors in an organization that undermine trust (HR decisions, excessive risk-management, etc.) whereas "Trust Dividends" (restoring retirement matches, empowering employees to make decisions, etc.) are those deposits that accelerate momentum in an organization and community. This is a keystone behavior and habit that is bedrock to strategy and execution.

Trust is better and more efficient than mere control. The challenge is that the webs of relationship relevant to the processes involving the health of entire populations are extensive and novel. In the state of New York, for example, the current process of "reinventing Medicaid" involves changing the relationship among current competing hospitals, which is hard enough given the billions of dollars at stake. Far more challenging is figuring out how to value and integrate hundreds of community based organizations that have critical roles in the social factors now recognized as crucial in shaping longer term outcomes for patients. All of those organizations have long related to the same people and operated in the same neighborhoods, but never in a model of shared risks, gains and outcomes. An old-fashioned system of highly controlled, rules-based compliance cannot possibly meet these challenges.

But how is it possible even to imagine a web of trusted relationships at such scale? The health of the community will not be achieved by including all the neighborhoods in the dominion, control and compliance of the hospital. Hospital leaders will not be the princesses or princes of their dominion managing their populations like the landed aristocracy managed passive feudal era peasants in order to satisfy the reimbursement logic. Hospitals and our leaders need to move across the moat, but with the best intentions of serving, not for purposes of control.

Thus, the third twisting of mindset is for leaders to move their organization towards understanding that it is literally out of (not in) control. As soon as we became liable for long term health dynamics of the large fraction of the humans living around us, we became subject to shared power with many others who control crucial nodes in the social networks affecting the choices of the people about their health and timing of treatment. We are not in control; but then neither is anyone else, so we should not be afraid. We remain the largest component of most community systems, capable of significant influence on those systems—as long as we don't try to control or "manage" them.

In our time of radical transparency, choice and connectivity, control is fractured and dispersed widely throughout the system. The advantage goes to those capable of embracing that complexity in their own institution and in the context of the larger community, by embracing large scale partnerships and by investing resources in long term goals that will help the whole system find its life.

Conclusion

All of these implications are equally true whether the institutional leader is focused on profit for shareholders, on taxpayers, or on a non-profit mission governed by a volunteer Board. It should be obvious, however, that mission-driven organizations have a powerful advantage in embracing the three leadership fundamentals presented here. We have—or should have—fewer distracting priorities that would make partnership with health-relevant organizations inherently difficult. And we have—or could have—internal alignment about the priorities of our own resources that would make the reallocation more logical (if not easier). We at least know why we are here and are glad that reason aligns nicely with what our most powerful stakeholders want (better health at larger scale at less cost).

The daily work of leadership in large institutions is about paying attention and signaling to the organization what is most important. Not just to one's direct reports, but to everyone who can see them, who notices what the leader is noticing and where they put their time, body and energy. Leaders of course cannot cease caring about the legal, regulatory and compliance issues that lend structure to quality and decency in healthcare. They are not free to make a margin that fails to pass industry standard audits. And they cannot remain within the old as if the new is not already breaking in.

How does one live between the old and the new? Technically, the leader helps the organization know how to recognize the things that will matter most on the journey forward and bring them into view alongside the metrics and methods that matter the most now. This makes for a more complex and less predictable, but still intelligible "balanced scorecard." It includes measures that allow us to be accountable for the increased priorities found in partnerships that would previously have been described as "external." And it includes entirely new roles and accountabilities on the edges of our organizations. Many of these are community oriented but are not designed just to be for "community benefit" as customarily defined in terms of compliance for non-profit tax purposes. Rather, they are designed to melt the wall so as to allow the sustained viability of the organization to thrive in more complex partnerships with a wider array of active partners. The leader's job is to notice all of that and to figure out how to create patterns of reporting and accountability so that the whole organization can be more self-conscious of its new role in a more complex relationship to community.

The first insight of Stakeholder Health remains the most challenging—embracing the social complexity of the individuals, including ourselves, and that of the component systems, including our own. Thus the first most basic quality the leader acting on these recommendations must embody is to take courage, and not be afraid of the future. That is the way that embodies the faith of the founders and not just their words, rules, HR policies or bylaws any more than we would want their outdated surgical tools and primitive anesthetics. Healthcare leaders know they are here for more than themselves. And they know they have more to work with than their own cleverness. In that sense, they are all faith-based, no matter who founded their institution. Fear makes us blind and slow; when we back into the community, we are surprised by its complexity and miss the opportunity to participate in its future. Setting fear aside allows us as leaders to find the path for our kind of institutions into the future. Optimistic uncertainty opens eyes for partners with intelligence, assets and energy with whom we can find our way.

REFERENCES

Franklin Covey and Covey Link LLC (2009). *Leading at the Speed of Trust*, Participant Manual, Franklin Covey and Covey Link : U.S.A.

Gunderson, G.R. with Pray, L. (2009). *Leading Causes of Life: Five Fundamentals to Change the Way You Live Your Life*, Abingdon Press: Nashville.

Mackey, J. & Sisodia, R. S. (2014). *Conscious Capitalism: Liberating the Heroic Spirit of Business*. Harvard Business Review Press: Boston, Mass.

McChrystal, S.A., Collins T., Silverman, D. & Fussell, C. (2015). *Team of teams : New rules of engagement for a complex world*. New York: Portfolio/Penguin Press.

Sisodia, R., Sheth, J. N., & Wolfe, D. (2014). *Firms of Endearment: How World-Class Companies Profit from Passion and Purpose*. Pearson Education: Upper Saddle River, New Jersey.

ACKNOWLEDGMENTS

We owe deep thanks to Michael Bilton of Dignity Health, Senior Director, Community Health and Benefit, San Francisco, CA, for his insightful editing and review of this chapter.

FULL AUTHORSHIP LISTING

Gary R. Gunderson, MDiv, DMin, DTh (Hon), Vice President of FaithHealth, Wake Forest Baptist Medical Center and Professor, Faith and Health of the Public, Wake Divinity School and Wake Forest School of Medicine, Winston Salem, NC

Teresa Cutts, PhD, Asst. Research Professor, Wake Forest School of Medicine, Div. of Public Health Science, Dept. of Social Sciences and Health Policy, Winston Salem, NC

Steve Scoggin, MDiv, PsyD, LPC, President, CareNet, Inc., Wake Forest Baptist Medical Center, Winston Salem, NC

Jerry Winslow, PhD, Vice President, Mission and Culture, Loma Linda University Health, Loma Linda, CA

Caroline Battles, MBA, Vice President, State Advocacy and Community Health, Ascension, St. Louis, MO

Thomas Strauss, PharmD, CEO Emeritus, Summa Health System, Akron, OH

For more information about this chapter, contact **Gary Gunderson** at e-mail, gary.gunderson@gmail.com or phone (336) 403-6861.

CHAPTER 4

Optimizing the Patient Encounter: Relational Technology that Integrates Social and Spiritual Domains into the Electronic Health Record

Dora Barilla, Eileen Barsi, Maureen Kersmarki, Monica Lowell,
with Mark Zirkelbach and Gurmeet Sran

Introduction: Health Policy & The Future of Information Technology

Much has changed in the health care arena since the World Health Organization's (WHO) broad definition of health was developed in 1948. (See Chapter 10 for in-depth review of that current definition.) Today, the United States health care system is undergoing a rapid transformation in the way care is being delivered through population health management and the formation of new accountable care and payment reform models.

According to the WHO the United States has the highest health care spending costs but the poorest health outcomes when compared to other industrialized nations. Our health care system is known for being inefficient, fragmented and expensive. Nevertheless, with the adoption of Health Care Reform and new financing methods, there are opportunities to become more efficient and effective in the way we deliver care and move to a payment model that rewards value and not volume.

The integration of socioeconomic information and environmental risk factors into the Electronic Health Record is an important aspect of improving community and patient health, and achieving health equity. The 2010 Affordable Care Act (ACA) *Health Information Technology for Economic and Clinical Health* provision has created an essential foundation for meeting these objectives through better methods of storing, analyzing and sharing health information (Beeuwkes, Blumenthal, Buntin & Sachin, 2010).

ACA sets forth three objectives for the U.S. health system commonly referred to as the Triple Aim: to improve people's health, lower health care costs, and provide better quality care (Bisgnano & Kenney, 2012). The Triple Aim calls for a shift in the delivery of care to consider the social, economic, spiritual and environmental factors that affect the health of an individual. Providers should understand not only a patient's medical condition but also have a clear understanding of the social factors and living conditions that may be influencing their health. As noted in our earlier monograph (Health Systems Learning Group, 2013), Stakeholder Health believes that equity should be added as the fourth aim, expanding the objectives to a Quadruple Aim.

As described in Chapter 2 on social determinants, this means that providers must consider what else is going on in their patients' lives. Is healthy food available to help control their diabetes? What housing conditions and local triggers are affecting their asthma? Is the neighborhood safe so that walking is an option to control hypertension? Can patients afford their medications? What are patient's physical needs and what community resources are available to support healthy living? What resources can help treat the patient in a holistic and effective way? What are the cultural and spiritual considerations that might influence medical interventions?

With 80% of poor health due to behavioral and social determinants, it becomes more and more crucial that providers optimize each patient encounter (County Health Rankings & Roadmaps, 2015). This can be made possible by the integration of physical, social and spiritual domains into the Electronic Health Record (EHR).

Fortunately, the shift towards incorporating the socioeconomic factors in the EHR is underway. The purpose of this chapter is to provide health care administrators and providers, policymakers, IT vendors and advocates with an overview of the importance of this much needed paradigm shift and the progress to date. We have included:

- An overview of the national organizations that have begun to integrate socioeconomic information and environmental risk factors into the EHR

- Technology challenges identified by Stakeholder Health members

- An overview of new models and promising practices

- A listing of potential domains to incorporate in the EHR

- Recommendations and a Call to Action.

Lastly, we view spirituality/faith as an important domain that must be embedded with all other domains with equal importance.

Overall, Stakeholder Health views the Affordable Care Act and the resulting policy environment as an opportunity to address the underlying causes of poor health in communities; make informed decisions to better align, integrate and leverage existing resources; and create partnerships with diverse stakeholders that will result in positive outcomes.

AHA's Second Curve of Population Health

The American Hospital Association (AHA) table above illustrates the differences in the First Curve (current system) and the Second Curve (necessary to meet the Quadruple Aim).

The Second Curve

As we move more deeply into health reform and the achievement of the Quadruple Aim, we find ourselves at a critical juncture. The American Hospital Association has said that "Hospital leaders need to develop strategies that move their organizations from the first curve, or volume-based environment, to the second curve, in which they will be building value-based systems and business models" (American Hospital Association, 2014). From now on, optimizing opportunities to improve individual and population health must include mature community partnerships and integrated health information technology.

The Causes of Health

As noted in Chapter Two, the *County Health Rankings* model of Population Health reinforces our understanding that the causes and management of disease are far more complex than the resultant illness itself (County Health Rankings & Roadmaps, 2015). The model identifies many factors that, if improved, can help make our communities healthier places to live, learn, work and play. It also weights the social determinants of health, reminding us that we must address factors outside the walls of the hospital to meet the health needs of patients and reduce the burden of cost, both human and financial, for them and for the health system.

Roadmaps to Health

WEB OF TRUST

According to the Roadmaps of Health, only about 20 percent of people's health status is related directly to Clinical Care (County Health Rankings and Roadmaps, 2015). The other 80 percent relates to health behaviors and the "social determinants" of health. With this in mind, Stakeholder Health members have identified four critical markers that can, and are beginning to erode the "old" boundaries between health care and health, and hospital and community. We believe that working in the context of these markers can produce tangible cost savings, and improve health outcomes and the quality of care.

1. **Socially Complex People in Socially Complex Neighborhoods:** We know that the most significant factors in determining health come from human interactions, health behaviors, and the social and physical environment. This knowledge demands that our Information Technology (IT) systems link the underlying factors (determinants) of a person's health to his/her environment.

2. **Larger Scale Partnerships:** It is crucial to identify and engage partners already invested in improving community well-being. Effective partnerships also call for IT systems that address and connect the value represented in these partnerships.

3. **Redesign the Connectivity:** Health systems face multiple data-sharing challenges (including HIPAA compliance) in creating a single identifier that would connect each patient with the appropriate community partners. Properly done, Health Information Exchanges (HIEs) could serve as sources of both patient data and community intelligence. The challenges that thwarted the first versions of HIEs could be employed as opportunities to rethink a new HIE framework for care coordination and genuine population/community health. For example, the recidivism rates of individuals presenting in the ED with substance abuse issues were daunting for a southern California hospital, not only because of the unresolved issues patients confronted, but also because their need for care was persistent and the hospital was not the optimal care provider beyond the perceived need for emergency care. Utilizing a health information exchange technology called CareConnect™, a new process of referral and case management to link individuals to community-based behavioral health

services filled the gap to make care coordination a reality. Ultimately, patients are better served and the demand for emergency room care by this vulnerable population is reduced.

4. **Better Aligned Incentives:** We need to know far better how to incentivize health systems to engage with patients more holistically.

ENHANCING WHOLE-PERSON CARE THROUGH TECHNOLOGY

As providers and community partners consider not only clinical needs but also the determinants that make a person healthy (or not), relevant information may be obtained through use of both the Health Information Exchanges and Electronic Health Record.

Individuals and patients can democratize the data by granting permission to share information with resource partners along the health continuum, which, as emphasized in other chapters, requires building and establishing trust. Geographic data and the implications of socioeconomic factors (social determinants) would be standard across all settings. A more holistic model of care can be achieved through connections with a community of providers, including family members.

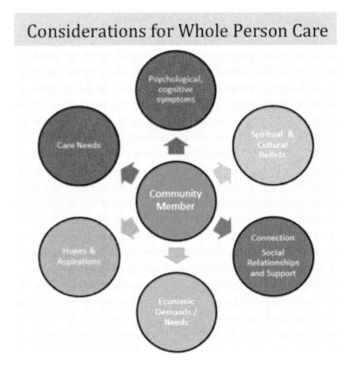

Considerations for Whole Person Care

THE STAKEHOLDER HEALTH INFORMATION TECHNOLOGY (IT) WORK GROUP

Stakeholder Health's earlier monograph on *Strategic Investment in Shared Outcomes: Transformative Partnerships between Health Systems and Communities* (Health System Learning Group, 2013) outlined our whole-person, whole-community vision with the intent of helping our partners strategically align their community investments.

Following the publication of the monograph, the Stakeholder Health IT Work Group, co-chaired by Dora Barilla, Dr.Ph., of Loma Linda University Health and Eileen Barsi of Dignity Health, set out through a series of subsequent meetings and discussions held from July 2013 to the present, to envision Information Technology that would ensure optimal care coordination in our communities.

Currently, the Electronic Health Record (EHR) technology that is widely sold (and, to some degree, required by the ACA's Meaningful Use provisions 1.0 and 2.0) does not begin to address the opportunities documented in the Stakeholder Health ensemble of practices noted in the 2013 monograph.

Those practices (see HSLG, 2013, page 15) focus directly on two interrelated groups: the people whom hospitals identify as the most challenging patients ("socially complex") as well as, the least desirable neighborhoods ("socially complex"); and large-scale partnerships that could align the requisite network of not-for-profit and faith-based entities that work in, and share hope for, these patients and neighborhoods.

Our IT Work Group quickly reached consensus that the current EHR format falls short in providing population health and neighborhood information and saw the need to make it more meaningful. Its members set out to create an IT framework that would optimize patient encounters by addressing not only physical health, but also the unaddressed issues that can negatively affect patients' and communities' health.

In discussing our IT needs in the context of "the complex patient" scenarios and in relation to various traditional and non-traditional partners along the health continuum, the same questions came up repeatedly:

1. How do caregivers know what resources are available in the community?

2. What services do the community partners provide?

3. How can we access these resources to optimize the health of an individual?

This dream of interconnectedness and robust IT systems to support it captured our imaginations. There has never been a greater moment to ensure the connectivity and validity of community assets. With the current Health Reform mandates we find ourselves at a new juncture, a time that points to the need for addressing health inequity and, ultimately, achieve better health outcomes. Sharing relevant information across the health care continuum is imperative and this can be done only in partnership with diverse stakeholders, including patients.

DATA FRAMEWORK FOR HEALTH EQUITY

A 1987 Institute of Medicine report entitled "Socioeconomic Status and Health: Closing the Gap" pointed out that as early as the 12th Century, people at the lowest socioeconomic levels had higher death and illness rates.

Over the last two decades, additional studies have generated an even clearer understanding of the disproportionate, unmet, health-related needs of vulnerable populations. Population health data have given us summary statistics and detailed information about specific health conditions.

This retrospective type of review, utilizing well-established principles of measurement and analysis, has also provided epidemiologic information about risk factors that have informed public health planning strategies and shaped health service delivery systems (Summarizing Population Health: Directions for the Development and Application of Population Metrics, 1998).

As such, consideration of not only the physical and clinical needs of individuals, but also of social needs and relevant environmental factors, must take place with prospective intelligence and predictive analytics. As yet, however, a comprehensive approach to addressing these unmet needs has not been realized.

The overarching objective of Stakeholder Health is to seize this opportunity, share the vision for the future, and act on the knowledge that we now have available. We believe, with the appropriately developed support and application of the information technology accessible today, that the potential to improve the health of populations and meet the goals of health care reform is unlimited.

THE INFORMATION TECHNOLOGY VISION

If traditional health care has primarily focused on the physical needs of a patient, we are now at a point of convergence in which we must also pay attention to the social needs of an individual and take into consideration the environmental risk factors that may negatively affect health. But the reality is that clinicians are likely to have neither the time to tend to both the physical and social needs in a limited office visit, nor ready access to the relevance of place and community resources for the health of the person s/he is treating.

To assist clinicians with ready access to tools that can provide resources and linkages when patient needs become known, Stakeholder Health would design a model based on a person's journey of health and needs and not only on hospital needs or traditional payer-specific segmentation. Imagine, then, during a patient assessment, if the providers considered the following questions:

1. What are the person's clinical needs?

2. What are the person's social needs?

3. Are the person's basic or fundamental needs being met?

4. What potential hazards lurk in the person's physical environment, the places he or she lives, works and plays?

Then, with the answers to those questions, imagine the resources that may open up. In this scenario, what would the various partners along the continuum need?

- **Individuals:**
  - Should be connected to resources and services in their own communities
  - Need education about their conditions and reasons why behavior changes may be required
  - May need information about the potential or actual health risks in their environments
  - May need community providers' support to work on their health improvement goals.
- **Non-Clinical Caregivers:**
  - May need more information from the patient, or assumed by the patient's socioeconomic status
  - Need to know community resources and the types of services provided near the patient's home
  - Need real-time connections to community-based resources in order to link immediate support to the individual at the point of care.
- **Community-based organizations:**
  - Need a connection to providers
  - Need the patient's relevant information in order to provide optimal support.

Ultimately, how can the individual, caregiver and community all be in alignment to ensure that appropriate interventions are occurring as needed? Clearly, there is a need for bi-directional communication between community-based organizations, clinical providers and non-clinical caregivers.

Finally, beyond provider assessments and/or primary care visits, how can IT help systems take the quantum leap from retrospective analysis (only) to prospective/predictive analytics? How can these systems provide tools that do not exist today but are vital to optimal care?

This IT challenge was vetted at meetings that brought together additional Stakeholder Health members from across the country. At the Washington DC gathering, participating staff from the Office of the National Coordination for Health Information Technology (ONC IT) included the Medical Director of Meaningful Use ONC IT. Among the issues raised were, "Who owns the information?" and, "How can it be democratized in a manner that will protect the privacy of an individual's health record while sharing what is relevant to members of those providing support or care in the community?" There was overall agreement that the inclusion of all aspects of health will result in more optimal care. And, though we may not achieve the ideal, we can certainly begin to make a more meaningful difference in population health through interoperability, health information exchanges, and the integration of socioeconomic variables that negatively affect health.

A Call To Action: Integration of Socioeconomic Information Into the Electronic Health Record (EHR)

Stakeholder Health is calling for the integration of socioeconomic information into the Electronic Health Record (EHR) and/or through Health Information Exchanges. We are offering another voice to the collective chorus that acknowledges the importance of this information in providing comprehensive whole-person care. Other voices include:

The following chart gives an overview of the ONC Strategic Plan, 2011-2015:

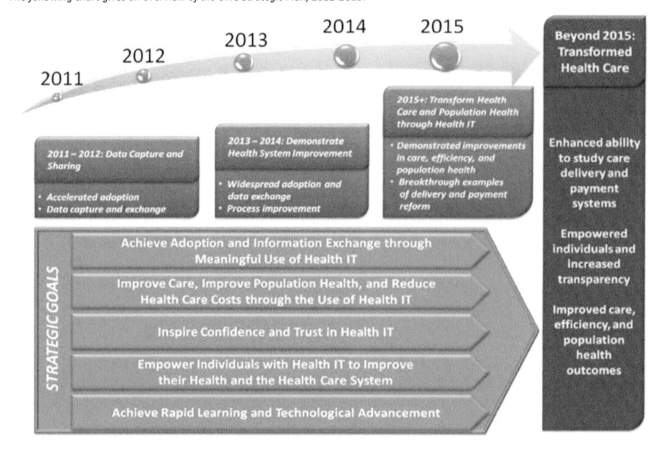

A. OFFICE OF THE NATIONAL COORDINATOR FOR HEALTH INFORMATION TECHNOLOGY (ONC)

Stakeholder Health has engaged staff from the Office of the National Coordinator for Health Information Technology (ONC) in this dialogue. The federal government's vision is "a health system that uses information to empower individuals and to improve the health of the population" and the ONC's mission is "To improve health and health care for all Americans through the use of information and technology," Dept. of Heath Information Technology, (2011).

Complementing the work underway by our government in its health IT strategy, Stakeholder Health is calling for a level of meaningful use that will make the EHR more potent in helping providers optimize patient encounters in addressing the full spectrum of factors that may be negatively influencing their health. This goal is not unlike one objective of the ONC, which is "to propose health information exchange and interoperability requirements that are more rigorous, so that patient information follows patients to the point of care and informs critical health decisions by health providers."

According to the Federal Health Information Technology Strategic Plan, in order to ensure that this type of exchange can take place:

• We must overcome barriers across geographies and among stakeholders (providers, laboratories, hospitals, pharmacies, behavioral health and patients).

• We must address additional barriers as identified in the Federal Health Information Technology Strategic Plan, such as an insufficient demand for electronic health information, the lack of a model for facilitating data exchange, security restrictions, and disparate federal, state and local policies that hinder the exchange of crucial information.

• Information exchange will require rigorous interoperability standards so that data can be used by multiple stakeholders.

B. THE AMERICAN HOSPITAL ASSOCIATION

In 2013, the American Hospital Association (AHA) Advocacy Agenda cited concerns about readmission measures and the methodology for payment penalties established in the Affordable Care Act (ACA) under P.L.111-148 and P.L.111-152 (American Hospital Association, 2013).

Specifically, the federal Hospital Readmission Reduction Program (HRRP) began imposing financial penalties on hospitals for "excess" (as compared to "expected") readmission levels on October 1, 2012. In incremental percentages, penalties can reduce hospital payments as much as three percent, with the initial three targeted conditions being myocardial infarction, congestive heart failure and pneumonia.

However, according to AHA's 2013 Advocacy Agenda, "the current readmission measures do not adequately adjust for socioeconomic factors." The agenda briefing also noted that "AHA has adamantly advocated that the Centers for Medicare and Medicaid Services (CMS) adjust the readmission measures to reflect socioeconomic differences in the patient populations served by different hospitals."

Substantial research has shown that readmissions are the result of many factors; some are within a hospital's control, and some are related to the lack of resources elsewhere in the community, such as: adequate numbers of primary care clinicians; access to pharmacies, home health services and rehabilitation services; transportation difficulties; and access to healthy eating alternatives. There is compelling evidence that safety-net hospitals and others serving large numbers of low-income individuals will have difficulty reducing readmissions due to the lack of certain resources in the communities they serve" (American Hospital Association, 2013).

C. UNITED STATES SENATE

In June 2014, Senators Joe Manchin (D-WV), Roger Wicker (R-MS), Bill Nelson (D-FL), and Mark Kirk (R-IL) introduced The Hospital Readmission Accountability and Improvement Act (Kirk, Nelson, Manchin & Wicker, 2014). This bipartisan legislation proposed an amendment to the Hospital Readmission Reduction Program (HRRP). The amendment would have required that CMS account for patient socioeconomic status when calculating risk-adjusted readmission penalties.

The sponsors noted that, all other factors being constant, socioeconomic conditions (such as poverty, low literacy levels, limited English proficiency, minimal social support, poor living conditions and limited community resources) very likely have direct and significant impacts on hospital readmissions. The bill also noted that including these factors would improve accountability and quality of care.

The bill did not become law, but it does signal raised awareness of the full range of health factors.

D. INSTITUTE OF MEDICINE OF THE NATIONAL ACADEMIES

In *Capturing Social and Behavioral Domains in Electronic Health Records: Phase 1*, an Institute of Medicine (IOM) report of the National Academies Committee identified 17 domains considered good candidates for inclusion in electronic health records (EHR). A second report, subtitled *Phase 2*, pinpointed 12 measures related to 11 of the initial domains (see sidebar on 12 Measures for Inclusion). The report considered the implications of incorporating the measures into all electronic health records (Institute of Medicine of The National Academies, 2014b).

The Committee identified certain domains related to neighborhoods and communities, and concluded that this information was potentially geocodable. If the EHR contains information about the geographic location (zip code or census block) where a person lives or works, that information could be linked to other databases to identify environmental conditions like air pollution or the availability of sidewalks, public transportation and healthy food (Institute of Medicine of The National Academies, 2014a).

Race/ethnicity, tobacco use, alcohol use, and residential address, education, financial resource strain, stress, depression, physical activity, social isolation, intimate partner violence, and neighborhood median household income.

The Committee charged with the development of the domains prioritized them in accordance with evidence on the association of health outcomes and the geographic locations. They concluded that there could be some utility for having the information in the EHR. Among the specifications considered, therefore, was the "usefulness of the domain as measured for decision making between the clinician and patient for management and treatment" (Institute of Medicine of The National Academies, 2014a).

This specification, in particular, limited those aspects of health for which management and treatment may not be within the realm of either participant.

Understandably, the IOM Committee's report concluded that some key measures were excluded if there were limitations in the ability of health providers to act upon the information presented. However, they also said, "Currently, the absence of social and behavioral determinants of health in EHRs limits the capacity of health systems to address key contributors to the onset and progression of disease. The addition and standardization of a parsimonious panel of social and behavioral measures into EHRs can help spur policy, system design, interoperability, and innovation to improve health outcomes and reduce health care costs" (Institute of Medicine of The National Academies, 2014a).

The IOM report affirms Stakeholder Health's belief that in order to support health beyond the traditional means offered yesterday, we must push beyond the boundaries of the EHR and explore the opportunities to strategically utilize data elements tomorrow.

According to the 2014 IOM report, "Capturing Social and Behavioral Domains in Electronic Health Records, "some domains reviewed but not selected were theoretically linked to health, but lacked an adequate evidence base to support routine collection of data.

"By limiting the recommended domains to those for which a reasonable evidence base exists, the committee is confident that the smaller set of domains and measures will result in the collection of crucial data for patient care, improvement of population health, and further expansion of the knowledge base to facilitate the development of precision medicine or other strategies for improving the health status of the U.S. population."

Challenges to the IT Vision

Before the vision of Stakeholder Health and others can be realized, a number of challenges must be addressed. One challenge is data availability. The Institute of Medicine study identified the need for research on the usefulness and feasibility of collecting social and behavioral data beyond that which is now collected. In addition, identification of interventions and treatments that effectively address the impact of social and behavioral determinants on health may generate the need to add new domains and measures in the EHR. Currently, there is no process for making such judgments (Institute of Medicine of The National Academies, 2014b, p. 16).

THE IMPORTANCE OF NON-CLINICAL DOMAINS

The November 2014 Institute of Medicine report, *Capturing Social and Behavioral Domains* and Measures in Electronic *Health Records: Phase 2*, noted that "EHRs have potential as essential tools for improving quality, increasing efficiency, and expanding access to the health system (Friedman, 2006; Friedman et al., 2010). They provide crucial information to providers treating individual patients, to health systems about population health, and to researchers about the determinants of health and the effectiveness of treatment. The inclusion of social and behavioral domains in EHRs is vital to all three."

TECHNOLOGY CHALLENGES IDENTIFIED BY STAKEHOLDER HEALTH AND IN THE IOM STUDY, "CAPTURING SOCIAL AND BEHAVIORAL DOMAINS AND MEASURES IN ELECTRONIC HEALTH RECORDS, PHASE 2, NOVEMBER 2014"

- **HIPAA** – Health information is protected by the federal Health Insurance Portability and Accountability Act of 1996, the Federal Health Information Technology Strategic Plan (HIPAA). HIPAA restricts the sharing of patient information by health care professionals. Certainly, we must vigorously protect patients (and the integrity of EHRs) from confidentiality breaches. Still, for EHRs to be optimized, we must collect data consistently across the country. This requires a commitment from all parties—including the patient—to sometimes allow access to sensitive personal data.

- **Interoperability** – Technology platforms that cannot "talk with one another" present one of the greatest challenges. Longtime users of EHRs, such as Denmark, New Zealand and Sweden, have benefited from the interoperable use of patient data. Practitioners and hospitals in those countries can access patient information—physician notes, examinations and prescribed medications—across the health system. This allows providers to plan across primary, secondary and long-term care settings (Gray et al., 2011).

- **Single Identifier (unique personal identifier used across multiple systems)** – EHR information on social and behavioral determinants could direct clinical utility in cases where this knowledge is relevant to diagnosis, treatment or prognosis. ACOs, perhaps, could best manage community health by using data systems that merge clinical data stored in EHRs with data from community information systems. These community systems often provide compositional and contextual information about the environments in which individuals reside, work and learn. Knowledge about the environmental factors that affect disease (and risk), as well as the distribution of community resources, may well become as important for managing patients' health as knowledge of clinical indicators like body mass.

  It is a strongly held opinion that a single patient identifier may be key to interoperability of the electronic health record to ensure appropriate care, reduce medical errors, and avoid duplicate tests; but concerns about privacy and identify theft have challenged the realization of that goal. On a business trip one of the authors found herself in need of emergency care for an episode of atrial fibrillation and was overwhelmed in a hospital by their need to know current medications, allergies and medical history. Though she realized how very important the information was to share, she was in a medical crisis and not thinking clearly. All of the information was on her health provider's system, but access to the information was not readily available on the out-of-town hospital system. Treatment was needed immediately. The value of interoperability and a single patient identifier became apparent to her personally in that moment of profound vulnerability.

- **Provider Education** – The inclusion of broader data in an EHR could foster better clinical care and enable information on the relationship between health determinants and treatment efficacy. Because most health care providers have been trained in clinical care (only), the integration of new EHR measures will require additional provider education.

Connecting with Community-Based Promising Practices

Several promising practices clearly demonstrate the benefit of shared information, including socioeconomic, environmental and relevant clinical information. Yet, with the explosion of data from various sources, the task of aggregating, evaluating and translating the *data* into meaningful *information* has remained a challenge. According to the federal Agency for Healthcare Quality and Research, the current health data infrastructure does not have the capability to translate data into usable information; this includes associated meta-data (Agency for Healthcare Research and Quality, 2014).

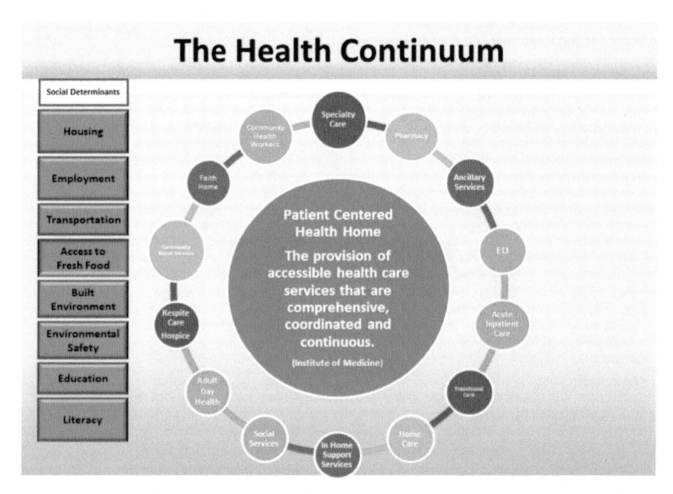

Democratization of information with relevance for support systems is key to achieving this level of sharing. This democratization would be empowered by patient permissions that allow different levels of information for support systems and interventions across the health continuum. The Health Continuum Sidebar, which includes the determinants of health cited earlier, begins to note the potential areas along the care continuum that Stakeholders Health IT members have identified and acknowledge may be a partial listing of community and related services.

Health systems can already collect and access an abundance of data at the community level or at the point of clinical contact, but this information is rarely considered in the treatment of disease—partly because the publicly available data and personal health information are not often connected. Further, the social and behavioral determinants of health are rarely incorporated into the EHR.

The time has also come for clinicians to ask not only, "What is the matter *with* you?" but also "What matters to you as an individual?" In other words, how do we begin to capture the *life aspirations* of the person in addition to meeting only the objectives of the health system? Health systems and clinicians must be equipped to understand the answers to these questions and collaboratively address the social needs of their patients and their communities. If not, the Quadruple Aim will not be realized.

Stakeholder Health's thoughtful health systems have long identified the need to address social determinants in the clinical setting, and recognize the opportunity to integrate the relevant vital information into the health record and into an appropriately considered plan of care. *(See The Health Continuum sidebar.)* They are eager for the technology that supports this endeavor in collaborative efforts to treat the physical, emotional and spiritual aspects of an individual. This cannot be done by the health system alone, but must include community partners. We will need the technology to support such collaborations. In September 2014, the Stakeholder Health IT Group and partners thus identified Promising Practices and new technologies that can connect *all* factors that contribute to health improvement. Among those highlighted were:

A. GEOGRAPHICAL INFORMATION SYSTEMS (GIS) TECHNOLOGY

GIS mapping identifies and helps navigate community resources as well as areas of disproportionate need. Incorporating GIS technology into the health care environment is an opportunity to give location a clear presence in the health of an individual and community (Esri, 2010). It also allows for a new data lens that can incorporate community data with individual data to inform providers of the patient's "place" or the environment—and its clinical relevance. GIS, in short, gives us the ability to focus on small geographic areas in which care can be delivered and managed with clinical value.

A number of health systems have begun the journey of incorporating GIS information, including Loma Linda University Health, Children's National Hospital, Adventist Health, and Duke University Health System. The benefits of utilizing GIS technology include:

- Geography becomes the common analytical denominator for linking individual and aggregate data to geographic place data.

- Internal hospital IT systems engineers can produce more accurate geographic information at modest costs. However, the most efficient long-term solution is to engage the assistance of their data system vendors.

- The GIS lens allows the provider and the individual to share the same view helping to bridge the understanding of health conditions.

Appropriating and utilizing externally generated data in real time (e.g., population change, health service demand, physician capacity and community resources) will require new analytical skills that are typically not present today in most health systems. Training will be crucial. It is also important to recognize, then, that "accountable care" requires systemic data changes. Both clinical and administrative Information must be historically consistent.

B. PROVIDER PERFORMANCE SYSTEM (PPS)

Under the federal Delivery System Reform Incentive Payment (DSRIP) program, states have a unique opportunity to advance delivery system and payment reform upgrades within their Medicaid programs. New York State's DSRIP initiative, for example, incorporates a broad set of health and social service providers, called Performing Provider Systems, to drive transformational delivery system integration. This could be a model for the nation.

The Medicaid Analytics Performance Portal (MAPP) is a performance management system that can also provide tools and performance management technologies to Provider Performance Systems in their effort to develop transformative DSRIP programs.

Community Commons is a web portal where data, tools and stories come together to inspire change and improve communities. The tool provides public access to thousands of layers of meaningful data, allowing mapping and reporting to users wanting to thoroughly explore community health.

Commons users can gain a deeper understanding of community assets and opportunities, and convey that knowledge through partnerships and collaboration. There is no charge for using Community Commons. A more in-depth review of this tool can be found in Chapter Six on Mapping.

D. COMMUNITY RX

Community Rx is a Chicago-based intervention designed to connect health care with self-care by engaging community navigators to help residents to identify health assets (Lindau, 2016). First, a 90-student MAPS Corps from Chicago's South Side uses cellphones to assess community assets. The assets are put into Health.eRx, through which Community Health Information Experts (CHIEfs) connect patients to community-based service providers and other social support resources. High school students map the assets of 26 communities in 12 zip codes. Chapter Six on mapping offers more detail on this program.

E. HEALTH LEADS

Health Leads allows clinics, physician offices and other providers to prescribe not only medications but also food, housing and heating assistance. Patients take their prescriptions to a designated help desk where volunteer Advocates (undergraduate college students) help them access community resources and public benefits. The impact of Health Leads is two-fold:

• The Health Leads program expands capacity to secure crucial non-medical resources. For example, the Dimock Center, a federally qualified health center (FQHC) in Boston, routinely screens every pediatric patient for basic resource needs. The physicians, nurses and social workers say that they feel empowered to ask "real" questions of their patients because they know Health Leads can help. An example is the patient who cannot pay his or her rent, or are running out of food at the end of the month.

• In 2012, 90 percent of Health Leads student graduates entered jobs or graduate studies in the fields of health or poverty.

Opportunities for Communities, Providers and IT Vendors

Communities, health providers and IT vendors have many opportunities to collaborate on IT systems that include community and social determinants in community health improvement efforts, e.g.:

1. The new IT system should be integrated into the existing IT systems and not be a separate portal.

2. Small geographic areas should become the context in which care is delivered and managed. Mapping of community assets such as primary care physicians, faith-based organizations, community centers, and farmers' markets can give providers and individuals a better understanding of the location of health assets near patient's home locations.

3. Data collection tools must include granular, census-tract-level data. Fitting data into more granular levels—neighborhood levels ideally as opposed to simply the county level—is challenging but necessary to making data relevant to the health of local communities.

4. Hospital data should be geocoded so that patients' home addresses have clinical relevance.

5. Public Health has multiple data sources, but we must define Public Health's new partnership role in the redesigned health system. We must also understand the data available, ways they share relevant data and information, and their organizational readiness in the world of the Quadruple Aim.

6. Health systems are hiring expensive people to code data, but they are not engaging health care staff to translate IT data into useful information. As hospitals build new business analytics infrastructures, we must adequately resource the business intelligence—not just add more data.

7. Who is the "they" that would bring together public health, hospital, and community?

8. How can data platforms be used to promote cross-sector health improvement initiatives in communities? The Federal Reserve, for example, is investing in community health improvement, but existing data structures and platforms do not support a collective approach to health improvement.

Very few health systems have realized any type of real-time information system that could provide a sense of what is actually happening, what is about to happen, or what actually happened.

Loma Linda University Health has created a Community Health Management System (CHMS) that incorporates GIS technology into their IT data platform. Their vision is one of real-time, geographically enabled, health utilization information that providers can use to influence resource utilization, patient care, and population health decisions. In effect, the CHMS introduced the concept of an "accountable-care ecosystem."

The data generated from this system has helped identify community hazards that trigger increased ER utilization and hospital readmissions for children with uncontrolled asthma. It has identified areas where patients do not have access to a pharmacy; the hospitals and clinics can now send the patients home with the necessary medications. CHMS also targets food deserts in which the hospital can help communities advocate for healthier food options.

CHMS has made "location" clinically relevant, and is being incorporated into the Loma Linda University Health system of care.

9. What are the viable options for health planning in communities? Health planners understand the questions and challenges they face, but communities may not have adequate data or information.

10. "Systems thinkers" must participate in data development. This work cannot be done in isolation. We need the data and information technology that support a health system's journey into our new future—and not hold us in the past.

11. Social Media may not be tightly controlled but as proven in models like PatientsLikeMe, Inc., can be much more effective in sharing community resources. If we shift the control over to the individual, and allow them to be in control, this alleviates the challenges posed by HIPAA. How can we use publicly available websites to register community resources and provide users with the logic to navigate based on their individuals needs or interests?

Identified Domains to Fulfill Our IT Vision

Stakeholder Health members recommended domains necessary for inclusion in the EHR that were consistent with those of the 2014 *Institute of Medicine (IOM) report entitled Institute of Medicine: Capturing Social and Behavioral Domains and Measures in Electronic Health Records*. While the data domains identified in the Stakeholder Health conversations were not vetted as thoroughly as those in the IOM report were, many of the Stakeholder Health domain categories paralleled those of the IOM and conversations throughout the field. While the IOM domains are not intended to serve as a final list, the table below includes the IOM's EHR domains and adds a spiritual domain to the list.

Socio-demographic Domains

- Sexual Orientation
- Race/Ethnicity
- County of Origin/U.S. born or non-U.S. born
- Education
- Financial resource strain
- Gender identity

Psychological Domains

- Health Literacy
- Stress
- Negative mood and affect (depression and anxiety)
- Psychological assets (conscientiousness, patient engagement/ activation, optimism, self-efficacy)
- Cognitive function in late life
- Psychological assets

Behavior Domains

- Dietary patterns
- Physical activity
- Tobacco use and exposure
- Alcohol use
- Abuse of other substances
- Sexual practices
- Exposure to firearms
- Risk-taking behaviors

Individual-Level Social Relationships & Living Conditions

- Social connections and social isolation
- Exposure to violence
- Social support
- Work conditions
- History of incarceration
- Military service
- Community and cultural norms

Neighborhoods and Communities

- Neighborhood and community compositional characteristics
- Socioeconomic and racial/ethnic characteristics
- Neighborhood and community contextual characteristics (air pollution, allergens, other hazardous exposures, nutritious food options, transportation, parks, open spaces, health care and social services, educational and job opportunities)

Spiritual Domain (not included in IOM report)

- Religious affiliation
- Place of worship/support
- Religious beliefs that could impact care
- Aspirations (what matters to you?)
- Spiritual screening (or assessment by a qualified health professional) and spiritual care

Stakeholder Health believes that the Spiritual Domain is a critical variable of overall health.

Recommendations/Call to Action

Stakeholder Health members are committed to working with community stakeholders and IT vendors to create the necessary technology to fulfill a vision of better health for individuals and communities. We are ready to begin a journey of collaborative learning on the following action items and invite you to join with us in these efforts:

1. **Create alignment** with health system data and community health data.

   - Location becomes clinically relevant and provides meaningful context for diagnosis, treatment and healing of patients.

   - The Community Health Needs Assessment (with additional, explicit focus on also making assets visible) becomes the new context for linking community to health systems overall strategy.

2. **Commit to documenting the issues and processes** involved in equipping a large health system to undertake a systemic adoption of analytical tools and techniques that will assist the health system in delivering on the promise of accountable care.

   - Perform geographical data audits on all data collection systems used within the health care system (HR, Medical Staff, Vendor, Visitors, etc.)

   - Benchmark the quality of all data before making improvements so that the benchmarks can be documented and communicated to management and data users (e.g., the percentage of unique addresses that can be verified at street level is one good measure of geographical accuracy).

- Inform health system IT vendors about the adequacy of on-going data quality efforts. Seek their assistance in integrating work-saving steps (across the entire workflow) that could be impacted by a bad or inaccurate street address (e.g., skip tracing, undeliverable bills, wrong service delivery address for a patient or visitor encounter, an employee hire, a medical staff office location or a health care-seeking consumer who has requested information from a web site).

3. **Build a community of learning** around health system geo-analytics that can increasingly and continuously support community health management and be capable of supporting daily operations.

   - Commit to documentation of the issues and processes that will equip a large health system to adopt analytic tools and techniques.

   - Develop a workshop for health system decision support and other analytics support professionals to understand the basics of geospatial information and learn how other organizations have leveraged these technologies.

   - Invite physicians with specialized training in geospatial sciences to teach clinical staff how geographically enabled information can be broadly deployed in practice settings to increase analytical precision at the population health and clinical decision-support levels.

   - Develop pilot demonstrations, document and share findings, and showcase best practices.

4. **Commit to moving beyond situational awareness.** The analytical needs of delivering a continuous and meaningful chain of care are far more challenging than simply reporting status at a given moment.

   - Data, including geographically enabled clinical data, must become actionable, and measurable in a relatively short time span (e.g., preventing undesirable readmissions, for example, cannot wait until all data is scrubbed). We must think like 911 operators who must make sure an ambulance goes to the "right" place—the first time out.

   - "Managing" community health requires a different analytical framework and a more refined way to describe exactness: how a community is defined geographically, its exact boundaries, and its service delivery pattern/network.

   - Traditionally, clinical data is thought to be of specific, necessary and immediate value to patients. At the same time, population health data is viewed as general, nice to know, and long-range. These contrasting perspectives no longer suffice when identifying the information needed to operate a large health system across a socially and culturally diverse, widely distributed "community."

   - The new data "voice" in health care will be about process, not just results. Improving the processes to create, deliver and understand data within the context of accountable care will require thoughtful and proactive modernization of the data, information systems, and workflows that underpin the organization.

5. **Make geographical accuracy a priority** in all internal systems: patient registration, medical staff credentialing, employee registration, vendor supplier registration, etc.

   - Add address verification and geocoding software as part of existing systems. For example, geographic standards already exist within HL7—Version 3.0. Implement it and require your system vendors to support the standard.

   - Create staff capacity to manage and evaluate the accuracy and usability of all geographic information. As with clinical coding, geography has requirements for historical consistency, data analysis, and guiding community care evaluations.

   - Incorporate community resources and their location to individuals as an integral part of the community of care.

- Drive out inefficient data-handling and data-linking inefficiencies. Implement automated systems to add geographic analytical value to existing data streams for both internal and externally generated data: EHRs, state vital event reporting, state and federal environmental reporting, etc. In contrast, spending time and money on ad hoc data cleaning efforts is inefficient and defeats the value of 24/7 systems.

6. **Work with existing IT vendors** to bring existing systems (and future systems) up to current geographical data accuracy standards **and be more inclusive of social determinants.**
    - Create briefing sessions for IT vendors. Focus on the need for more accurate address verification and geocoding workflows.
    - Create documentation supporting IT vendor needs for specific requirements concerning geographical standards, including address verification and geographic information software conventions and techniques.

7. **Commit to partnering with governmental entities** to engage in:
    - Open advisory committees with opportunity for public comments.
    - Feedback and input for rulemaking groups regarding IT policies.
    - A back-up mandate for public input.
    - Partnerships for the joint development of recommended IT capabilities.
    - Work with public health entities to share community health data.

8. **Work with IT to connect providers** to accessible and current databases of community resources.
    - Explore development of real time bio-directional system with feedback loop.
    - Track health changes/outcomes post connection to community based services.
    - Consider a common site for resource information, e.g., CDC Community Health Improvement Navigator (CHI Navigator).

9. **Commit to having a single patient identifier** that traverses all IT source systems to ensure that a patient's longitudinal record of care across the clinical and community space is maintained.
    - Work with regional HIE to enforce the maintenance of a universal identifier (UID).
    - Ensure EHRs, billing systems, community settings have access to this UID.

Conclusion

Health care finds itself at a crossroad; it is no longer business as usual. There are many factors that influence an individual's health outside of traditional health care settings. Incorporating knowledge about a patient's spiritual aspirations and both the socioeconomic and environmental risks must be part of the standard of care and incorporated into the Electronic Health Record and included as a part of the data incorporated into health systems overall strategy. We need to create the appropriate connections for our health systems and the community to ensure quality of care is provided to all. It is time to re-think how we share relevant information across the health care continuum that protects the individual's privacy while providing the highest quality of care. In one of Stakeholder Health's face-to-face meetings, members thus dreamed without inhibition about their IT vision, and compiled a list of questions in multiple categories to help inform innovators and vendors working on IT solutions (see below). SH hopes that these clarifying questions might activate others working in the IT improvement space to envision and create the optimal EHR.

Stakeholder Health pledges to work with national organizations like the American Hospital Association, the Institute of Medicine, the Association of American Medical Colleges, faith-based groups, politicians/legislators, advocates and medical IT vendors to increase awareness to move the industry to accept this important and much needed shift in the delivery of care.

Our members view the Affordable Care Act and the current policy environment as an opportunity to: address the underlying causes of poor health in communities; make informed decisions to better align, integrate and leverage existing resources; and create partnerships with diverse stakeholders that will result in positive outcomes.

WHAT DO WE NEED?

COMMON MEASURES
- What is "standard" socioeconomic data? Is there a set of common, core measurements?
- What "standard" socioeconomic data do we need?
- Where does this data currently "live"? How do we gather it?
- What are the standard elements of shared EHR and Public Health data?
- What are the common denominators for data relating to shared causes?
- How do we capture data around social and cultural barriers (bias, distrust, etc.)?
- How do we re-frame and examine hospital disparities data?

DATA VALIDITY
- How do we identify gaps in data relevance?
- How do we make the data real-time and relevant to the clinical intervention?

BI-DIRECTIONALITY
- How do we make data bi-directional so we can connect pre- and post-acute services to a consolidated EHR?
- How do we ensure the validity of bi-directional data?
- How do we create data reciprocity between the health system and the community?
- How can data systems help hospitals work more closely with Public Health?

SECURITY
- How do we ensure the security of bi-directional data?
- Which key elements of the EHR could be shared for population health purposes, e.g., what would be of value?
- Who "owns" the data?

C-SUITE VALUE
- How do we display infographics and dashboards that are meaningful to health system executives?
- How do we use data to create C-Suite value and support for the incorporation of publically available data into the EHR?

COMMUNITY
- How do we create data value for the communities we serve?
- How can shared data provide opportunities for resource alignment?
- How can shared data provide opportunities for shared investments?
- How do we garner feedback for course correction?
- How do we educate all data users?
- How do we align faith and education resources with other partners?

SOCIAL RETURN ON INVESTMENT (SROI)
- How do we capture the social value of such a data platform?
- How do we calculate SROI opportunities for all partners?

REFERENCES

Agency for Healthcare Research and Quality. (2014). Data for Individual Health, Publication No. 15-0006-EF.

American Hospital Association. (2013). Advocacy Agenda: Transforming the Health Care Delivery System. Retrieved from http://www.aha.org/content/13/2013-advocacy-agenda.pdf.

American Hospital Association. (2014). Your Hospital's Path to the Second Curve: Integration and Transformation. Retrieved from http://www.aha.org/research/cor/paths/index.shtml.

Bisognano, M. & Kenney, C. (2012) *Pursuing the Triple Aim: Seven Innovators Show the Way to Better Care, Better Health, and Lower Costs.* San Francisco: Jossey-Bass Publishers.

Buntin, M., Beeuwkes, J., Sachin H. & Blumenthal, D. (2010). Health Information Technology: Laying the Infrastructure for National Health Reform. Retrieved from http://content.healthaffairs.org/content/29/6/1214.full.

County Health Rankings & Roadmaps. (2015). Our approach. Retrieved December 4, 2015, from http://www.countyhealthrankings.org/our-approach

Dept. of Heath Information Technology. (2011). Federal Health Information Technology Strategic Plan, 2011-2015. Retrieved from www.healthit.gov/sites/.../final-federal-health-it-strategic-plan-0911.pdf.

Esri. (2010). GIS for asset and facilities management. Efficient management of assets, interior space, and the building life. Redlands, CA: Author.

Health Systems Learning Group. (2013). *Strategic investment in shared outcomes: Transformative partnerships between health systems and communities*. April 4, Washington, D.C.

Institute of Medicine of The National Academies. Social and Behavioral Health Domains. (2014a). Capturing Social and Behavioral Domains and Measures in Electronic Health Records: Phase 1. March, 2014 pgs. 7 Preface, 17 Summary, 34, and Section 1-4. Retrieved from http://www.nap.edu/catalog.php?record_id=18709.

Institute of Medicine of the National Academies (2014b) Capturing Social and Behavioral Domains in Electronic Health Records: Phase 2, November 2014. Retrieved from http://www.iom.edu/Reports/2014/EHRdomains2.aspx Finding 7-3, pg. 16, Section 1-4, Section 1-6, Section 1-8,9.

Manchin, J., Wicker, R., Nelson, W., & Kirk, M. (2014). The Hospital Readmissions Program Accuracy and Accountability Act. Retrieved from https://www.aamc.org/download/382516/data/thehospitalreadmissionsprogramaccuracyandaccountabilityactbills.pdf.

University of Chicago Medicine. (2016). Associate Professor of Obstetrics/Gynecology and Medicine-Geriatrics: Stacy Tessler Lindau, MD, MAPP. Retrieved from http://www.uchospitals.edu/physicians/stacy-lindau.html.

University of Wisconsin Population Institute. (2014). County Health Rankings & Roadmaps. Retrieved from http://www.countyhealthrankings.org/our-approach.

ACKNOWLEDGMENTS

More than 45 health care systems participated in the Stakeholder Health learning that produced these insights. The collective wisdom of these conversations and learning are shared throughout this document.

FULL AUTHORSHIP LISTING

Dora Barilla, DrPH, President, HC2 Strategies, Inc. and Executive Leader, Community Investments, Providence Health and Services, Tacoma, WA

Eileen Barsi, GC, Population Health and Community Benefit Consultant, formerly with Dignity Health, San Francisco, CA

Maureen Kersmarki, BA, Director, Community Benefit & Public Policy, Adventist Health System, Orlando, FL

Monica Escobar Lowell, BA, Vice President of Community Relations, UMass Memorial Health Care, Worcester, MA

Mark Zirkelbach, MSPSA, Chief Information Officer, Loma Linda University Health, Loma Linda, CA

Gurmeet Sran, MD, MS, Medical Director of Health Analytics & Data Science, Dignity Health, San Francisco, CA

For more information about this chapter, contact **Eileen Barsi** at e-mail, eileen.barsi@gmail.com or phone, (650) 438-7877.

CHAPTER 5

Navigating for Health

Nancy Combs, Kimberlydawn Wisdom, Dominica Rehbein, Catherine Potter and Joan Cleary, with Loel Solomon, Nada Dickinson, Teresa Cutts, Ameldia Brown, and Monica Lowell

"Serving as a community health worker is being a resource to help ease some of the stressors in people's lives. We are a bridge of support that brings our clients to the road of their success."

- Nada Dickinson,
Community Health Worker, Detroit

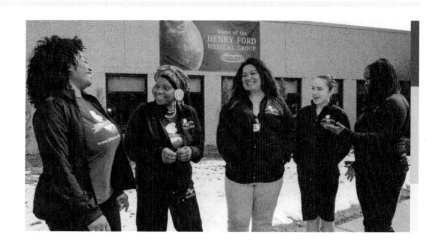

A DAY IN THE LIFE OF A COMMUNITY HEALTH WORKER
Nada Dickinson, a community health worker (CHW) since 2011, is on a team with four other CHWs, all of whom have key roles within the Women-Inspired Neighborhood Network: Detroit. The WIN Network is a collaboration among four Detroit health systems, public health agencies, universities and more than 40 community partners to reduce Detroit's high infant mortality rate. Nada also serves as a health insurance navigator at Henry Ford Health Medical Center-Hamtramck, in a culturally diverse, largely underserved neighborhood north of downtown Detroit. Throughout this narrative, you will see the CLOCK icon to mark a moment in Nada's average day—although she assures us that no day is "average" in the life of a CHW!

Navigation is More than a Compass
We'll begin by asking this key question: "Why is navigation important in health care today?" In today's complex health environment many people struggle to find the health care services they need. Even highly educated people with comprehensive insurance may struggle to understand and successfully negotiate our fragmented system when facing a health crisis or needing other services. People from marginalized communities or those in poverty may be even less able to find or access the care they need. As a result, many organizations have recognized the need for navigation to improve health care access and to connect patients with the social services necessary to truly optimize health.

Navigators of many types may be hired to support strategies in the name of "population health," a real challenge in light of aging demographics, an epidemic of chronic disease and disparate health outcomes among subgroups. This broadly used term is built into the Institute for Healthcare Improvement's Triple Aim (Berwick, Nolan, & Whittington, 2008), which we have repeatedly expanded to the Quadruple Aim or Triple Aim+ (HSLG, 2013). To help achieve Quadruple Aim goals, we can provide navigation services that are particularly critical to patients facing barriers related to poverty, culture, language, literacy, isolation, mistrust, disability, geography and other such factors.

Due to their experience and training, many navigators are equipped to work across a variety of health-related sectors. In the population health environment, navigators can assist with insurance enrollment,

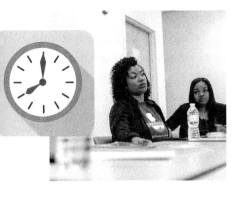

8 A.M. Coffee in hand, Nada arrives at her office and sits down to check email. Over the weekend, she's received contact info for 73 community members who have reached out to the CHWs for help getting enrolled in Michigan's expanded Medicaid program. "Many of these callbacks will be brief," Nada says, "but you never know when someone will have more complex health needs that will require a longer conversation. My team members and I will divide up the calls to address everyone's concerns." Collecting the information, she heads off to her weekly CHW Team huddle.

connecting people with health care services, locating and connecting clients with social supports, interpreting treatment plans, making follow-up appointments and contributing to research projects. Many worker types include navigation as one of their core competencies, and some exclusively serve in a navigator capacity.

The following describes some of the many types of navigators, with examples of the settings where they may be found, and one example of their work duties.

Title	Examples of Settings	Examples of Navigation (specific to worker type)
Care Coordinator	Hospital, Health System, or Care Delivery Setting	A nurse or social worker helping a cancer patient understand her treatment plan and make optimum use of health system resources
Health Navigator	Community-Based Organization	A worker in a social service setting who helps community members with insurance enrollment
Community Health Worker	Community Based Organization or Health System	A lay person, with unique skills and community connections, who helps community members find and connect with needed services
Promotora	Community Clinic	A lay person who does outreach and education on behalf of a clinical team, including home visits, to Spanish-speaking patients (often considered one of the major titles under the broad "CHW umbrella")
Faith Community Nurse	Church or other Faith Community	A nurse (often a volunteer) who helps congregation members find needed services and maintain their health
Peer Support Specialist	Community Mental Health Agency	Lay person with personal experience in the mental health system, helping someone else in the early stages of recovery, to find housing and meet other basic needs
Navigator	Primary Care Team	A bachelor's level worker who works in a team-based care setting, helping patients address social needs and connect with community resources
Doula	Home	A lay person, with special training in childbirth and postpartum care, who helps a new mom find supplies needed to care for an infant

Navigation is rarely enough for people with complex health needs or those struggling with weighty basic issues of food, housing, and violence. Ongoing support and the ability to address larger issues—not only with a compass, but with trust and companionship for the journey that comes from shared culture or shared life experience—are often needed.

Community health workers (CHWs) are particularly well suited to play this more comprehensive role. As members of the communities they serve, they are intimately familiar with the barriers and challenges facing people with complex medical and sociocultural needs. Through them, we will see what frontline health workers can accomplish, as navigators but also as clinical team members, neighborhood-based mentors or guides, and powerful agents of measurable community and systems change. We will find it easier to envision a health care system, where the term "population health" is understood and embraced by all—even for the most challenged, vulnerable communities.

Below, we will further examine the work of CHWs to show the impact and potential for addressing population health, and we will also highlight other navigation models—all best practices in their own right—in sidebars. Look for the Best Practice icon to learn more.

In summary, in today's complex health system, navigators of various types are needed to help individuals connect with resources to help them live healthier lives, but in our current environment, simple navigation is often not enough. Community health workers go "beyond the compass" through their relationships with patients and clients over time, evidence-based outcomes, and connectedness to clinical and community settings, illustrating the highest potential for frontline navigators working for population health.

How Community Health Workers contribute to the Triple Aim+

Reduced per capita costs
- Improved utilization of preventive services
- Reduced use of ED
- Improved birth outcomes

Improved quality and the patient experience
- Improved utilization of preventive services
- Improved care transitions
- Improved patient activation

Improved population health
- Improved chronic disease management
- Better connections with social services and supports
- Culturally appropriate health education

Improved health equity
- Reduced infant mortality
- Improved asthma control
- Better language access
- Increased knowledge of local community needs

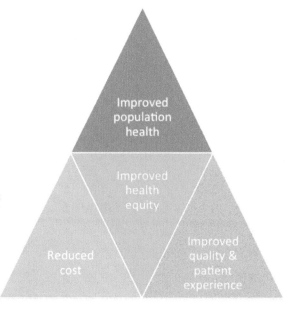

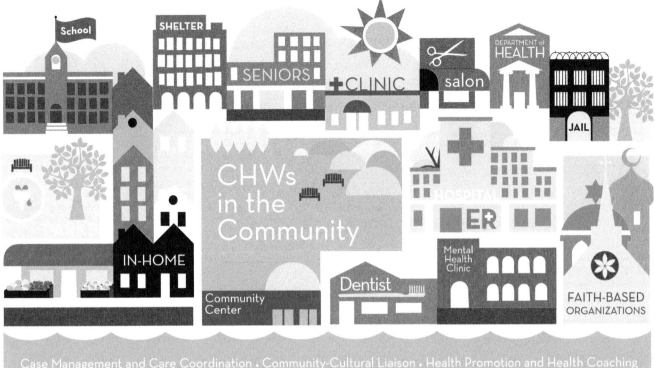

CHWs in the Community

School · SHELTER · SENIORS · CLINIC · salon · DEPARTMENT of HEALTH · JAIL · IN-HOME · Community Center · Dentist · Mental Health Clinic · HOSPITAL ER · FAITH-BASED ORGANIZATIONS

Case Management and Care Coordination · Community-Cultural Liaison · Health Promotion and Health Coaching
Home-based Support · Outreach and Community Mobilization · Participatory Research · System Navigation*

*Matos S, Findley S, Hicks A, Legendre Y, Do Canto L. Paving a path to advance the community health worker workforce in New York State: a new summary report and recommendations. CHW Network of New York City, 2011

Minnesota Community Health Worker Alliance

Used with permission from the Minnesota Community Health Worker Alliance

"As Henry Ford continually addresses the Triple Aim of improving population health, enhancing patient experience and outcomes, and reducing per capita cost of care, we see community health workers as playing a pivotal role. We invest in CHWs because we know they help us make a difference where our patients live their lives and make their daily health choices. And as the Triple Aim+ embraces Equity as its fourth component, our CHWs are already there—at the key juncture where clinical and community work converges to reduce health disparities. At Henry Ford we like to say we are 'All For You'—our patients and community. There is no better personification of this than the community health worker."

- Nancy Schlichting, CEO, Henry Ford Health System, Detroit

Advancing the Triple Aim+ or "Quadruple" Aim

We first ask how CHWs can help our organizations work toward achieving the "Quadruple Aim" or "Triple Aim+," adding the critical dimension of equity to the Triple Aim (Achieving the Triple Aim, 2015). In working to simultaneously improve the quality and experience of care, improve population health, and reduce the per capita cost of health care, health systems are finding that CHWs play an important role in achieving all these goals. CHWs' history and trusted connections with underserved communities uniquely equip them to reduce health disparities, while their deep community understanding (language and culture) allows them to serve as effective brokers between their communities and the broader healthcare setting. Here we highlight key evidence of how CHWs contribute to achieving the Triple Aim+.

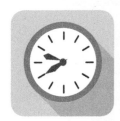

9:40 A.M. Nada is gathering up materials for the group prenatal care class she will help lead later this morning when the phone rings. It's a fellow CHW who's active in the Michigan Community Health Worker Alliance, (MiCHWA), the statewide CHW advocacy organization. Next week, Nada will join her colleague and other CHWs from across the state, along with health plan and health system decision makers and representatives of the Michigan Department of Health & Human Services. This ad hoc group is working to develop a payment model so that CHWs can be funded through Medicaid. Nada and her colleague check in on details for the summit, then Nada heads to the clinic classroom to set up for the prenatal group visit.

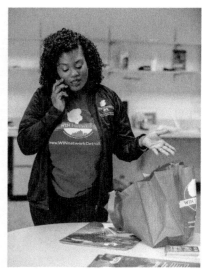

Reducing Per Capita Costs

As the healthcare system continues to take on increasing responsibility for the costs and outcomes of their patients, healthcare providers, health plans and purchasers are seeking care delivery improvements that lower costs and offer a positive return on investment. The Institute for Clinical and Economic Review (ICER) completed a rigorous review of the evidence on value of CHWs and found that, compared to usual care, CHW programs resulted in significantly improved outcomes and reduced healthcare costs, in part due to their ability to fill an important gap in services (ICER, 2013). Healthcare professionals are directed to provide care "at the top of their license." This creates space in the care team for CHWs to address some of the patient's basic needs such as scheduling healthcare appointments, connecting with available community resources and applying a health care provider's recommendations in daily life. Integrating CHWs into care teams as experts in addressing these needs is a cost-effective way to ensure these needs are met (Felix, Mays, Stewart, Cottoms, & Olson, 2011).

Cost savings can be realized in various ways, including improved utilization of preventive health care services, reduced waste such as missed appointments, decreased overall costs for group visits, and avoided high-cost services. For example, CHWs working through the Arkansas Community Connector Program (ACCP) assisted individuals in setting up home and community-based services that could meet their needs instead of their moving to a costly long-term care facility. This reduced per-participant Medicaid spending by 23.8 percent on average, and generated $2.619 million in savings over a three-year period (Felix, et al., 2011).

For a health care organization, savings may come in the form of fewer emergency room visits, pre-term births or admissions/readmissions. In Baltimore, home visits by CHWs to low-income patients with diabetes and hypertension reduced their visits to the emergency department by 40 percent. The Children's Hospital of Boston Community Asthma Initiative reduced emergency visits by 65 percent and hospitalizations by 81 percent, and the success of this initiative led to the inclusion of CHWs on the team of providers in a bundled payment arrangement with the state's Medicaid plan (CHWA, 2013).

In a matched cohort study of enrollees in Molina Health, a Medicaid managed care plan in New Mexico, an assessment of the economic impact of a CHW intervention on high-risk patients found a sustained ROI of at least 3:1 (Johnson, Saavedra, Sun, Stageman, Grovet, Alfero, Kaufman, 2011). Molina's corporate office thus expanded this model from New Mexico to all states where it has a Medicaid contract. Using frequent ED visits to identify high-risk patients, CHWs provided home visits for needs assessments, appointment support and reminders, health literacy support and education, advocacy, equipment and supplies. Using claims data to evaluate the program, the team found that costs decreased from the pre-program period in both groups. Compared to a similar group that received no CHW services, there were significantly greater reductions in ED use, hospitalization, and both narcotic and nonnarcotic prescriptions, with an annual cost reduction of $3,003 per patient (Johnson, 2011).

Return on investment for CHWs can also be measured from the societal perspective. Improving health outcomes for groups of patients increases their economic productivity in a community. This includes wages earned, taxes paid and reduced urgent care use. A 2012 study conducted by the St. Paul-based Wilder Foundation found that for every dollar invested in CHW cancer outreach, society receives $2.30 in benefits, a return greater than 200% (Hardeman & Gerrard, 2011).

10 A.M. Twelve women at similar stages in their pregnancies have arrived for this group prenatal care session with a certified nurse midwife, medical assistant and Nada. The women receive their prenatal care together and learn about important practices for their prenatal health. Nada, who is making home visits to each participant, co-facilitates the session, and shares resources. "I really enjoy spending time with these women," says Nada. "We have some common experience, and I can guide them toward services near where they live. It's also great to work in partnership with the clinical team," she adds. Having this connection to a trained health professional who is familiar with their circumstances puts the group members at ease.

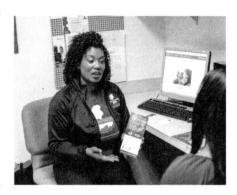

Improving Quality and the Patient Experience

As patient-centered medical homes and behavioral health home models are established across the country, team-based, patient-centered approaches for organizing care and services are receiving greater emphasis. These models focus on care coordination, patient goal-setting and activation, coaching, and community-clinical linkages in order to help achieve the Quadruple Aim.

Integrating CHWs as part of these teams improves the effectiveness of the models and accessibility to community members. An increasing number of studies demonstrate the dramatic impact they can have on health care quality (as measured by the National Committee for Quality Assurance or NCQA, and the HealthCare Effectiveness Data and Information Set, HEDIS). For example, statistically significant increases in breast cancer screening rates have been noted when CHWs working in primary care practices reached out to women via phone, mail, or home visits. They offer support and education, meet women at the screening sites, provide needs assessments and address financial, coverage and transportation barriers. Women accessing these CHW services were three times as likely to receive mammograms as those not engaged with CHWs (Achieving the Triple Aim, 2015).

CHWs can also be deployed within clinical teams to improve care transitions and reduce hospital readmission rates with considerable potential value to providers especially in light of payment models that assign penalties for high readmission rates. The IMPaCT (Individualized Management for Patient Centered Targets) community health worker model developed by the University of Pennsylvania Health System is a good example. IMPaCT is a standardized, scalable CHW model that includes clear guidelines for hiring, supervision, integration into care teams, and work planning for CHWs. In this model, CHWs began working with patients early on during their hospital stay to set patient-identified goals for recovery. Through regular ongoing contact and follow-up post-discharge, patients receiving the CHW intervention showed improved rates of timely follow-up care, increased rates of patient activation and reduced rates of multiple readmissions (Kangovi, Mitra, Grande, White, McCollum, Sellman, Shannon & Long, 2014).

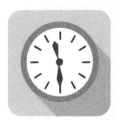

11:30 A.M. Nada arrives at Kayla's address in Detroit's Osborn neighborhood, on a street where half the houses are boarded up. Kayla, 26 and in her first trimester, has recently signed up for group prenatal care. She and her energetic toddler are currently are staying with Kayla's older sister until they can afford their own place. "We call this situation 'couch-homeless,'" Nada says quietly as we wait for Kayla to answer the door. It's the first time Nada has met with Kayla so she walks through the standard first-visit protocol. "Kayla, it's so great to meet you, and I look forward to our getting to know each other better," Nada says. "What are your major concerns today?"

"I'm really worried about how we can pay the heating bill," Kayla responds. "What if we get a shutoff notice?" Right there, Nada dials United Way 2-1-1 and puts Kayla on the phone to talk to one of their trained counselors who assures her they can work out a payment plan.

Immediate crisis averted, Nada reminds Kayla about her group prenatal care visit coming up next week. She then arranges for free transportation through Kayla's Medicaid health plan. She shares helpful tools: a brightly illustrated book on having a healthy pregnancy, a directory of community resources, and last but not least, links to the WIN Network: Detroit website and Facebook page, replete with resources and upcoming events. Together they look at opportunities to connect with other WIN Network: Detroit members. Nada hands Kayla her cell number and contact info for the WIN Network. Lastly, they work out action steps that Kayla agrees to accomplish in the next week, and set a time for Nada's next check-in.

"Developing a trusting relationship with Kayla is first and foremost," says Nada upon leaving. "My assistance to her is guided by her priorities for her and her family. Kayla also is worried about getting her own place. We'll work on affordable housing options next."

Improving Population Health

Community health workers are significant assets to a community for the prevention and management of chronic diseases, as well as tireless advocates for community development. They are thus also allies and key partners in addressing the socioeconomic and behavioral risk factors of patients.

For example, in the prevention and early identification of chronic disease, Access El Dorado (ACCEL) includes public and private agencies that work with vulnerable populations to connect community members with existing local services, particularly health insurance (AHRQ, 2011). CHWs from participating agencies help participants navigate the array of services. Besides a more coordinated experience for families, the participation of a variety of organizations, including social services and health care, allows for outcomes data from all sectors to be collected and analyzed together (CHWA, 2013). This approach also allows stakeholders to see the link between health education or connection with a medical home, and averted emergency visits or other costs due to prevention.

A survey of community health centers in Massachusetts found that the task of assisting with chronic disease management is another primary focus of many CHWs (Achieving the Triple Aim, 2015). As trusted resources, CHWs may be the first to learn about symptoms a patient with a chronic disease is experiencing and can enable them to access primary care at the appropriate time. Further, CHWs have more opportunities to understand the unique challenges a patient is experiencing in managing their chronic disease and can assist them in problem-solving (CHWA, 2013).

At the most upstream level, CHWs can impact social determinants such as employment, food insecurity or homelessness (CHWA, 2013). This occurs both through direct referrals to needed resources for individual clients and through policy change. Through building relationships with community organizations, CHWs keep up with services available and how to access them. Through community "asset mapping," a participatory endeavor, community members identify what they view as assets in their neighborhoods and, as members of the neighborhoods, CHWs contribute to this process and can use information about strengths and gaps in resources to advocate for policy change (City of Healthy Neighborhoods & Buildings, n.d.).

Improving Health Equity

Factors such as culture, language, literacy, income, disability, and geographic location often create barriers to achieving ideal health status in our increasingly diverse U.S. population. We are challenged to confront and eliminate these health inequities, which shorten life expectancy, impair health and well-being, and reduce the ability of many Americans to lead productive lives (Disparities, n.d.). In the context of such inequities, which are unjust and costly for individuals, communities and society, the American Public Health Association, the Centers for Disease Control and Prevention, the Institute of Medicine and other leading health authorities all endorse and recognize the key contributions that CHWs can make to reducing health disparities (Smedley, Stith, & Nelson, 2003).

First, CHW programs designed for chronic disease management will more frequently work with communities negatively impacted by poverty and other social determinants where people are more likely to develop chronic diseases (Achieving the Triple Aim, 2015). Second, as members of those communities, CHWs tend to have a deep and thorough understanding of the communities they serve that helps them better communicate issues, promote healthy options and problem-solve with patients, resulting in more acceptable recommendations.

Here we highlight three projects that illustrate how CHWs are reducing health disparities:

* There is no more glaring or troubling health disparity than infant mortality, a sentinel health indicator or barometer of a community's health. In Detroit between 13 and 15 babies per thousand live births do not survive until their first birthday—among the highest rates in the U.S. (Infant Mortality, 2016) and almost three times that of the state's non-Hispanic white babies (Infant Mortality by Race, 2016). A game-changing public-private partnership in Detroit—which includes competing health systems—is making promising headway in addressing this crisis.

The WIN Network: Detroit, a program of the Detroit Regional Infant Mortality Reduction Task Force facilitated by Henry Ford Health System, employs CHWs to support women at high risk for preterm, low-birth weight infants. In the three neighborhoods where

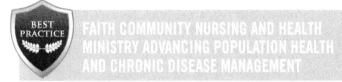

BEST PRACTICE — FAITH COMMUNITY NURSING AND HEALTH MINISTRY ADVANCING POPULATION HEALTH AND CHRONIC DISEASE MANAGEMENT

Partnering with Faith Community Nursing (FCN) and Health Ministry is a key community benefit strategy for Henry Ford Health System (HFHS) as it addresses chronic disease management, population health, and lifestyle improvement. Aligning mutual goals has allowed Henry Ford Macomb Hospital, one of five HFHS hospitals, to achieve many positive health outcomes.

In one transitions-of-care project targeting heart failure patients, unpaid FCNs were able to achieve decreases in physician, ED and hospital visits by 70%, 50% and 29% respectively over a 24-month period. Similarly, successful results were documented in a clinic for low-income uninsured and newly insured clients with diabetes management. In 2014, the average A1C change was a decrease of 5.7% (N = 38) and in 2015 the average A1C was decreased by 5.9% (N=29).

FCNs and their teams have been instrumental in the planning and rollout of the systematic approach to advance care planning for end-of-life. They account for 25% of the documented outcomes of HFHS advance care planning efforts (classes, conversations initiated, advance directives completed). Faith Community Nursing also is leading the implementation of the health system's Diabetes Prevention Recognition Center activities. In seven months, 17 coaches were trained and 6 classes implemented.

The commitment and quality of the FCNs and health ministers is what allows such rapid deployment of this complex program. HFHS also communicates on behalf of the national network using the documentation system. Over three years, FCNs and Health Ministers from 23 different networks in 25 states have documented 78,086 individual interactions, 1,587,070 group participant contacts for education, screenings and support groups, and $4,818,454 group cost savings and cost avoidances.

its CHWs have been working since 2012, there have been no infant deaths among more than 364 mothers enrolled in the program. WIN Network also has enrolled 1,518 non-pregnant women who are connected with and learn about resources that focus on healthy living, family planning, stress management, budgeting, nutrition and physical activity. WIN has also trained more than 438 local health providers on the health equity framework and social determinants of health. It is expanding its model to introduce group prenatal care for obstetric patients at Henry Ford, and beginning in spring 2016, CHWs are co-facilitating the sessions with groups of 12-15 patients and Henry Ford nurse midwives.

- Across the U.S., asthma disparities challenge many low-income communities where costly and preventable suffering continues as a result of substandard housing with patients often landing in busy hospital emergency rooms. Effective use of trained CHWs as home visitors can substantially improve asthma outcomes and reduce costs, as Krieger, Takaro, Song, Beaudet and Edwards (2009) show. They document the work of the Seattle-King County Healthy Homes II Project, which serves low-income, multi-ethnic communities, and conclude that CHW home visits coordinated with support from asthma nurses in the clinic increased symptom-free days and improved caregiver quality of life.

- CHWs also help health systems implement the National Culturally and Linguistically Appropriate Services (CLAS) Standards of the U.S. Office of Minority Health while improving outcomes for diabetes and other chronic diseases (Office of Minority Health, n.d.). As one of multiple examples, a culturally competent pilot study known as the Promotora-Led Diabetes Prevention Program (PL-DPP) used promotoras as intervention facilitators for a group of 20 Latina women in Chicago who were at risk for diabetes. The participants—socioeconomically challenged with limited access to health care services—engaged in a 12-month lifestyle intervention by a Spanish-speaking promotora. Eighteen of them attended at least half of 24 sessions. After a year, a mean loss of almost 11 pounds or 5.6% of initial body

 A HEALTHCARE HERO IN MEMPHIS

Joy Crawford Sharp is an exceptional Community Health Network navigator, the first place-based population health navigator in the Methodist Le Bonheur Healthcare (MLH) system in Memphis, Tenn. She was born and lived her early years in zip code 38109, the poorest in Memphis, where MLH first identified in 2010 that they had high levels of charity care, anticipating the Affordable Care Act.

Joy, hired early in 2013, literally "hit the ground running," establishing alliances with trusted locals like "Big Dog" who gave her explicit instructions on staying safe in the neighborhood, as well as local pastors, and neighborhood youth, many of whom were unemployed. To date, her most important job has been serving as the point person for the Cigna-funded "Wellness without Walls" initiative, which spun out of what the community said they needed: better access to healthcare.

MLH leadership, seeking a more innovative approach than building brick and mortar clinics, in 2013 began offering a "Shall Not be Called Health Fair" held regularly at the local community center. Joy personally followed up with every person who had needs or outlying values on screenings at those events, which grew to reach more than 1,700 people. She found herself engaging in tasks as diverse as locating hearing aids, finding adoption agencies for pregnant teenagers, or counseling a 16-year-old girl frequently hospitalized for intractable gastrointestinal disease who just wanted to graduate from high school.

Joy's efforts led to early overall reductions in charity care (reported in the 2013 Health Systems Learning group monograph). Although charity care had increased 35% from 2010-2011, overall charity care costs dropped 6.9% from 2011-2012, with costs in zip code 38109 dropping an astounding 8.9%. Of course, the most important "metric" is that persons who stay out of the hospital have much improved quality of life. Joy and the team continued in 2014 to focus on frequent utilizers in 38109—97 people, most of whom had at least 3 co-morbid conditions (Congestive Heart Failure, Diabetes Mellitus, Chronic Obstructive Pulmonary Disease, Chronic Renal Disease). By November, charges for those persons had dropped by 43% (Nelson, Rafalski, Bailey & Marinescu, 2014).

She sees her job as a ministry and feels blessed to be able to provide such hands-on care to so many, addressing the social determinants of health that truly drive avoidable health care costs and readmissions. Her efforts have been so important on the ground that the Memphis Business Journal acknowledged Joy with the 2015 "Healthcare Hero" award.

weight was reported, along with pre-post reductions in blood pressure, LDL cholesterol and insulin levels. Participants also reported high program satisfaction (O'Brien, Perez, Alos, Whitaker, Ciolino, Mohr & Ackermann, 2015).

In sum, CHWs can "stand in the gap" to link clinical and community resources for their clients and, as members of clinical teams, provide a culturally competent, intrinsically trustworthy bridge while also helping clinicians increase patient engagement in a treatment plan. Because time with the doctor can be very brief, CHWs help by following up with the patient to assess for health literacy and understanding of a plan, listen for core concerns that could impede self-management, and offer ongoing support that can favorably impact health outcomes.

By bridging important gaps in services, helping manage chronic diseases among patients, improving preventive screening rates, reducing readmissions and improving patient satisfaction—all aspects in achieving the original Triple Aim—CHW programs generate savings for providers, payers and society as a whole. Lastly, community health workers' knowledge about and connection with the neighborhoods they serve make them powerful advocates for policy change and key players in improving health equity, the critical fourth or Quadruple Aim.

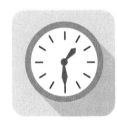

1:30 P.M. Nada arrives back at the office with a sandwich she's grabbed in route. She ensures Kayla's pregnancy info file is up to date. Additionally, she sets an alert for the day she will follow up with Kayla to see how she is progressing. "Planning and organization are key in a job like mine," she reflects.

Now, Nada will start working on a phone call queue of community members who have recently connected with the WIN Network. Among these contacts is a young woman who is interested in joining the Co-Captains Club. The Co-Captains Club is a way to expand the WIN Network and empower the young women who have worked with the program in the past. Co-Captains are trained in groups by WIN Network CHWs to host informational meetings where they talk to their friends and family about physical and mental health, family planning and other issues impacting the community. This training empowers the Co-Captain to be a resource for her network of friends and family and supports her along the way. Nada enrolls the new caller in the upcoming Co-Captains training the following week.

The next message is from Tara. Nada explains that Tara has gestational diabetes and was having trouble affording the foods that will help keep her blood sugar in check. "We connected with Detroit's Food Assistance Program which, so far, has helped Tara stay out of the ED," Nada said. But today, Tara was calling because her local grocery doesn't consistently stock the foods approved by the assistance program. Nada helps Tara find the name and contact information for the grocery store manager to ask about the inconsistent food stock. "Please call me back after you talk with him," Nada says. "We'll figure this out."

Standardized Training: Benefits and Challenges

Health systems need to know how to find trained CHWs in their community. They also need to know what steps to take if they wish to send persons for CHW training and what the key considerations are for starting a CHW program in their own organizations. As CHWs continue to gain recognition for their role in impacting the Quadruple Aim, full integration into health systems they are helping to transform is likely to require more formalization and standardization of this workforce.

CHWs and other lay frontline navigators historically have been trained on the job, with emphasis on learning about local resources, understanding practices and guidelines of their employers, and occasional continuing education opportunities, often narrowly focused in response to specific funding opportunities. Now regional training programs in several cities and states put greater emphasis on teaching for core competencies using effective and proven adult education methodologies. Community-based organizations, public health departments, or CHW associations have led the movement toward standardized training and in some states, community colleges or universities have taken on the task of creating more formal training curricula.

The benefits of more defined and structured training for CHWs are substantial. Credentialing or certification becomes possible, with greater opportunities for career advancement and portability of skills. Through credit-based foundational programs in post-secondary schools, such as Minnesota's model statewide curriculum, CHWs gain an educational pathway towards an associate or bachelor's degree and matriculation in other health professions. The Minnesota CHW Alliance has found that CHWs are often the first in their families to pursue higher education. In successfully completing the certificate program, they provide the inspiration and know-how for relatives and members of their communities to access education beyond high school and experience employment opportunities and health co-benefits associated with education and better income.

Improving the consistency of training programs also facilitates evaluation and research, which in turn builds the evidence for and credibility of the workforce, while standardized training supplies an important prerequisite for sustainable funding given that payers want to know that the workforce is competent to provide covered services.

This also raises some important issues. CHWs are trusted members of the communities they serve and are recruited for their lived experience, communication skills and local knowledge, but many have less formal education than other health care professionals, while those from marginalized communities may confront barriers to completing training programs. Registration requirements that inadvertently leave out certain groups including immigrants may be an issue. So too, training costs can be a barrier—though scholarships, employer tuition payment benefits, and school financial aid can be used to address potential financial barriers to CHWs achieving higher education.

Across the country, work has been under way for several years to define, create, and standardize various aspects of the CHW role, including training, certification, scope of practice and payment models. The National Academy for State Health Policy (NASHP) maintains a comprehensive listing of certification programs (www.nashp.org/state-community-health-worker-models). Some states, including Florida and Ohio, have created certification programs linked to other credentialing boards, such as nursing or behavioral health professionals. Massachusetts, Oregon and Rhode Island have built independent bodies to guide and approve the certification process for CHWs. Certification typically involves completion of an approved training program, criminal background check, a written application and professional references as well as a fee. Recertification often requires proof of continuing education among other provisions.

Though the process may vary from state to state, establishing a set of core competencies is one important prerequisite. These were first documented in the National Community Health Advisor Study published in 1998. Seven roles were identified: cultural mediation, health education, building individual and community capacity, connecting people with services, informal counseling and social support, advocacy, and direct service (e.g., taking blood pressure or administering other screening exams with sufficient training and supervision). Currently, a multi-state effort is underway to expand the list of core competencies and update the list to reflect new and emerging roles related to health reform, such as participating in community health needs assessments.

While the body of evidence supporting the effectiveness of CHWs continues to grow, work also is under way to develop a set of common metrics and indicators of success. Measures such as return on investment and reduced utilization of high-cost services may be effectively applied to CHW programs, but these programs also provide opportunities to measure more nuanced outcomes such as increased health knowledge, levels of empowerment, or quality of life of program participants. Such measures, though not yet common, may be exactly the indicators necessary for guiding responses to health disparities and the social determinants of health.

As meaningful standards continue to develop at the national, state or local level, CHWs themselves need to be part of the process. State CHW associations or networks are growing and deserve support and recognition. Likewise, their members need support to continue to bring their knowledge and energy to the work ahead, including training programs, curriculum development, and inclusion as faculty. This practice recognizes CHW expertise while creating career advancement opportunities for experienced CHW's. As the popular CHW slogan says, "Nothing about us without us!"

To find out if your state has a CHW alliance or association and to get involved at the state or national level, visit the webpage for the American Public Health Association (APHA) CHW Section at: www.apha. org/apha-communities/member-sections/community-health-workers.

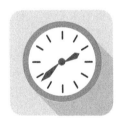

2:37 P.M. Nada makes it through most of her planned phone calls for the day when the clinic's front desk rings her. A patient who had just walked into the clinic needs to talk about health insurance enrollment as they do not have a health plan in place. Nada grabs her laptop and goes to meet with the patient in the office conference room. She confirms with the patient that he does not already have an application for Medicaid filed with the state and then proceeds to help complete his application. After informing him what to expect next in the application process, Nada learns the patient has not activated his online patient health portal, or MyChart, account. Nada helps the patient activate his account and learn how to utilize it.

Stakeholders and Partners

CHW stakeholders are richly diverse—from health plans to federally qualified health centers, from private health systems to federal, state and local public health; from banks to blight fighters; from accountable care organizations to foundations and faith-based partners. Their aims and the community context shape a variety of models through which CHWs are employed, deployed and funded. For example, CHW teams may be hired by an insurance organization to address needs of high-utilizer patients, or they may become part of an accountable-care strategy to fill gaps in services provided. The table opposite matches nationally embraced CHW core competencies with stakeholders who have the potential to benefit from engaging them.

Community health workers not only are touch points for population health in a hospital's ability to build and engage in meaningful community partnerships but help support the triennial IRS requirement for non-profit hospitals and health systems to perform Community Health Needs Assessments (CHNAs) and post their actionable and measurable CHNA Impact Plans. From stakeholder surveys to community-based partnerships that address assessed health needs, CHWs can help build the relationships that make programs effective and sustainable.

HEALTH LEADS AT KAISER PERMANENTE

As one key element of its work to address the social needs of its members and the communities it serves, Kaiser Permanente (KP) has developed a strategic partnership with Health Leads, a pioneering nonprofit that connects patients with community resources through a variety of interventions including on-site help desks staffed by volunteer students using highly reliable, constantly refreshed local resource directories. Initially piloted in a KP pediatrics practice and a public safety net hospital in Northern California, Health Leads is now being deployed in multiple KP medical centers in its Southern California region. In that region, a variety of different models are being tested that integrate KP and Health Leads operations in order to screen, refer and close social need gaps. The goal is to reach approximately 5,000 patients in the first phase, with a focus on patients expected to be high utilizers of healthcare based on predictive analytics. This is one of more than 30 social needs programs and pilots being implemented across Kaiser Permanente's service areas as part of its broader Total Health strategy—a strategy that focuses on addressing the drivers of health beyond the walls of its hospitals and medical office buildings.

As of January 15, 2016, the KP/Health Leads Community Resource Hub had proactively called 412 predicted high utilizer members, 181 picked up, and 117 participated in screening. Of 117 screened, 81% (95) reported at least one social need! This preliminary data shows a much higher prevalence of social needs in health care settings than prior reports indicated. It further illustrates the importance of the coordinated effort for KP Southern California members. A systematic approach to screening and resource navigation could lead to decreased utilization, decreased total costs of care, improved self-management of chronic conditions, increased patient satisfaction and greater member retention.

"Effective engagement of individuals most at risk for poor health outcomes calls for a collaborative approach among multiple stakeholders— and it's often CHWs and other frontline workers who supply the connective tissue."
- Kevin Barnett, DrPH, MCP, Public Health Institute, Oakland, California

CHW Core Competencies (from C3 Project)	Stakeholders
Cultural Mediation among Individuals, Communities, and Health and Social Service Systems	Payers, health systems and other providers, Accountable Care Organizations, social service agencies, government agencies such as public health, human services, education and housing; Federally Qualified Health Centers, State Innovation Models; health policy/health service researchers; policymakers; professional associations and trade associations; community/neighborhood organizations; faith-based organizations; K-12 schools; community colleges and other post-secondary schools; foundations, community/economic development, employers/business community and more.
Providing Culturally Appropriate Health Education and Information	
Care Coordination, Case Management, and System Navigation	
Providing Coaching and Social Support	
Advocating for Individuals and Communities	
Building Individual and Community Capacity	
Providing Direct Service	
Implementing Individual and Community Assessments	
Conducting Outreach	
Participating in Evaluation and Research	

From The Community Health Worker Common Core Project (C3)

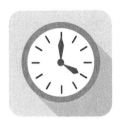 **4 P.M.** Nada updates the office records for each of the phone calls she has made and starts a teleconference with a community agency, Matrix Human Services, to learn more about their youth programs. "It's important that we CHWs develop and maintain good working relationships with the organizations that serve members of our community," she explains. "When an organization offers a new service or a new director is hired, I call to connect and to be sure they are providing the most up-to-date information about WIN Network, as well."

Toward Sustainability

As the clear value that CHWs bring to the healthcare team becomes increasingly evident, opportunities for programs and health care organizations to identify more sustainable funding are being explored across the country. Most CHW programs have depended on grant and contract funding in the past. Narrow categorical guidelines, coupled with discontinuous support, have led to unstable CHW jobs and unpredictable, sporadic access to CHW services. While philanthropic dollars will continue to be vital for start-up costs, research and evaluation, and infrastructure development, more sustainable funding sources for CHW services are needed. A variety of existing and potential funding sources outlined by the National Fund for Medical Education at the University of California San Francisco Center for the Health Professions (now Healthforce Center) at University of California, San Francisco includes grants and contracts, government support, health plan/insurance payment, companies with a diverse workforce and consumer self-pay (Dower, Knox, Lindler, & O'Neil, 2006).

Healthcare reform has also created a variety of CHW payment methods such as federal innovation funds and Medicaid dollars. CHWs show the greatest value in serving low-income populations that are Medicaid-eligible. Additionally, around the U.S., Medicaid expansion has extended access to thousands of previously uninsured persons who are now able to obtain coverage. Medicaid policies can drive interest by private payers and a greater number of providers (Rush & Mason, 2015).

As one example, the Michigan Community Health Worker Alliance (MiCHWA) has led efforts to convene payers, providers and state administrators in a series of highly effective stakeholder forums that include CHWs in promoting standardized training, and developing implementation and payment models in tandem with the state's new requirement that Medicaid managed care hire or arrange for CHWs. Henry Ford Health System, Spectrum Health, St. John Providence and other Michigan health systems are also deeply involved in these efforts. Other examples include (Rush & Mason, 2015):

- **State Plan Amendments.** Minnesota has CMS authority through a State Plan Amendment (SPA) to provide Medicaid coverage for CHW services specific to diagnostic-related patient education, both individual and group.

"Community health workers in the U.S. and in countries around the world, such as Brazil, India, Kenya, Liberia and South Africa play a growing role on the frontline in addressing the world-wide epidemic of chronic disease which disproportionately affects underserved communities experiencing health barriers related to income, literacy, access and other issues. Strategic philanthropic investments hold potential to broaden the adoption of high impact, sustainable CHW models—particularly when in partnership across key stakeholders such as governments and nonprofits. As a field, moving from time-limited grant support to proactive partnerships that elevate well-integrated CHW approaches is an important marker of success and key to empowering communities for better health."

- Paurvi Bhatt, MPH, Senior Director, Global Access, Medtronic Foundation

- **Medicaid Managed Care Organizations.** Several states have taken steps to ensure that Medicaid managed care plans include CHWs in contracting arrangements. As noted, beginning in 2016 in Michigan, the state Medicaid agency requires that all managed care plans maintain a ratio of at least one CHW for every 20,000 enrollees. In New Mexico, CHW services are included in the list of Medicaid benefits, and Medicaid contracts must encourage CHW care coordination.

- **Preventive Services Rule.** In July 2013, CMS published a rule change in the Federal Register which allows state Medicaid programs to pay for qualified non-licensed providers such as CHWs to deliver approved preventive services that are recommended by a physician or other licensed practitioner. Some view the Preventive Services SPA as a way for states to sustain CHW initiatives that are initiated with federal and state demonstration funds.

- **Medicaid Waivers and Reform Initiatives.** Most state strategies for covering CHW services are through waivers such as 1115a demonstration programs. Exciting health reform initiatives underway in many states through the CMS State Innovation Model (SIM) awards include policy and financial support for CHW models such as Oregon's Coordinated Care Organizations and Minnesota's Accountable Communities for Health. Patient-centered medical homes and healthcare homes in many states incorporate CHWs as members of patient-centered teams, some with per member per month funding that can help cover CHW care coordination services.

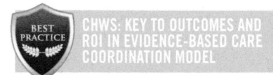

CHWS: KEY TO OUTCOMES AND ROI IN EVIDENCE-BASED CARE COORDINATION MODEL

To date, Medicare does not yet regard CHW services as a covered benefit. However, Massachusetts' One Care Program for beneficiaries that qualify for both Medicare and Medicaid ("dually-eligible") include specific services that can be provided by CHWs (Communication, MA Dept. of Public Health). In some states, community benefit funds from charitable hospitals underwrite CHW programs. Hospitals can use the results of their required community health needs assessments to identify gaps that CHWs can effectively address. And while opportunities for CHW employment are burgeoning in the healthcare sector, CHWs also work in community-based settings such as schools, affordable family and senior housing, and other settings where there is potential to tap different funding streams.

The outlook for CHW financing is favorable in the context of new payment reform models, including bundled payment and global financing. Already, we are seeing volume-based payment for healthcare services replaced by value-based purchasing arrangements. State and private payers will continue to invest in programs such as these as they simultaneously manage costs and provide

Recognized by the federal Agency for Health Research and Quality (AHRQ), the Pathways Community HUB model is designed to identify the most at-risk individuals within a community, connect them to evidence-based interventions, and measure the results. This "Find-Treat-Measure" approach emphasizes the importance of tracking health and social service interventions at the individual, agency and regional level using common metrics. Each "Pathway" begins with a frequent need of the at-risk population, identifies appropriate interventions to address the issue and, upon completion of the interventions, measures the outcome. Payment is based on completing the Pathway.

The Pathways model originated with the Community Health Access Project (CHAP) in Richland County, Ohio. Co-founders of CHAP, Drs. Mark and Sarah Redding, developed the HUB with an initial focus on preventing low birth weight babies. Pathways identified for this at-risk group included: education, depression, prenatal care and housing. A Pathway is complete when an identified problem is addressed, and a patient may pursue several Pathways, based on their situation. Key to the model's success is the trusted and trained CHW who navigates the patient along the Pathway.

Since this model began 14 years ago, CHAP has designed, tested and implemented 20 core pathways and created the community HUB infrastructure. With endorsement and replication of this model by AHRQ and support from The Kresge Foundation, a certification process for community HUBs now is in place. Programs have expanded to new states and have also been adapted to address other high-risk populations, such as individuals with chronic disease. Evaluation of this model has found return on investment to be $5.59 for every dollar spent on the program. Tools and technology in support of the HUB model are available through Care Coordination Systems, Inc., headed up by Dr. Sarah Redding.

the best outcomes for patients. If effectively focused and operated, CHW programs hold promise to help providers, organized as ACOs or in other risk arrangements, to help achieve key metrics on which the new value-based financing methods are based. At a fall 2015 meeting of policymakers convened by the National Academy for State Health Policy, a federal official observed that "incorporating CHWs into team-based models of care has the potential to augment CHWs' role in emerging value-based and bundled payment models and minimize the reliance on grant funding to support CHW initiatives" (Clary, 2015).

More than ever, greater diversity of CHW funding is beginning to replace dependence on limited grant and contract funds that has impeded the growth of the CHW work force. Under health reform, states are funding CHWs through State Innovation Model (SIM) Initiatives, 1115 waivers, Accountable Care Organizations and advanced primary care initiatives. Looking to the future, innovative payment policies and mechanisms that reward value and equity hold promise for stronger CHW integration and financing.

For a national map summarizing CHW financing policies and developments by state, see: www.nashp.org/state-community-health-worker-models.

Why the Time is Now

For so many compelling reasons, health navigators have a crucial and evolving role in health care today. Indeed, navigators improve health by addressing the cascade of non-medical factors that get in its way. Exemplifying the most robust of navigator roles, community health workers provide more than a compass—they extend important population heath-management efforts beyond clinic walls into neighborhoods where health happens, where people "live, learn, work and play" (Hecht, 2010). CHWs stand in the gap, connecting the dots between clinic and community to support the Quadruple Aim goals of population health, improving quality and the patient experience, reducing cost, and achieving health equity.

Interest in CHWs and other types of health

"As health policy, research and practice are becoming increasingly focused on improving the health of populations and addressing social determinants of health, Community Health Workers (CHWs) may be just what the doctor ordered."

- *Health Affairs, January 16, 2015*

"The policy and financial climate are ideal for expanded use of CHW programs. We must take advantage of this historic opportunity in order to create high-quality programs that measurably improve health in high-risk populations"

- *Shreya Kangovi, MSHP, Assistant Professor Perelman School of Medicine at the University of Pennsylvania, Executive Director, Penn Center for Community Health Workers*

navigators has grown exponentially in response to health reform and new complexities in the health care system. This includes powerful demographic shifts that will continue to shape healthcare delivery and finance, such as a rapidly growing 65+ year-old cohort and an increasingly diverse younger population with cultural, linguistic, socioeconomic and other challenges to good health. More and more, health systems, public health agencies, payers and other stakeholders are recognizing the key contributions that CHWs can make in addressing these social determinants. As enthusiasm and evidence for CHWs grow, initiatives to standardize their training also are burgeoning across states—improving opportunities for certification, inclusion on clinical teams, and benchmarking for outcomes and effectiveness. CHWs can also produce a manifold return on investment—with an ROI of up to and exceeding fivefold for each dollar spent. Built into government payment models and commercial coverage, CHW programs will become sustainable over time, no longer grant-dependent.

In our high-tech age, on-the-ground relationships remain the indispensable key to sure and sustainable population health improvement. CHWs and other health navigators use the tools of technology—such as social media, real-time community resource databases, online reporting and measurement

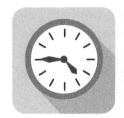

4:45 P.M. Nada adds to her team's "asset map," with its list and location of services and key contacts available to community members. "People sometimes think that poor communities only have needs," Nada says, 'but there are a lot of assets here, too. You just have to get to know the neighborhoods and the people in them."

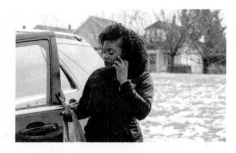

Nada ends her day sharing with her supervisor the progress she has made on the phone call queue. She responds to e-mails and checks her calendar for tomorrow. "Serving as a community health worker is being a resource to help ease some of the stressors in people's lives. We are a bridge of support," Nada says, "that brings our clients to the road of their success."

platforms—as important supports. But these tools cannot replace the value of walking with someone on their journey. Hope never happens on the internet alone, or in a medical record. It happens at the intersections where people come together with the care that is right for them—accessible, patient-focused, health literate, culturally competent, high-quality, and equitable. And it's eminently more likely to happen when people—especially but not exclusively in vulnerable populations—can see, embrace and embark on a clear road forward, connecting to other people and existing resources that empower them to achieve the healthiest, best life possible for themselves and their families.

REFERENCES

Achieving the Triple Aim: Success with Community Health Workers. (2015, April/May). Retrieved February 05, 2016, from http://www.mass.gov/eohhs/docs/dph/com-health/com-health-workers/achieving-the-triple-aim.pdf.

Agency for Health Research and Quality (AHRQ). Innovation Profile: Program Uses "Pathways" to Confirm Those At-Risk Connect to Community Based Health and Social Services, Leading to Improved Outcomes. (2001). Retrieved February 05, 2016, from https://innovations.ahrq.gov/profiles/program-uses-pathways-confirm-those-risk-connect-community-based-health-and-social-services.

American Public Health Association (APHA). Community Health Workers. (n.d.). Retrieved February 05, 2016, from https://www.apha.org/apha-communities/member-sections/community-health-workers.

Berwick, D., Nolan, T., & Whittington, J. (2008). The Triple Aim: Care, health, and cost. *Health Affairs*, 759-769.

Centers for Disease Control and Prevention. Health Disparities and Inequality Report. MMWR 2011; 60(Suppl):1-109.

California Health Workforce Alliance (CHWA). Taking Innovation to Scale. (2013, December). Retrieved February 05, 2016, from http://www.chhs.ca.gov/PRI/_Taking Innovation to Scale—CHWs, Promotores and the Triple Aim—CHWA Report 12-22-13 (1).pdf.

City of Healthy Neighborhoods & Buildings. (n.d.). Retrieved February 05, 2016, from http://www.sanantonio.gov/Health/HealthyLiving/HealthyNeighborhoods.aspx.

Clancy, C., Munier, W., Crosson, K., Moy, E., HoChaves, K., Freeman, W., & Bonnett, D. (2012, March). *National Health Care Quality Report 2011* [PDF]. Department of Health and Human Services.

Clary, A. (2015, December 07). Community Health Workers in the Wake of Health Care Reform: Considerations for State and Federal Policymakers—NASHP. Retrieved February 05, 2016, from http://nashp.org/community-health-workers-in-the-wake-of-health-care-reform-considerations-for-state-and-federal-policymakers/.

Davis, K., Stremikis, K., Squires, D., & Schoen, C. (2014, June). Mirror, Mirror on the Wall: How the Performance of the U.S. Health Care System Compares Internationally, 2010 Update. Retrieved February 05, 2016, from http://www.commonwealthfund.org/publications/fund-reports/2010/jun/mirror-mirror-update.

Diaz, J. (2012, June). Social return on investment: Community Health Workers in Cancer Research. Retrieved February 05, 2016, from http://www.wilder.org/Wilder-Research/Publications/Studies/Community%20Health%20Workers%20in%20the%20Midwest/Social%20Return%20on%20Investment%20-%20Community%20Health%20Workers%20in%20Cancer%20Outreach.pdf.

Disparities. (n.d.). Retrieved February 06, 2016, from http://www.healthypeople.gov/2020/about/foundation-health-measures/Disparities.

Dower, C., Knox, M., Lindler, V., & O'Neil, E. (2006). Advancing Community Health Worker Practice and Utilization: The Focus on Financing. Retrieved February 05, 2016, from http://healthforce.ucsf.edu/publications/advancing-community-health-worker-practice-and-utilization-focus-financing.

Felix, H. C., Mays, G. P., Stewart, M. K., Cottoms, N., & Olson, M. (2011). Medicaid Savings Resulted When Community Health Workers Matched Those With Needs To Home And Community Care. *Health Affairs*, 30(7), 1366-1374.

Goodwin, K., & Tobler, L. (2008, April). Community health workers: Expanding the scope of the health care delivery system. Retrieved February 05, 2016, from http://www.chwcentral.org/community-health-workers-expanding-scope-health-care-delivery-system.

Hardeman, R., Gerrard, M.D. (2011, June). Community Health Workers in the Midwest: Understanding and developing the workforce. Retrieved February 05, 2016, from https://www.wilder.org/Wilder-Research/Publications/Studies/Community%20Health%20 Workers%20in%20the%20Midwest/Community%20Health%20Workers%20in%20the%20Midwest%20-%20Understanding%20and%20 Developing%20the%20Workforce,%20Full%20Report.pdf.

Hecht, B. (2010). Health Starts Where We Live. Robert Wood Johnson Foundation. Retrieved February 07, 2016, from http://www.rwjf.org/en/library/research/2010/10/health-starts-where-we-live.html.

Infant Mortality. Kids Count Data Center. Michigan League for Public Policy. (2016). Retrieved February 08, 2016, from http://datacenter.kidscount.org/data/tables/1637-infant-mortality?loc=24.

Infant Mortality by Race. Kids Count Data Center. Michigan League for Public Policy. (2016). Retrieved February 08, 2016, from http://datacenter.kidscount.org/data/tables/21-infant-mortality-by-race?loc=1#detailed/2/24/fase/36,868,867,133,38/10,11,9,12,1,13 /285,284.

Institute for Clinical and Economic Review (ICER). Community Health Workers: A Review of Program Evolution, Evidence on Effectiveness and Value, and Status of Workforce Development in New England. (2013). Retrieved February 05, 2016, from http://cepac.icer-review.org/wp-content/uploads/2011/04/CHW-Draft-Report-05-24-13-MASTER1.pdf.

Institute of Medicine: U.S. Health in International Perspective Shorter Lives, Poorer Health. (2013, January). Retrieved February 05, 2016, from http://iom.nationalacademies.org/Reports/2013/US-Health-in-International-Perspective-Shorter-Lives-Poorer-Health.aspx.

Johnson, D., Saavedra, P., Sun, E., Stageman, A., Grovet, D., Alfero, C., Kaufman, A. (2011). Community Health Workers and Medicaid Managed Care in New Mexico. *Journal of Community Health*, 37(3), 563-571. Retrieved February 5, 2016.

Kangovi, S., Grande, D., & Trinh-Shevrin, C. (2015). From Rhetoric to Reality—Community Health Workers in Post-Reform U.S. Health Care. *New England Journal of Medicine*, 372(24), 2277-2279.

Kangovi, S., Mitra, N., Grande, D., White, M. L., Mccollum, S., Sellman, J., Long, J. A. (2014). Patient-Centered Community Health Worker Intervention to Improve Posthospital Outcomes. *JAMA Internal Medicine*, 174(4), 535.

Krieger, J., Takaro, T. K., Song, L., Beaudet, N., & Edwards, K. (2009). A Randomized Controlled Trial of Asthma Self-management Support Comparing Clinic-Based Nurses and In-Home Community Health Workers. *Archives of Pediatrics & Adolescent Medicine*, 163(2), 141. Retrieved February 7, 2016.

Massachusetts Dept. of Public Health. (n.d.) Communication, List of Covered Services for Members Enrolled in a One Care Plan. Retrieved from http://www.mass.gov/eohhs/docs/masshealth/onecare/services-covered-by-one-care.pdf

Matos, S., Findlay, S., Hicks, A., Legendre, Y., & Do Canto, L. (2011). Paving a path to advance the community health worker workforce in New York State [Minnesota Community Health Worker Alliance]. Retrieved February 7, 2016, from http://successwithchws.org/asthma/ wp-content/uploads/sites/3/2015/02/CHWs-In-the-Community1.pdf.

National Academy for State Health Policy (NASHP). State Community Health Worker Models—NASHP. (2015). Retrieved February 07, 2016, from http://www.nashp.org/state-community-health-worker-models/.

Nelson, K., Rafalski, E. Bailey, S. & Marinescu, R. (2015). Managing Rising-Risk Patients in a Value-Based World. 2015 Congress on Healthcare Leadership.

O'Brien, M. J., Perez, A., Alos, V. A., Whitaker, R. C., Ciolino, J. D., Mohr, D. C., & Ackermann, R. T. (2015). The Feasibility, Acceptability, and Preliminary Effectiveness of a Promotora-Led Diabetes Prevention Program (PL-DPP) in Latinas: A Pilot Study. *The Diabetes Educator,* 41(4), 485-494.

Office of Minority Health. U.S. Department of Health and Human Services. Think Cultural Health—CLAS & the CLAS Standards. (n.d.). Retrieved February 07, 2016, from https://www.thinkculturalhealth.hhs.gov/Content/clas.asp.

Pathways: A system designed to produce positive outcomes and impact health disparities [PDF]. (n.d.).

Phalen, J., & Paradis, R. (2015, January 16). How Community Health Workers Can Reinvent Health Care Delivery In The US [Web log post]. Retrieved February 5, 2016, from http://healthaffairs.org/blog/2015/01/16/how-community-health-workers-can-reinvent-health-care-delivery-in-the-us/.

Redding, S., Conrey, E., Porter, K., Paulson, J., Hughes, K., & Redding, M. (2014). Pathways Community Care Coordination in Low Birth Weight Prevention. *Journal Maternal Child Health*, 19(3), 643-650.

Rosenthal, E.L et al. (Nov 2, 2015). C3: The Journey towards a United Consensus. PPT presented at American Public Health Association 2015 Annual Meeting.

Rush, C. (2015, October 15). Creating a Policy Infrastructure for Community Health Workers: Four Domains and Four Dilemmas. Lecture presented at National Academy for State Health Policy Convening.

Rush, C., & Mason, T. (2015, November 4). *Strategies for Integrating CHWs into Health Care Teams: Financing Options Under Medicaid.* Lecture presented at APHA Annual Conference, Chicago.

Smedley, B. D., Stith, A. Y., & Nelson, A. R. (2003). *Unequal treatment: Confronting racial and ethnic disparities in health care.* Washington, D.C.: National Academy Press.

Snapshots: Health Care Spending in the United States & Selected OECD Countries. (2012, April). Retrieved February 05, 2016, from http://kff.org/health-costs/issue-brief/snapshots-health-care-spending-in-the-united-states-selected-oecd-countries/.

RESOURCES

The following is a select sample of the many resources, tool kits, publications and guides for planning, implementing and evaluating community health worker programs. Many of the resources listed here have more extensive resource lists included in their publications. This list is not intended to be inclusive and Stakeholder Health is not specifically endorsing these resources, but providing them as a starting place to learn more.

CHW TOOL KITS

Behavioral Health Leadership Institute CHW Tool Kit:
http://bhli.org/communityhealthworkertoolkit.shtml. This toolkit and reference is specifically designed for CHWs with a focus on mental health and substance use disorders within primary care settings.

Best Practice Guidelines for Implementing and Evaluating CHW Programs in Health Care Settings:
http://www.sinai.org/sites/default/files/SUHI%20Best%20Practice%20Guidelines%20for%20CHW%20Programs.pdf.
This extensive report includes evidence-based guidelines on how to launch and evaluate a CHW programs in health care settings, from Sinai Urban Health Institute in Chicago, IL.

Building a CHW Program: The Key to Better Care, Better Outcomes and Lower Costs:
http://www.nursing.virginia.edu/media/2014-06-27_BCHWP.pdf. This publication is geared to the nurse executive in hospital and integrated health settings with accountabilities for starting and overseeing CHW initiatives.

Centers for Disease Control (CDC) CHW Toolkit:
http://www.cdc.gov/dhdsp/pubs/chw-toolkit.htm. This compilation of evidence-based research supports the effectiveness of CHWs for use by state health departments and other organizations.

Penn Center for CHWs Tool Kit:
http://chw.upenn.edu/tools. This tool kit provides extensive materials and guidelines for hiring, training, supervising and measuring CHWs in health care settings, using the IMPaCT model.

Rural Health Information Hub CHW Tool Kit:
https://www.ruralhealthinfo.org/community-health/community-health-workers. This 8-module guide is designed to help rural health providers evaluate opportunities for developing a CHW program and provide resources and best practices developed by successful CHW programs.

Success with CHWs for Asthma Care Providers:
www.successwithchws.org/asthma. Web-based resource to help asthma care providers learn about and implement CHW strategies.

Success with CHWs for Mental Health Providers:
www.successwith chws.org/mental-health. Web-based resource to help mental health providers learn about and implement CHW strategies.

STATE COMMUNITY HEALTH WORKER ASSOCIATIONS

Many states, cities, counties and regions have developed CHW associations to promote the workforce, contribute to policy development, share resources, provide professional development opportunities, and advocate for CHWs in general.

California Association of Community Health Workers: http://www.cachw.org/.

Community Health Worker Network of New York City: http://www.chwnetwork.org/.

Michigan Community Health Worker Alliance: http://michwa.org/.

Minnesota Community Health Worker Alliance: http://mnchwalliance.org/.

New Mexico Community Health Workers Association: http://nmchwa.com/.

Ohio Community Health Workers Association: http://www.med.wright.edu/chc/programs/ochwa.

Oregon Community Health Worker Association: http://orchwa.org.

ADDITIONAL RESOURCES

Addressing Chronic Disease through Community Health Workers: A Policy and Systems Level Approach:
   http://www.cdc.gov/dhdsp/docs/chw_brief.pdf. A policy brief that includes recommendations for integrating CHWs into community-based chronic disease prevention efforts

Care Coordination Systems:
   http://carecoordinationsystems.com/. Website of the Community Pathways HUB model developer, Dr. Sarah Redding.

Centers for Disease Control Policy and Systems Change to Expand Employment of CHWs: E-Learning Course:
   http://www.cdc.gov/dhdsp/pubs/chw_elearning.htm. Online self-paced course to acquaint stakeholders and others with the CHW field.

CHW Central: www.chwcentral.org. An online resource for International CHW programs.

Community Health Workers: Expanding the Scope of the Health Care Delivery System:
   \Community Health Workers\Research & Data\Community Health Workers- Expanding the Scope of the Health Care Delivery System.pdf. A publication of the National Association of State Legislatures about state policy issues related to CHWs.

FULL AUTHORSHIP LISTING

Nancy Combs, MA, Director of Community Health, Equity & Wellness, Henry Ford Health System, Detroit, MI

Kimberlydawn Wisdom, MD, MS, Senior Vice President of Community Health & Equity and Chief Wellness & Diversity Officer, Henry Ford Health System, Detroit, MI

Dominica Rehbein, MHA, MPH, Administrative Fellow, Henry Ford Health System, Detroit, MI

Catherine Potter, MA, Program Manager, Safety Net Partnerships, Kaiser Permanente, Portland, OR

Joan Cleary, MM, Executive Director, Minnesota Community Health Worker Alliance, St. Paul, MN

Loel Solomon, PhD, Vice President for Community Health, Kaiser Permanente, Oakland, CA

Nada Dickinson, Community & Neighborhood Navigator, Henry Ford Health System, Detroit, MI

Teresa Cutts, PhD, Asst. Research Professor, Wake Forest School of Medicine

Ameldia Brown, MDiv., BSN, RN, Manager, Faith Community Nursing Network, Henry Ford Macomb Hospital

Monica Lowell, BA, Vice President of Community Relations, University of Massachusetts Memorial Medical Center, Worcester, MA (reviewer)

For more information about this chapter, contact **Nancy Combs** at e-mail, ncombs1@hfhs.org or phone, (313) 874-6625.

CHAPTER 6

Community Asset Mapping: Integrating and Engaging Community and Health Systems

Teresa Cutts and Ray King with Maureen Kersmarki, Kirsten Peachey,
Jason Hodges, Sherrianne Kramer and Sandy Lazarus

Community asset mapping can be a crucial component for forging meaningful and useful partnerships between health systems and communities. This chapter describes the history and specifications of select asset-based mapping methodologies, existing mapping tools, as well as their potential integration into the federally mandated Community Health Needs Assessments (CHNAs). The potential use of mapping findings to build, nurture and enhance community health improvement efforts will be explored, as well as key strategies and considerations in use of these processes. Lastly, case studies are used to illustrate how asset mapping can be leveraged to build meaningful clinical-community partnerships with health systems.

Overview

Numerous forms of participatory community asset "mapping" frameworks or methodologies have been used for decades and exist in many iterations. They range from Participatory Rural Appraisal in the 1970's (Chambers, 1980) to the work of Kretzman and McKnight (1993) in the early 1980's to more current approaches, such as those used by the National Association of City and County Health Organizations' (NACCHO) Mobilizing for Actions through Planning and Partnerships or MAPP process (NACCHO, 2015), the African/International Religious Health Assets Mapping Programme Models (ARHAP, 2006), and Dr. Jeffrey Brenner's hot spotting in Camden, NJ (Gawande, 2011).

Most early asset mapping models were developed by community development, public health or community psychology practitioners and researchers but were of little interest to health systems. However, recent Affordable Care Act mandates and Internal Revenue Service (IRS) requirements that not-for-profit hospitals must conduct meaningful Community Health Needs Assessments (CHNAs) and incorporate those findings into their strategic planning and community benefit efforts, have commanded the attention of health system leaders. Community asset mapping models are ideal for augmenting this requirement, as well as for pushing healthcare upstream by encouraging health systems to move outside their walls (Gunderson & Cochrane, 2012).

Community Asset Mapping: Definition and Models/Frameworks

The following section draws heavily on the work of South African colleagues, for whom community asset mapping is a set of practices that provides communities with multiple opportunities to identify and mobilize previously unrecognized but existing strengths and capabilities (Kramer, Amos, Lazarus, & Seedat, 2012). It is defined as "a process of documenting the tangible and intangible resources of a community by viewing the community as a place with strengths or assets that need to be preserved and enhanced, not deficits to be remedied" (Kerka, 2003, p. 3). These resources may belong to an entire community, or they may be specific to individuals, groups or organizations within communities (Rossing, 2000). A key characteristic of community asset mapping is its participatory nature (Kramer et al., 2012). Ideally, it reflects the principles embedded in Community Based Participatory Research (CBPR), which aims to develop and foster genuine partnerships between community members and researchers, demonstrated by co-learning, capacity building, mutual benefits, and long-term commitment to achieving equity (Wallerstein & Duran, 2006). Select, recommended models and frameworks are discussed below.

ASSET BASED COMMUNITY DEVELOPMENT (ABCD)

The Asset Based Community Development (ABCD) model, derived from the work of Kretzman and McKnight (1993), is often viewed as the seminal mapping approach (see tools and resources at http://www.abcdinstitute.org/). As stated by our ARHAP colleague, the late Reverend Steve De Gruchy, it is predicated on the notion that "one can't build a community based on what one does not have." In the introduction to their ABCD guide, Kretzman and McKnight (1993) describe the model as a "community-building path which is asset-based, internally focused and relationship driven."

Aimed originally at harnessing a community's own resources against poverty (Mathie & Kearney, 2001), ABCD encourages and empowers grassroots leadership and capacity building locally (Kramer et al., 2012). This approach has been shown to be successful in many settings, including the US and other countries (Mathie & Cunningham, 2008). However, it is important to note that very different objectives may be accomplished in each setting. In this respect, poverty needs to be understood in various ways: absolute deprivation is often easier to work with in the ABCD model as there is a sense of everyone being "equally" poor, whereas relative deprivation, where competition rather than cooperation is more likely, makes it more difficult. In the experience of our South African colleagues, ABCD and other asset mapping models are more successful in rural areas (often absolutely deprived) than in urban ones (usually relatively deprived), which may or may not be generalizable beyond South Africa. Nonetheless, ABCD's principles and exercises are valuable beyond a focus on poverty and they are foundational to and often incorporated into other mapping models (e.g., Building Communities of Shalom).

MOBILIZING FOR ACTION THROUGH PLANNING AND PARTNERSHIPS (MAPP)

Mobilizing for Action through Planning and Partnerships (MAPP) is described as "a community-driven strategic planning process for improving community health" (NACCHO website). MAPP was developed by NACCHO and the Public Health Practice Program Office at the Centers for Disease Control and Prevention (PHPPO/CDC). It is a web-based tool/process/framework that enables local public health agencies (LPHAs) and communities to assess and improve community health (Pullen et al., 2005; http://www.naccho.org/topics/infrastructure/mapp/).

Facilitated by public health leaders, the MAPP framework is a collaborative process that helps communities strategically identify and prioritize health issues, assets and resources. It aims to collectively improve the health of the community, as well as the performance of the local public health systems. Seven elements critical to MAPP success include: systems thinking, dialogue, shared vision, data to inform the process, partnerships and collaboration, strategic thinking and celebration of successes (Journal of Public Health Management and Practice, September/October 2005; NACCHO, 2015). MAPP is "... an interactive process that can improve the efficiency, effectiveness, and ultimately the performance of local public health systems" (NACCHO, 2015), and is suggested by the Public Health Accreditation Board (PHAB) as a standard for assessment and planning. This is achieved with multi-level processes, data triangulation, mixed methods approaches, and partnering with multiple stakeholder systems. Although there is much variation in how the MAPP process is being implemented, there is increasing emphasis on integrating MAPP into health system CHNA efforts.

Six steps with four critical assessments in the MAPP Process are noted in the diagram below (from the NACCHO website, http://www.naccho.org):

- Step 1: Organize for Success/Partnership Development
- Step 2: Visioning
- Step 3: Four MAPP Assessments: Community Health Status Assessment (CHSA), Community Themes & Strengths Assessment (CTSA), Local Public Health System Assessment (LPHSA), Forces of Change Assessment (FOCA)
- Step 4: Identify Strategic Issues
- Step 5: Formulate Goals and Strategies
- Step 6: Action Cycle Plan

Mobilizing for Action through Planning and Partnerships

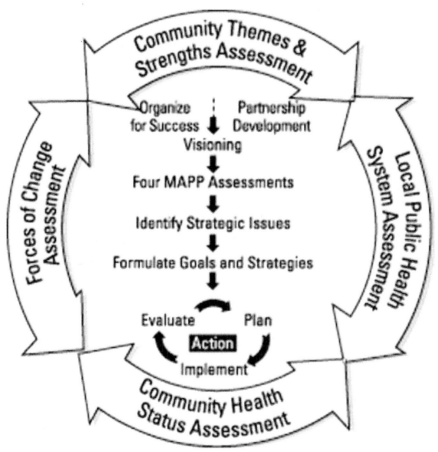

Further MAPP implementation and cost details are found in the Implementation sidebar below.

MAPP IMPLEMENTATION DETAILS (from MAPP Handbook, http://www.naccho.org/topics/infrastructure/mapp/upload/mapp_handbook_fnl.pdf)

Timeline to Implement: 18 months is suggested timeline (MAPP Handbook, pp. 22-23).

Product Generation and Sharing: Numerous reports are generated and the focus is on sharing transparently on websites and through other media (e.g., hard copy of early draft reports, regular meetings with community partners to discuss findings). Specifically, four assessment reports under the MAPP process provide the foundation for the Community Health Improvement Plan (CHIP). Regularly collected data from the CDC, local and state health departments, and other organizations are also critical, and are found on public websites.

Staffing Required: A key dedicated full-time staff planner is critical for "success" of the MAPP process, as related by Pullen et al. (2005). Administrative assistant and epidemiologist services will be needed, at least part-time. A robust group of community partners/volunteers representing sectors of the local public health system is also necessary to insure a diversity of input is included throughout the process.

Training Required: Yes. NACCHO provides free online resources and training in the form of webinars and social networking, in addition to a comprehensive MAPP Guidebook. Most of these are located here: http://www.naccho.org/topics/infrastructure/MAPP/TAwebcasts.cfm. Additionally, sponsored in-person MAPP training is available for a registration fee of $1,500 for NACCHO members or $2,000 for non-members. However, local health department staff can apply for a scholarship to waive the registration fees (http://naccho.org/topics/infrastructure/mapp/framework/mapp-trainings.cfm). These meetings are held over 2-3 days typically somewhere in the DC area. Lodging and transportation are not covered by the scholarship.

Estimated Costs: Not fully known, but the MAPP Handbook suggests covering personal, contractual, meeting space, equipment, travel, supplies, printing and postage costs. Personal estimates from key leaders in local public health departments suggest a minimum of $150K for the full process (covering a minimum of two FTEs: coordinator and administrative type staff persons) and dissemination of reports.

Suggested Frequency to Repeat/Update: Once every 5 years.

Aligned with CHNA: Yes, often MAPP serves as a key component in partnership with local health systems who are undertaking the CHNA process.

Strengths: Thorough asset-based and strongly participatory process that is well-known, easily comparable across different states and counties, used to certify public health departments by the Public Health Accreditation Board and an integral part of public health infrastructure, used extensively since 2000.

Challenges: The process is lengthy, has limited flexibility in implementation and can be costly for under-resourced public health departments. Commonly identified areas for community health improvement focus often seem redundant and face-valid to participants, especially given the expense and work required to undertake MAPP as prescribed. Maintaining community engagement throughout the lengthy process is a challenge. Reports generated and local public health project undertakings are secondary to goals and reporting, and may not have obvious utility for health systems in their strategic CHNA efforts.

Contact: NACCHO MAPP Toolkits and Resources www.naccho.org/topics/infrastructure/mapp

The work of the African Religious Health Assets Mapping Programme (ARHAP, now the International Religious Health Assets Mapping Programme or IRHAP), in existence since 2002, reflects transdisciplinary thinking at the intersection of faith and community health (Cochrane et al., 2011). The various ARHAP/IRHAP tools described below were derived from a deep bench of both academic theory and practice models. The qualitative data captured from using ARHAP/IRHAP models is an excellent supplement to hospital CHNA efforts, especially in terms of involving community in strategic planning for focus areas.

The original Participatory Inquiry into Religious Health Assets, Networks and Agency (PIRHANA) tool was developed in response to a World Health Organization (WHO) request/RFA in 2005-06 to "map" the religious or faith assets in at least two countries in sub-Saharan Africa experiencing the HIV/AIDS pandemic (De Gruchy et al., 2011). The model drew deeply from four basic domains of work: participatory rural appraisal (Chambers, 1980), appreciative inquiry (Cooperrider & Srivastva, 1987), ABCD (Kretzman and McKnight, 1993) and Paulo Friere's Liberation Theology (Friere & Shor, 1987). PIRHANA's main architect was Reverend Steve De Gruchy, PhD (1962-2010) of the University of KwaZulu-Natal, South Africa. The grounded theory of the work was established by implementing the PIRHANA process in Zambia and Lesotho, which resulted in the original PIRHANA manual (De Gruchy et al., 2007). There are four processes included in PIRHANA: GIS, participatory mapping, leadership engagement and deeper case studies (see http://www.irhap.uct.ac.za for more details).

Key differentiators between PIRHANA and its subsequent hybrids (see below for details) are the focus on both tangible (e.g., clinic and services on a map) and intangible factors (e.g., the way that care is delivered in a clinic), as well as a focus on the types and extent of relationships between healthcare seekers and providers in a given area. These differences are illustrated through individual and group exercises, including spidergrams, or social network maps. Two separate workshops (one for health seekers and one for health providers) are held and then detailed findings are reported back to both groups and any interested community members within a 4-6 week timeframe. PIRHANA also builds on a progressive logic of earlier exercises in its process. For health seekers, the maps drawn early on and entities designated as important on those maps are used for subsequent ranking exercises. Identifying exemplary individuals and organizations and teasing out characteristics which define that exemplary status has also been a signature of the ARHAP mapping processes. Also, in keeping with its community development DNA, this model seeks to make grassroots voices audible to policy makers, as well as empowering those agents on the ground to set their own agendas and strengthen sustainability (De Gruchy et al 2011).

The PIRHANA process was piloted in the U.S. in Memphis, TN, where staff were trained and eight PIRHANA workshops conducted from 2007-2008 (Cutts, 2011). Emory University staff from the Interfaith Health Program also developed hybrids of the original participatory inquiry model to map adolescent sexual health (PIRASH) in both South Africa and the U.S. South, as well as to conduct general asset mapping in Kenya (Blevins et al, 2012).

In 2009, the Community Health Assets Mapping for Partnership or CHAMP was adapted from PIRHANA. CHAMP focused more on long-term partnerships with community than PIRHANA originally could in Zambia and Lesotho, with a stronger emphasis on both engaging community and continuing to develop and sustain relationships. The CHAMP language also shifted the focus from the more narrow "religious health assets" (RHAs) to "community health assets" of which RHAs are a subset. This is necessary where religion is not as ubiquitous nor as holistically experienced as in many African contexts, and it avoids the danger of thinking solely of faith communities or congregations versus broader community organizations and assets.

CHAMP was refined and developed further in South Africa in 2009 for the South African Hospice and Palliative Care Association (HPCA) by Reverend Steve De Gruchy, PhD and his team. HPCA staff were trained to conduct CHAMP-Palliative Care (CHAMP-PC) workshops and subsequently rolled out CHAMP in nine districts, with such success that the Primary Care districts of South Africa have explored various uses of the model (Kramer et al., 2012). U.S. Teams have also been trained in CHAMP in Buffalo, NY (local Area Health Education Centers or AHEC and faith community coalition) and Chicago, IL, engaging the Center for Faith and Community Health Transformation, Advocate Healthcare, the University of Chicago and others (Cutts & Peachey, 2014).

CHAMP ACCESS TO CARE

CHAMP Access to Care was developed by Cutts and others and piloted in Memphis (2011) and North Carolina (2012-2015) in response to a need for health systems providing care to vulnerable populations to better align and leverage existing assets. CHAMP Access to Care focuses on promoting dialogue between both health seekers and providers to identify local tangible and intangible assets and gaps in care, and results are often incorporated into hospital CHNA processes. A good example of how intangible assets are identified and used can be seen in the four North Carolina CHAMP Access to Care workshops conducted with the Hispanic community in Forsyth County in July 2014 (Cutts et al., 2016). Findings from these workshops are being used to establish improved policies for care of Hispanic persons in local safety nets (e.g., changing sliding scale guidelines, building trust with providers, promoting delivery of more respectful care). The key focus is building trustworthy partnerships between both health seekers and providers to improve care quality and access, particularly by engaging leaders of local safety net organizations.

CHAMP SPECIALTY MAPPING

CHAMP has also been used in Memphis for specialty efforts to map elder care (2009) and behavioral health services (2010), as well as a System of Care project (2010-2012), in which youth were trained to conduct GIS and participatory mapping workshops. Additionally, North Carolina recently adapted it as CHAMP-Food Pathways. This process makes visible common ways that community members adapt to and work toward food security and to better align provider services (Cutts & Jensen, 2015). See sidebar below for more details on the PIRHANA, CHAMP and other hybrids of these models.

SCRATCHMAPS

SCRATCHMAPS (Spiritual Capacities and Religious Assets for Transforming Community Health by Mobilization Males for Peace and Safety) is another hybrid of the PIRHANA/CHAMP models, developed as a research study led by Professors Sandy Lazarus and Mohamed Seedat. This CBPR study was designed to answer the question, "How can mobilizing spiritual capacities and religious assets promote

SCRATCHMAPS

How can the mobilization and leveraging of spiritual capacities and religious assets promote safety and peace, particularly in relation to young men, in specific communities in South Africa and the USA?

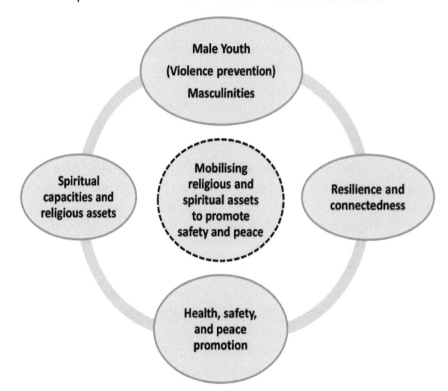

safety and peace, particularly through the promotion of positive forms of masculinity?" Based at the Violence, Injury and Peace Research Unit (South African Medical Research Council and the University of South Africa), the study compared workshop findings from Erijaville, South Africa, and Memphis, TN.

The project included the mapping of spiritual capacities and religious assets as part of creating a community-based intervention to decrease inter-personal violence among young men of color (Lazarus et al., 2014). Community members and service providers in both South African and U.S. sites identified common intangible factors that promote peace and safety. These included personal values and behavior (such as love, compassion and prayer), family relationships (such as family socialization, care, role modeling, and peer guidance or sharing from peers versus family members), and community connectedness (such as trust and leadership), all with strong implications for prevention (Cutts et al., 2016, accepted for publication).

A recently published concept paper explored the central elements in this project (Cochrane et al., 2015), including spiritual capacity, religious assets, masculinities and violence prevention, and health promotion. It also addressed the concept of Leading Causes of Life (Gunderson with Pray, 2009), including resilience and connectedness as components of health and safety promotion (see figure above, reproduced with permission, from Cochrane et al., 2015).

COMMUNITIES OF SHALOM

Another example of an explicitly faith-based model of mapping with CHNA relevance is the Communities of Shalom model (Communities of Shalom, 2015) or SHALOM ZONES. SHALOM ZONES were initiated by the General Conference of The United Methodist Church (UMC) in response to

Timeline to Implement: 2 day-long workshops (one for health seekers or community members, one for health service providers), with a minimum 90-minute follow-up meeting within 4-6 weeks post workshops. Note that SCRATCHMAPS requires a full-day "Action Planning" workshop beyond a simple report follow up.

Outputs/Product Generation and Sharing: 2 reports from workshops, enhanced and validated GIS maps and PowerPoint with summary information for follow up meeting. Reports transparently posted on website after follow up meeting, with select number of hard copies of reports produced for participants.

Staffing Required: 8 staffers per meeting (minimum of 2 facilitators, 2 scribes, 2 photographers and 2 "runners").

Training Required: Yes. IRHAP staff suggest two days of theory and preparation, then running a seeker/community members and service provider workshop and follow up meeting, as training package.

Estimated Costs: To run a set of workshops: $2,500 total ($1,500 for workshop supplies, report production and printing costs; $250 each for each workshop host site, for a total of $500; meals for participants, $500). This does not include training costs.

Suggested Frequency to Repeat/Update: Once every 3 years.

Aligned with CHNA: Yes, the qualitative data captured is an excellent supplement to hospital efforts, especially as regards community involvement in strategic planning for focus areas.

Aligned with MAPP: Yes, the qualitative data captured is an excellent supplement to MAPP efforts.

Strengths: Great community engagement strategy and springboard for future involvement of community members; excellent platform for long-term strategic work of trust repairing and trust building in communities and creating a foundation for CBPR.

Challenges: Somewhat rigid and lengthy structure that requires extensive training to conduct and a good deal of human resources to implement. The workshops entail moderate costs.

Contact Person(s): For CHAMP, CHAMP-Access to Care or CHAMP-Behavioral Health, Teresa Cutts at cutts02@gmail.com; for SCRATCHMAPS, Naiema Taliep at naiema.taliep@mrc.ac.za; CHAMP-Food Pathways, Mark Jensen at mjensen@wakehealth.edu

the civil uprisings in Los Angeles in 1992 that followed the "not-guilty" verdict for the police officers involved in the beating of Rodney King. According to their website (www.CommunitiesofShalom.org, 2015), seven local United Methodist churches (representing African American, Korean and Caucasian communities) came together to create the first "Shalom Zone" to work on systemic issues and rebuild a community devastated by racial conflict, riots, violence and social injustice. The model combines ABCD with community organizing and faith-motivated coalition building.

Shalom Zone Training entails completing seven sessions of online or onsite training in the strategies and skills of ABCD. It also includes biblical reflection on Jeremiah 29:1-12, reflecting on how ancient exiles from Jerusalem learned to "seek the shalom" of the community to which they had been sent, knowing that "if Babylon prospers, they too would prosper." Applying the biblical principles of Shalom (health, wholeness, well-being, shared prosperity) as well as mapping local assets across ethnic, cultural and religious lines of difference, it has resulted in an ecumenical network of local churches and other community-based coalitions focused on community health and a higher quality of life. Currently, there are shalom zones in over 20 Annual UMC Conferences in the USA, as well as in Haiti, Northern Ireland, Malawi and Uganda (www.CommunitiesofShalom.org, 2015).

Though Methodist in origin, Communities of Shalom work is ecumenical and inclusive of other faith traditions. It focuses on community health, immigration reform, decreasing youth violence, conflict transformation, after-school education, and economic community development as well as more traditional ministries of care for the poor (www.CommunitiesofShalom.org, 2015). Previously housed within Global Ministries of The United Methodist Church from 2008-2014, the Shalom Initiative was based at Drew University, where it was supported by the Shalom Resource and Training Center on campus. While it is still affiliated with Drew Theological School and its curriculum remains incorporated into its Doctor of Ministries program and summer internships, Communities of Shalom today offers basic and specialized training and support through its certified National Trainers and online through NorthwindInstitute.org (M. Christensen, Personal Communication, November 23, 2015; see sidebar for details).

COMMUNITIES OF SHALOM: IMPLEMENTATION DETAILS

Timeline to Implement: Minimum 7-week (42 hours) training on 7 strategies of community development, the asset mapping process, and biblical reflection on relevant texts that illustrate Shalom principles.

Outputs/Product Generation and Sharing: Platform for community development efforts; program development and implementation.

Staffing Required: Voluntary association with no paid staff.

Training Required: Yes. Online Shalom course offered through Northwind Institute, and onsite Shalom Training offered by certified regional and national trainers affiliated with Drew Theological School, http://communitiesofshalom.org/online-shalom-course.

Estimated Costs: $150 for 8-week online course and/or contracted on-site training.

Suggested Frequency to Repeat/Update: NA.

Aligned with CHNA: Yes, could be a faith-based collateral addition to CHNA process.

Aligned with MAPP: Yes, can be useful to guide phases of the MAPP process from faith-based perspective.

Strengths: On-line training is easily accessible and relatively low cost for users to train to develop their own Shalom Zone focused on sustainable community development vs. simple mapping of assets.

Challenges: Time commitment requirements and training are substantial. Program is tied to biblical mandates and ministry principles, so the Shalom approach will primarily resonate with people of religious faiths, probably primarily Christian (although interfaith in intent).

Contact Person(s): Michael Christensen, Ph.D. at shalommaster@gmail.com

Another version of mapping, often used by health systems as part of CHNA efforts, focuses on using hospital records to track patients to their homes and is termed "hot spotting." Jeffrey Brenner, MD, and his colleagues at the Camden Coalition of Healthcare Providers (Gawande, 2011) popularized hot spotting in the health system arena, where they GIS-mapped the addresses of hospital patients who were high utilizers of the emergency department, and discovered that many were clustered in a series of high-rise apartments in Camden (Gawande, 2011). Memphis Colleagues in the Congregational Health Network (CHN), a partnership between over 600 congregations and Methodist Le Bonheur Healthcare (MLH), and the business and strategic development staff of MLH took this patient hot spotting model a step further in what they titled "participatory hot spotting" (Cutts et al., 2014). Persons identified as high utilizers through the electronic medical record were engaged on the ground in target zip code 38109 through relationships among those persons, local church members and clergy, including focus groups, home visits and training programs. A place-based navigator, Joy Crawford Sharp, was also involved (her story was shared in Chapter 5), and the outreach effort saw decreases in the need for charity care services from 2010-2012 (AHRQ, 2013) among the residents of the targeted zip code.

Tools for Community Mapping

A variety of tools and databases exist to aid in community mapping efforts, some of which are described briefly below.

The most basic of mapping tools is the one that most of us use on our cell phones daily: Geographic Information Systems (GIS). Used for community mapping, GIS combines location data with both quantitative and qualitative information and allows one to visualize, analyze and report information through maps and charts (Kramer et al., 2012; Esri, 2010). This is often easier to grasp and interpret than numerical, tabular or narrative formats (Kramer et al., 2012). GIS "...are computer based systems for the integration and analysis of geographic data," but also serve as an "enabling technology" that allows other methodologies, like MAPP, to model spatial data "where people live and the environments they experience" (Cromley & McLafferty, 2002, p. 340).

Previously, highly specialized Mapping Laboratories (heavily funded at local universities) were required to create even basic maps. However, by the mid-2000s, technology had improved to the extent that such labs were no longer needed and much more nimble models of mapping assets were available through Esri and other vendors (e.g., Just Maps, GoogleMaps). Esri, founded in 1969 (http://www.esri.com/about-esri/history), was an early pioneer that helped develop GIS as the commonly used tool it is today. MapObjects, Esri's first component-based software, became its first platform for publishing maps on the Internet in 1996, and in 1997 Esri reached a milestone with the release of ArcGIS Explorer, providing GIS for everyone. The desktop settings, in which hardware, software and data are on local networks, can require significant investment in terms of finances and training staff. The company released ArcGIS Online in 2012, a cloud-based mapping system for organizations that offers collaboration tools for cataloging, visualizing, and sharing geospatial information. ArcGIS 10, now in version 10.4, also debuted at that time, enabling users to deliver any GIS resource as a web service, and putting geographic information in the hands of more people. The cloud-based GIS, although increasingly accessible, and often free, may offer less functionality in creating layered maps.

The power of GIS for participatory asset mapping lies in its ability to enable users to visualize and explore geographic (or spatial) components in combination with communities' context/interpretation of the data. Many of the participatory mapping models described above rely on GIS-generated data to augment or provide a foundation for their particular methodologies. For example, PIRHANA and CHAMP models build on existing GIS maps, which are then "validated" by participants (De Gruchy et al., PIRHANA manual, 2007).

CDC COMMUNITY HEALTH IMPROVEMENT NAVIGATOR

The Community Health Improvement (CHI) Navigator, developed by the Centers for Prevention and Disease Control (CDC), is vital for both community members and health systems, and was first made available to the public in 2015. Information on the CHI Navigator was excerpted from an interview with the CDC's Denise Koo, with her permission. The CDC developed the CHI Navigator (www.cdc.gov/CHInav/) in response to the passage of the Affordable Care Act (ACA) and its section 9007 regarding Community Health Needs Assessment for Charitable Hospitals following a request for technical assistance from the Internal Revenue Service (IRS).

CDC staff first worked with IRS to help shape the initial guidance and Final Rule, but quickly realized that resources and tools were vitally important to help translate the regulation into implementation strategies that could truly affect the health of the community. CDC then created the CHI Navigator (www.cdc.gov/chinav/) as a unifying framework and source of tools and resources to be used by hospitals, health systems, public health agencies, community organizations, and other stakeholders interested in improving the health of their communities.

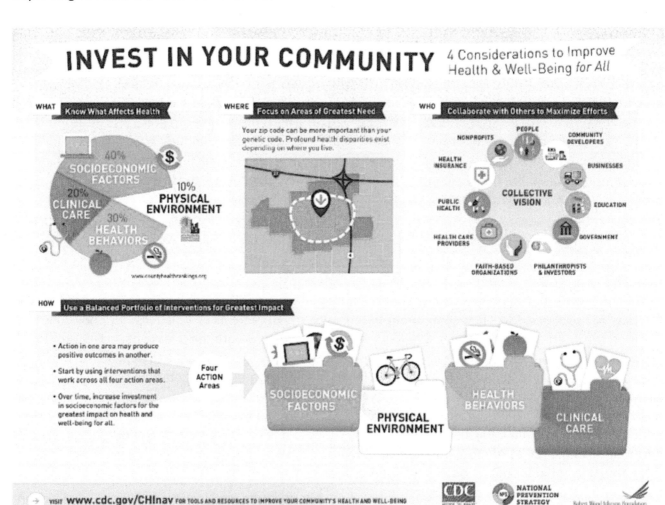

83

The CHI Navigator differs from other, similar resources in several ways. Its signature infographic (see above) provides an evocative visual tool that facilitates dialogue about what affects health, where to focus one's efforts, with whom to collaborate, and how to have the greatest impact on health. This infographic has been downloaded an average of 150 times a week since the site went live in May 2015, in addition to being an exceedingly popular handout at meetings.

The CHI Navigator provides succinct, focused examples of health systems collaborating with others outside of the health care field, but still identifies strategies that address bottom-line outcomes important to the health care system (such as decreased admissions or readmissions, decreased emergency room visits, and increased per-patient per-month cost savings). These stories show the importance of collaborative partnerships crucial to the new value-based healthcare system.

There are numerous tools in the marketplace and on the Internet, but many of them are just extremely long lists. The CHI Navigator tools section "curates" these tools. The CDC carefully reviewed hundreds of tools to find those that both conceptualized and operationalized some key concepts. The tools are also presented to the user in a community health improvement—process framework that provides some sense of what each tool offers and exactly where to go for the appropriate guidance (not only the general URL for the tool, but what section or page).

The unique CHI Navigator search engine pulls together evidence-based interventions from multiple sources for specified high volume, high impact conditions underlying the leading causes of disease and death. Many people do not know that individual-source databases exist, much less, how to comb through them for focused interventions that target their desired risk factor. CDC has done the work of identifying these sources, reviewing interventions from them and adding useful filters or tags to make it easier for users to find those that work that they might consider using with their partners (see sidebar below for more details about the Navigator tool).

CHI NAVIGATION TOOL IMPLEMENTATION DETAILS

Timeline to Implement: Only time required to review the website and use tool; estimated 1-2 hours maximum.

Outputs/Product Generation and Sharing: Free website: www.cdc.gov/CHInav. Can help health systems create their own plan, adapting resources and programs that have been used in other settings.

Staffing Required: Local staff reviews website or partnerships explore together.

Training Required: None specifically, but webinars are archived to expedite use (e.g., at www.stakeholderhealth.org and http://CommunityCatalyst.org).

Estimated Costs: Free.

Suggested Frequency to Repeat/Update: NA.

Aligned with CHNA: Yes, tool/site was developed to aid in creating more robust CHNA processes.

Aligned with MAPP: Yes, can be useful to guide phases of the MAPP process.

Strengths: Free and easily accessible for all users; aligned with ACA and IRS thinking about creating CHNAs and community benefit plans that are robust and useful. Looks at various social determinant domains beyond usual health system programming.

Challenges: Offers prototypical best practices and ROI when available for programs in other settings. May be difficult to generalize that information to other settings and apply to those settings.

Contact Person(s): Denise Koo, MD, MPH at dxk1@cdc.gov or healthpolicynews@cdc.gov

Hospitals and health systems can use the CHI Navigator's examples, framework and tools to strengthen their partnerships with public health and other partners, conduct needs assessments, and develop community health improvement plans collaboratively. They can use its database to identify evidence-based interventions for population management plans or community health implementation strategies, move their partnership from planning to action and, in the end, improve community health and well-being. The Navigator also includes quotes from the *IRS Final Rule on CHNAs for Charitable Hospitals* (2015) that underscore the connection to hospital community benefit work (although we believe that much of the CHI Navigator can be helpful for all of their work, especially as we move to a value-based healthcare system).

COMMUNITY COMMONS

Community Commons, managed by the Institute for People, Place and Possibility, the Center for Applied Research and Environmental Systems, and Community Initiatives, is a website for data, tools, and stories to inspire change and improve communities (www.communitycommons.org/about/). Run by a dedicated team from a wide variety of backgrounds, it provides public access to thousands of meaningful data layers. The data allows mapping and reporting capabilities that thoroughly explore community health, and focuses on three domains: blending the art and science of change and making meaning of the data and tools; making public data available with easy-to-use visualization tools: and, bringing deep expertise and broad experience in coaching, training and supporting local and national change efforts. Driven by Kaiser Permanente, other partners include the Robert Wood Johnson Foundation, the American Heart Association, CDC and the University of Missouri.

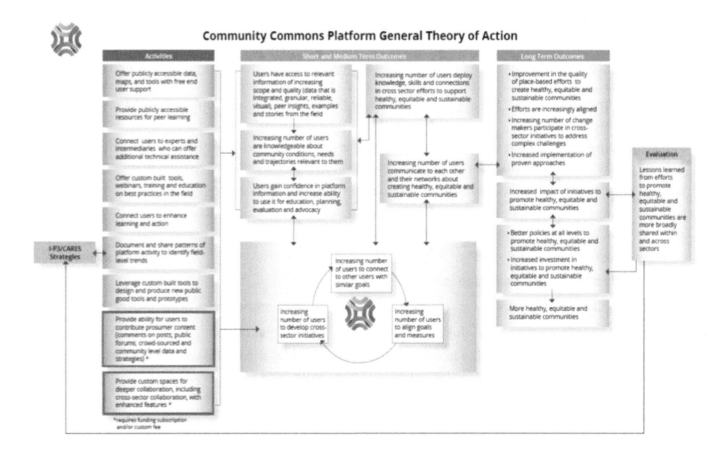

The goal of Community Commons is to increase the impact of those working toward healthy, equitable, and sustainable communities by helping users access tools to gain a deeper understanding of community assets and opportunities, and to use data visualizations to convey that knowledge through partnerships and collaboration (http://www.communitycommmons.org/about/, 2015). The Commons works best when those collaborations create and implement plans of action and return their knowledge of what works and what does not back to the greater Commons' community. The sidebar above offers a visualization of the Community Commons Platform for their general theory of action.

Users of Community Commons can build maps down to census tract level, and focus on the different "channels" of economy, education, environment, equity, food and health. Additionally, users can build a comprehensive CHNA, identify populations without health insurance, identify mortality data by certain conditions (e.g., heart disease), and construct a "vulnerable populations footprint."

COUNTY HEALTH RANKINGS & ROADMAPS WHAT WORKS FOR HEALTH (WWFH)

The County Health Ranking Roadmaps (CHR&R) has been briefly described in earlier chapters, but one of its key tools that can be used for mapping is What Works for Health (WWFH). Developed by the University of Wisconsin Population Health Institute in collaboration with the Robert Wood Johnson Foundation, WWFH is an on-line tool to help find policies, programs and systems changes that affect the factors that we know make communities healthier places to live, learn, work and play (WWFH one pager, 2016; found at https://countyhealthrankings.org/what-works-for-health). WWFH contains ratings of intervention effectiveness, literature summaries and implementation resources for over 360 policies and programs. The site can be searched by keyword (e.g., obesity) or browse by health factor (e.g., Community Safety), decision maker (e.g., Business) or evidence rating. WWFH also offers expected beneficial outcomes, key points from relevant literature, examples of toolkits and other resources to help move toward action steps and an indication of the strategy's likely impact on disparities. Lastly, WWFH not only includes policies and programs that hospitals or health systems might want to consider to help improve greater community health, but also summarizes evidence-based approaches to improving the value of clinical care.

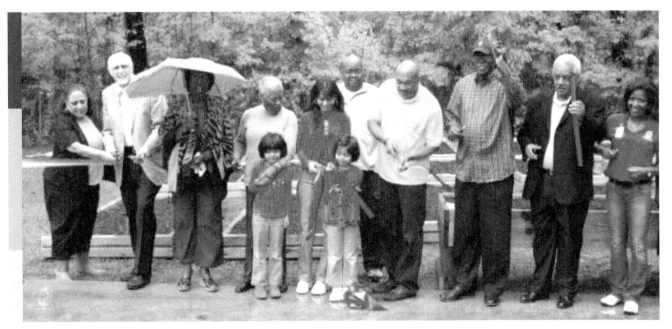

Community Members featured on RWJF County Health Rankings & Roadmaps and What Works for Health Website (used with permission from RWJF)

Key Strategies and Considerations

We now shift focus to key strategies and considerations that relate to the planning, implementation and utilization of asset mapping, particularly at the intersection between health systems and community partnerships. We begin with a series of case studies on how CHNAs can be better integrated with community asset mapping efforts to enhance health systems strategic planning and long-term work.

CHNAS, "MAPPING ASSETS" AND HEALTH SYSTEM STRATEGY

Multi-sectoral collaboration, shared outcome goals, improved health, and health equity are all aspirations, as well as "healthy communities" tools for hospitals and community partners to integrate broad community needs into hospitals' strategic planning by deeply listening to community members and incorporating that "learning" into their ongoing work. Often, these tools are not top priority for hospitals. The pressing issues of providing quality care, readmissions and overuse of Emergency Departments can spawn internal efforts to manage disease—without consideration of the factors that cause poor health and chronic conditions. Traditional projects measure the effectiveness of clinical projects but are not applicable to evaluating investments in population health, social determinants and community health improvement.

The ACA requirement for broad CHNAs gives hospitals the keys to the healthy communities "tool box" and a path to broad, strategic thinking around health improvement. Carefully conducted CHNAs look at disease and mortality rates, but also identify the "determinants" of health in communities, especially those with high rates of disease (CDC, 2013). But these same assessments can also map or make visible the assets often not seen by health systems that are key building blocks in strengthening community health. In this sense, the terminology of "needs" assessment falls short for, as we have stressed in the models discussed above, "assets" (especially those held by communities themselves, whether latent or actively utilized) are as important if not more important than needs. An asset focus can better and more sustainably empower community members and instill hope.

A dynamic example of building on the CHNA can be seen in Adventist Florida Hospital's work with the Bithlo community in Florida (reported initially in the HSLG Monograph, 2013, p. 30). Florida Hospital in Orlando, part of the 44-hospital Adventist Health System in 10 states, is also part of a broad coalition called the Bithlo Transformation Effort. Bithlo is a semi-rural community of 8,200 residents just miles from Orlando, the "Happiest Place on Earth." After 80 years of generational poverty, Bithlo residents still endure high unemployment, substandard housing, minimal public transportation, and high illiteracy rates. Drinking water (from shallow wells) is tainted by rust and carcinogens from an eight-acre illegal landfill, sixteen junkyards and an old gasoline leak.

Not surprisingly, Bithlo has high rates of diabetes, heart disease, asthma, low birth weight babies, and depression. Many residents appear "non-compliant" with diet, medication adherence, exercise, and so on, but the reality is that health and health care are people's least concerns. Their issues revolve around basic needs: food, clothing and shelter, and they often lack access to venues that make healthy choices easier to make.

A small 501c3 called United Global Outreach (UGO) began work in Bithlo in 2010. Residents, through a participatory mapping process, had identified education, housing, transportation, the environment, health care, basic needs and sense of community as their most urgent challenges. Florida Hospital joined the Transformation Effort in 2010.

"Hospitals typically focus on health care and are used to leading community projects," said Lars Houmann, Florida Hospital CEO. "This commitment is different. Health care will not be our primary focus," he continued. "Instead of health care only, we will join with UGO and other community partners to address the deeper issues identified by Bithlo residents," (L. Houmann, Personal Communication, April 26, 2016).

With support from Florida Hospital and other partners, Bithlo now has a town center with a private school, public transportation, library, GED program, and a community garden. A community health center and other partners offer primary care, mental health, dental and vision services. There is a plan for environmental cleanup and clean water. The hospital contributed some dollars but more importantly, engaged its community, business, education and faith partners in the Transformation Effort.

The Bithlo Transformation Effort is an example of a hospital moving outside of its walls to address social health determinants. There is recognition that good health is based on a complex interaction of factors that contribute to hospital utilization, improved outcomes and improved conditions in the broader community. CHNAs challenge all hospitals to recognize that good health is not as simple as diabetes education or blood pressure checks. Rather, health foci must be strategically driven by data, needs and assets, and contextualizing the lives of those served in our respective communities.

Similarly, Advocate Health Care used the CHAMP model with BroMenn Medical Center in Bloomington/ Normal, IL, to bring together their congregational network, faith leaders and service providers to identify how faith communities are contributing to the health and well-being of people in the community. Across four workshops with community members, faith leaders, congregation members and service providers, the common theme was a desire for strong, diverse, connected communities. All participants thought that one of the main ways that faith-based entities could help foster health and wellness was by leading efforts to build community among residents. Health seekers wanted to know each other better and wanted communities to be safe and welcoming for all people, while providers wanted to come together more regularly to connect and network. This information will be incorporated into Advocate's regional Community Health Needs Assessment and help inform the implementation planning process.

Other examples include Tacoma, WA, where two competing health systems (Multi-Care Health Systems and Catholic Health Initiatives [CHI] Franciscan Health) have joined together to work on achieving health equity in Pierce County. Led by the Northwest Leadership Foundation and their Leaders in Women's Health community network, some of whom are African-American and Hispanic breast cancer survivors, this group is undertaking CHAMP Access to Care in 2015-16 to supplement the critical health equity work already being done by the Tacoma Pierce County Health Department and their Community Health Improvement Program (CHIP). The group will focus on three of the most vulnerable Pierce County neighborhoods, which coincide with the areas the health department identified through key hotspot mapping foci on health and other disparities.

NON-INSTRUMENTAL COMMUNITY ENGAGEMENT

Besides being a critical part of ongoing CHNA assessments, community asset mapping can be seen as a specific form of community engagement (Kramer et al., 2012). However, with the push to make CHNAs more relevant (via the federal mandate mentioned earlier), hospital leadership may fall into the trap of using both CHNAs and other mapping efforts as a means to "check the box" on their community engagement strategies or delivery of community benefits. Such leaders, who focus on harvesting and "using" community intelligence without a commitment to building genuine and trustworthy partnerships, can damage fledgling collaborative efforts.

This is the reason why our colleagues in the ARHAP/IRHAP group stress that its PIRHANA and CHAMP methods should not be used instrumentally or as an end unto itself (Cochrane & Gunderson, 2012). Instead, community asset mapping must be viewed as a first step or "springboard" to engage community partnerships that integrate both hospital and community assets. Hospital leaders must see that community members are agents capable of shaping their own contexts with the use of appropriate and available resources (De Gruchy et al., 2007; Kramer et al., 2012).

Indeed, as we will share later in this chapter and in Chapter 8 (outlining the financial impact), we see community asset mapping as a critical first step to building viable and sustainable health systems and community partnerships that have demonstrated true impact in improving disparity, healthcare utilization and finances. In addition, finding synergies between community asset mapping efforts and internal "mapping" of health system data and indicators provides a very rich data set that can be leveraged strategically to inform program development, plan initiatives, allocate resources and evaluate progress.

ADDRESSING HISTORICAL TRAUMA

In addition to becoming an integral aspect of health system CHNAs, strategic planning and implementation efforts, community asset mapping is also useful in exploring historical trauma through truth telling, reconciliation and community healing, and trust building. This is especially apparent where fractured relationships among marginalized communities, health systems or other power brokers negatively affect services and delivery.

"Historical trauma" is a term first used by Brave Heart and DeBruyn (1998). It draws on the literature of Jewish holocaust survivors (Brown-Rice, 2014) and links the current problems facing the Native American people (among others) to the "legacy of chronic trauma and unresolved grief across generations" enacted on them by the European-dominant culture (Brave Heart & DeBruyn, 1998, p. 60). Historical trauma, transferred to subsequent generations through biological, psychological, environmental and social means, is thought to result in cross-generational cycles of trauma (Sotero, 2006).

Historical trauma is present in virtually all communities (Mohatt, Thompson, Thai & Tebes, 2014), and is also particularly relevant to the understanding of community health disparities in minority populations, which are often made visible in CHNAs. Health systems, sadly, have sometimes been anchor institutions either complicit with or actively engaging in those traumatic events (CDC, 2013). In Memphis, for example, mapping exercises unearthed a widespread distrust of the hospital system, particularly among older members of the African-American community who held the belief that "a hospital is where you go to die," (Personal Observation, Teresa Cutts, 2013). In Forsyth County, North Carolina, the academic health system's history included running a decades-long eugenics program until 1973, through which both poor whites and blacks were involuntarily sterilized (Begos, Deaver, Railey & Sexton, 2012). Marginalized communities' long memories of such medical injustices rendered the academic medical hospital worthy of distrust, a place where persons are "experimented upon," to be used only as a last resort. Such distrust is dislodged only by new, credible and trustworthy actions.

Historical trauma can also extend beyond hospitals to supposedly trusted agents in the community. In Chicago, mapping efforts in two low-income African American communities (in July 2011) unveiled a strong dynamic of mistrust, collective grief and disappointment in institutions that were meant to serve the community. The church was also a source of mistrust; participants noted that even clergy could be agents of abuse as well as complicit with power and political systems. The CHAMP process opened a powerful space for people to name and reflect on their experiences, and engage in a social analysis of their context. This experience led organizers to adapt the workshops to include ritual space to acknowledge wounds as well as to name those things that are whole and good in the community.

While the CHAMP process has helped make visible these past injustices and sets the stage for a dialogue to rebuild trust, we recognize that holding a few workshops will not repair decades of historical trauma and unjust actions. Nonetheless, asset-mapping workshops can signal that this is a "new day" in which the health system (and other community support services) begin to own their past unjust acts and make efforts to reconcile with the community. Often these efforts coincide with long overdue state restitution programs, such as that related to eugenics in North Carolina (Mennel, 2014). Stakeholder Health believes that speaking truth to power, while acknowledging past injustices and authentically attempting to rebuild trust between health systems and communities, is essential for both health and equity in general (Health System Learning Group, 2013). This has been particularly evident where community members have had direct access to, and engaged in dialogue with, local health system providers in a more active and mutually accountable fashion.

BUILDING MUTUAL ACCOUNTABILITY BETWEEN HEALTH SYSTEMS AND COMMUNITY MEMBERS

Mutual accountability between health systems and communities has been most evident in sites where the mapping process led to internal health system policy changes, as well as energizing and mobilizing community members as active participants in self-management of chronic diseases, in addressing neighborhood problems, and in improving the educational and workforce status. Additionally, mapping efforts in some instances have resulted in improved healthcare utilization or community indicators. In Memphis, for example, based on the education that health seekers identified as needed, the Congregational Health Network (CHN) developed 14 training programs (Care at the End of Life, Mental Health First Aid, Navigating the Healthcare System, Hospital Visitation, Cancer, Medicine and Miracles, Chronic Diseases You Can Live With, etc.) offered over 7 weeks; over 4,000 persons have taken the programs. These events have helped empower congregational and community members both to care for their own and their peers' health more actively and to begin to build trust with providers (Cutts, 2011).

These trainings, coupled with the work of Paula Jacobs and her team at Methodist North Hospital (MLH), also resulted in a decrease in disparity in sudden cardiac death in African Americans in Memphis (Cutts, Jacobs & Bounds, 2013). As part of the Aligning Forces for Quality (AF4Q) work on race and ethnic disparity, Paula's team was charged with establishing an ideal clinical practice for cardiac disease. Although the hospital achieved this goal in treating Congestive Heart Failure (96%) and Acute Myocardial Infarction (100%)—rates which were the highest of 8 sites—the work also unearthed the fact that African-Americans were dying at twice the rate of Whites in its Emergency Department. CHN leaders then engaged the CHN Liaison Advisory Council (a self-organizing group of women who serve as "gatekeepers" of CHN's interaction with researchers and other community agents and organizations) and CHN members to tap into community wisdom about why these death rates were so high.

Findings from the CHN members were then used to improve both community and medical staff education, led to simplification of discharge materials for cardiac patients, and to co-branding and teaching of those modules in CHN Chronic Disease sessions. These combined efforts helped MLH decrease its disparity in sudden cardiac death among African-American persons at its Methodist North hospital by 16 % between 2010 to 2012 (Cutts, Jacobs & Bounds, 2013). Additionally, CHN and community members have begun their own efforts to create community gardens, reclaim and take over ownership of blighted properties, and work as a group to apply for state level funding to maintain these properties. These examples have taught health system leaders and staff the value of community members in activating and engaging partners in improving their individual and community-level health.

CREATING A FOUNDATION FOR COMMUNITY-BASED OR ENGAGED RESEARCH

Community asset mapping also creates a foundational platform for Community Based Participatory Research or CBPR (Wallerstein & Duran, 2006). CBPR, in its best iteration, can build trust, focus on long-term and sustainable partnerships and help design, implement and conduct research, with equal voices in terms of determining shared risks, benefits and allocation of resources across communities, academics and health systems (Sandy & Holland, 2006). Lessons about how best to conduct and implement CBPR with cultural sensitivity and strong ethical standards (Burhansstipanov & Schumacher, 2005) can make asset mapping a potent investment in long-term, authentic health system and community partnerships.

An example of such efforts comes from Dr. Stacy Tessler Lindau and her team from South Side Health and Vitality Studies at the University of Chicago, (http://uhi-dev.uchicago.edu/what-are-south-side-health-and-vitality-studies). This group has developed the innovative "Community Rx" program that connects patients in doctors' offices and clinics with community health resources in Chicago's South Side in order to help patients stay healthy, live independently and manage disease, while supporting local businesses and organizations. Funded by a 2012 Centers for Medicare & Medicaid Health Innovation Award, their system processes patient data and prints out a "Health-eRx" for patients, including a customized map and list of health and social resources in their community. The initiative includes MAPS Corps (Meaningful Active Productive Science in Service to Communities), the engine that powers Health-eRx, by training and employing local high school students to map a community's health assets (Lindau, 2014). The South Side Health and Vitality Studies, in partnership with Chicago Health Information Technology Regional Extension Center (CHITREC) and the Alliance of Chicago Community Health Services, developed the MAPS Corps system through which data is captured via smart phones with web-enabled applications called "MapApp" (http://healtherx.org/mapscorps/about-mapscorps).

Every summer, local youth go out on foot in the neighborhood to identify and update existing (and often inert and outdated) community resources data. MAPS Corps student researchers continuously update this electronic database of community health resources, which is shared publicly and linked to the electronic health record database of local safety net providers. This partnership, leveraging healthy local resource "prescriptions" for primary care patients and a mapping program run by student researchers, uniquely builds relationships and trust, refreshes resource listings, and engages local youth to validate the information on the resource maps that Dr. Lindau's team uses in primary care settings (Lindau, 2014). This partnership model, which nurtures trust, creates the foundation for a pipeline for a future workforce and aids the career development of youth of color embedded in this community.

DATA GATHERING, USE AND SHARING ACROSS STAKEHOLDERS

Another unique example illustrating how data and community asset mapping methodologies can be used to integrate data sets across public and community health initiatives and health systems, while also engaging community members, is seen in the work of King and others (2016, submitted for publication). King and his team have developed a Community Health Record Project in Shelby County, TN, supported by the CDC's Division for Heart Disease and Stroke Prevention. This work builds upon the electronic health record (EHR) in hospitals, the personal health record (PHR), and the University of Wisconsin-Madison Population Health Institute's Mobilizing Action Toward Community Health (MATCH) county level tools, standardized information and measures, and guidance for improving population health. While the MATCH system (Kindig, et al., 2010) web-based County Health Rankings tool integrates a broad array of health information for end-users to characterize a county's health and make comparisons over time to others and the nation, there is a missing piece.

The Community Health Record (CHR) (King et al., 2016, submitted for publication) aims to provide relevant and timely information to help end-users with health-related decision-making. The principal difference between the CHR and other systems is that it proposes to integrate and presents standardized multi-stakeholder information at community levels ranging from the address to census block, census track, neighborhood and/or zip codes. Moreover, the CHR is communally owned and therefore requires a significant social component to initiate and sustain collaboration and information exchange among stakeholders. The goal is to inform, target, monitor and evaluate a portfolio of community health interventions, recognizing that these issues can be simultaneously addressed across the spectrum of health by multiple groups. Collectively, these efforts provide a foundation for health care, public health and community partners to better understand and manage the health of their population.

The CHR Framework (illustrated here) is a multi-tiered, multi-stakeholder model to facilitate CHR development. It describes an iterative and participatory process for achieving collaboration and information exchange between healthcare, public health and community organizations. Identifying key concepts and a technical infrastructure to facilitate CHR development, its aims are to: 1) enable meaningful collaboration, 2) facilitate a shared approach, 3) build workforce and infrastructure capacity, and 4) establish a new way of doing business that enables the transformation of community health data into information and information into knowledge to aid decision makers in collectively improving population health. Although still in its early development phase in Shelby County, TN, the

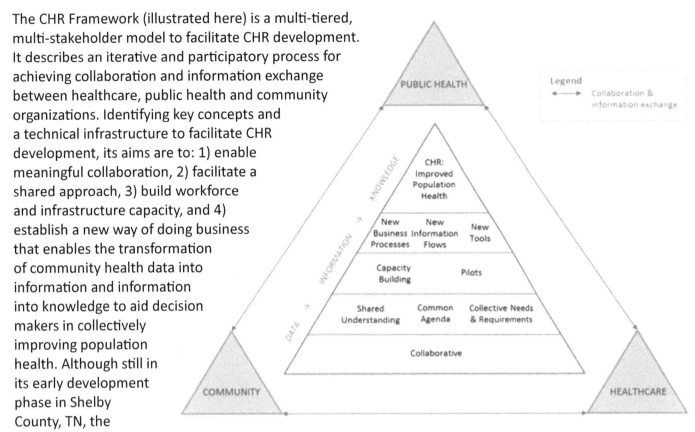

CHR model has great potential to make data more useful to a variety of stakeholders in ways that can truly transform community health.

MAKING GRASSROOTS VOICES HEARD BY POLICY MAKERS

Lastly, community asset mapping also makes grassroots "voices" audible to those who influence health policy. The 2014 Forsyth County mapping of Hispanic seekers and providers described earlier in this chapter (Cutts et al., 2016) generated information that highlighted the need for, and expediting the development of, a healthcare identification card for undocumented persons, so that they could legally obtain necessary prescription medications. These mapping findings were critical in engaging local governmental officials and in enlisting two competing health systems in providing health ID cards to undocumented Hispanics. The first FaithAction ID drive, held in Forsyth County on Jan. 8, 2016, attracted 580 undocumented persons seeking a picture ID. It was supported by both local health systems, city police and sheriff department staff, as well as a nearby coalition that produced the ID cards; unprecedented trustworthiness was demonstrated by those participants. Keeping elected officials invested in providing this form of justice in healthcare for undocumented people is especially critical in North Carolina, where an anti-immigrant focus has grown in the past several years (White & Gill, 2015).

Reports from those mapping workshops have also been incorporated into several other vital initiatives, such as the Latino Migration's Project of Building Integrated Communities, which is designed to better integrate immigrants into local North Carolina communities (White & Gill, 2015).

Summary

Stakeholder Health strongly promotes the use of the community asset-mapping models shared in this chapter (or some hybrid of them). The models are strong vehicles for building and strengthening a system of health outside hospital walls, even as they are integrated with CHNAs as part of health system strategic planning. Further, such mapping also aids in fostering mutually accountable partnerships, dealing with historical trauma, building trust and promoting equity and justice in health and healthcare, and in general.

We deeply suspect that those health systems that can intentionally de-center their own power base in the community, as well as actively listen and partner with community members, will in the future be the most successful in their efforts to improve healthcare upstream and reduce their charity care margins. Implementing such mapping efforts can result in positive social return on investment for systems that care for vulnerable populations but need to view their own landscape with fresh eyes. This process can instill hope for overall health improvement and social justice-focused change via truly transformative partnerships.

REFERENCES

Agency for Healthcare Research and Quality. (2012). Service Delivery Innovation Profile: Church-Health System Partnership Facilitates Transitions from Hospital to Home for Urban, Low-Income African Americans, Reducing Mortality, Utilization, and Costs. Retrieved from https://innovations.ahrq.gov/profiles/church- health-system-partnership-facilitates-transitions-hospital-home-urban-low-income.

Begos, K., Deaver, D., Railey, J., & Sexton, S. (2012). *Against their will: North Carolina's sterilization program*. Apalachicola, FL: Gray Oak Books.

Blevins, J., Thurman, S., Kiser, M. & Beres, L. (2012). Community Health Assets Mapping: A Mixed Methods Approach in Nairobi. In *Mapping, Cost, and Reach to the Poor of Faith-Inspired Health Care Providers in Sub-Saharan Africa: Strengthening the Evidence for Faith-inspired Health Engagement in Africa*, Volume 3, The World Bank: Washington, D.C.

Brave Heart, M. Y. H., & DeBruyn, L. M. (1998). The American Indian Holocaust: Healing Historical Unresolved Grief. *American Indian and Alaska Native Mental Health Research*, 8(2): 60–82.

Brown-Rice, K. (2014). Examining the Theory of Historical Trauma Among Native Americans. *The Professional Counselor*, Oct. Retrieved from http://tpcjournal.nbcc.org/examining-the-theory-of-historical-trauma-among-native-americans/

Burhansstipanov, L., Christopher, S., & Schumacher, S. A. (2005). Lessons Learned From Community-Based Participatory Research in Indian Country. *Cancer Control: Journal of the Moffitt Cancer Center*, 12(Suppl 2): 70–76.

Bushe, G.R. (2011) Appreciative inquiry: Theory and critique. In Boje, D., Burnes, B. and Hassard, J. (eds.) *The Routledge Companion To Organizational Change* (pp. 87¬103). Oxford, UK: Routledge.

Chambers, Robert. (1980). Rapid rural appraisal: Rationale and repertoire. *IDS Discussion Paper, No. 155* Brighton: IDS, University of Sussex.

Cochrane J.R. & Gunderson, G. (2012). *Mobilising religious health assets for transformation*. The Barefoot Collective. Retrieved from http://www.barefootguide.org/barefoot-guide-3.html.

Cochrane, J. R., Seedat, M., Lazarus, S., Suffla, S., Taliep, N., & Shochet, I. (2015). *Conceptualizing religious assets, spiritual capacity, masculinity and violence in the context of peace and safety*. Position Paper. University of Cape Town, International Religious Health Assets Programme; Medical Research Council-University of South Africa Violence, Injury and Peace Research Unit; Hearts of Men Cape Town.

Cooperrider, D.L. & Srivastva, S. (1987) Appreciative inquiry in organizational life. In Woodman, R. W. & Pasmore, W.A. (eds) *Research In Organizational Change And Development, Vol. 1*: 129- 169. Stamford, CT: JAI Press.

County Health Rankings & Roadmaps. (2016). State Health Gaps. Retrieved April 5, 2016, from https://countyhealthrankings.org/what-works-for-health).

Cromley, E.K. and McLafferty, S. (2002). *GIS and Public Health*. USA: The Guilford Press.

Cutts, T. (2011). The Memphis Congregational Health Network Model: Grounding ARHAP Theory. In: *When Religion and Health Align: Mobilizing Religious Health Assets for Transformation*. Pietermaritzburg: Cluster Publications: 193-209.

Cutts, T., Jacobs, P. & Bounds, C. (2013). Improving Cardiovascular Disparity through Community-Based Partnerships: The Memphis ModeL: Methodist North Hospital and Congregational Health Network (CHN) Case Study. Presented as invited workshop at the Rhodes Disparity Conference, March 7, Memphis, TN.

Cutts, T.F., Rafalski, E., Grant, C., Marinescu, R. (2014). Utilization of Hot Spotting to Identify Community Needs and Coordinate Care for High-Cost Patients in Memphis, TN. *J of Geographic Information Systems*, 6: 23-29. Retrieved from http://www.scirp.org/journal/jgishttp://dx.doi.org/10.4236/jgis.2014.61003.

Cutts T. & Peachey K. (2014). "Community Health Asset Mapping: Building Sustainable Networks of Community Health Partners." Forum presented on behalf of Stakeholder Health, Feb. 5, 2014.

Cutts, T. & Jensen, M. (2015). *Community Health Assets Mapping Partnership-Food Pathways: Forsyth County*. A follow-up presentation made to food seekers and providers, July 30; Winston Salem, NC, Wentz Memorial United Congregational Church.

Cutts T., Langdon S., Rivers Meza F., Hochwalt B., Pichardo-Geisinger R., Sowell B., Chapman J., Batiz Dorton L., Kennett B. & Jones M.T. (2016). Community Health Asset Mapping Partnership Engages Hispanic/Latino Health Seekers and Providers. *North Carolina Medical Journal*, May/June, 77(3),160-167.

Cutts, T., Olivier, J., Lazarus, S., Taliep, N., Cochrane, J., Seedat, M., van Rennan, R. Hendricks, C. & Carlese, H. (2016). Community Asset Mapping for Violence Prevention: A Comparison of Views in Western Cape, South Africa and Memphis, USA. Accepted for publication in the *African Journal of Safety Promotion*.

De Gruchy, S., Matimelo, S., Jones, D., Molapo, S., Olivier, J., Germond, P., Thomas, L. (2007). *PIRHANA: Participatory inquiry into religious health assets, networks and agency for health seekers and health providers*. Practitioner's workbook, version 6. South Africa: PIRHANA.

De Gruchy, S., Cochrane, J. R., Olivier, J., & Matimelo, S. (2011). Participatory inquiry on the interface between religion and health: What does it achieve and what not? In J. R.Cochrane, B. Schmid, & T. Cutts (Eds.), *When religion and health align: Mobilising religious health assets for transformation* (pp. 43–61). Pietermaritzburg, South Africa: Cluster.

Esri. (2010). *GIS for asset and facilities management. Efficient management of assets, interior space, and the building life*. Redlands, CA: Author.

Esri website. (2015). Retrieved http://www.esri.com/about-esri/history.

Freire, P. and Shor, I. (1987). *Pedagogy for liberation*, New York: Bergin and Garvey.

Gawande, A. (2011). The hot spotters: can we lower medical costs by giving the neediest patients better care? *New Yorker*. Jan: 40-51.

Gunderson, G.R. with Pray, L. (2009). *Leading Causes of Life: Five Fundamentals to Change the Way You Live Your Life*. Nashville: Abingdon Press.

Gunderson, G. R. & Cochrane, J. R. (2012). *Religion and the health of the public: shifting the paradigm*. New York: Palgrave MacMillan.

HealtheRx website. (2015). Retrieved from http://healtherx.org/.

Health System Learning Group (HSLG) (2013). *Strategic Investment in Shared Outcomes: Transformative Partnerships between Health Systems and Communities*, April 4, Washington, DC.

Internal Revenue Service. (2015). IRS Final Rule on CHNAs for Charitable Hospitals. Retrieved from https://www.irs.gov/Charities-&-Non-Profits/Charitable-Organizations/New-Requirements-for-501(c)(3)-Hospitals-Under-the-Affordable-Care-Act.

Journal of Public Health Management and Practice. (2005). Entire journal focus on MAPP, September/October.

Kerka, S. (2003). Community asset mapping. *Trends and Issues Alert*, (47). ERIC Clearinghouse on Adult, Career, and Vocational Education, Columbus, OH.

Kindig DA, Booske BC, Remington PL. (2010). Mobilizing Action Toward Community Health (MATCH): metrics, incentives, and partnerships for population health. *Preventing chronic disease*. 7(4):A68. PubMed PMID: 20550826; PubMed Central PMCID: PMCPMC2901566.

King RJ, Garrett, N, Kriseman, J, Crum, M, Rafalski, EM, Sweat, D, Frazier, R, Schearer & Cutts, T. (2016). A Community Health Record: Improving Health Through Multisector Collaboration, Information Sharing, and Technology. Manuscript submitted for publication.

Kramer, S., Amos, T., Lazarus, S., & Seedat, M. (2012). The philosophical assumptions, utility and challenges of asset mapping approaches to community engagement. *Journal of Psychology in Africa*, 22(4), 537-546.

Kretzman J.P. & McKnight, J.L. (1993). *Building Communities from the inside out: A Path Toward Finding and Mobilizing a Community's Assets*. Evanston, IL: Institute for Policy Research, pp. 1-11.

Lazarus, S., Naidoo, AV, May, B., Williams, LL, Demas, G., & Filander, FJ. (2014). Lessons learnt from a Community-Based Participatory Research Project in a South African rural context. *South African Journal of Psychology*, 44(2): 147-159.

Lindau, S. (2014). Community Rx: Connecting Health Care to Self-Care. An invited presentation to the Stakeholder Health Forum Series, September, http://stakeholderhealth.org/events/.

Mathie, A., & Kearney, J. (2001). Past, present and future: Educating for social and economic change at the Coady International Institute (Occasional Paper Series, No. 1). Antigonish, Nova Scotia: St. Francis Xavier University, Coady International Institute.

Mathie, A., & Cunningham, G. (2008). *Mobilizing assets for community-driven development. Participant manual*. Antigonish, Nova Scotia: St. Francis Xavier University, Coady International Institute.

MapsCorps website. (2015). http://healtherx.org/mapscorps/about-mapscorps.

Mennel, E. (2014). Payments Start for N.C. Eugenics Victims, But Many Won't Qualify. National Public Radio, Oct. 31, 2015 broadcast. Retrieved from http://www.npr.org/sections/healthshots/2014/10/31/360355784/.

Mohatt, N. V., Thompson, A. B., Thai, N. D., & Tebes, J. K. (2014). Historical trauma as public narrative: A conceptual review of how history impacts present-day health. *Social Science & Medicine (1982)*, 106, 128–136. http://doi.org/10.1016/j.socscimed.2014.01.043

National Association of City and County Health Organizations (NACHO) (2015). Mobilizing for Action through Planning and Partnerships: Achieving Healthier Communities through MAPP, A User's Handbook. Retrieved from http://www.naccho.org/topics/infrastructure/mapp/upload/mapp_handbook_fnl.pdf.

Pullen, N. C., Upshaw, V. M., Lesneski, C. D., & Terrell, A. (2005). Lessons from the MAPP demonstration sites. *Journal of Public Health Management and Practice*, 11(5): 453-459.

Rossing, B. (2000). *Identifying, mapping and mobilizing our assets*. University of Wisconsin–Madison, School of Human Ecology, Madison, WI.

Sandy, M. & Holland, B. (2006). Different worlds and Common Ground: Community Partner Perspectives on Campus-Community Partnerships. *Michigan Journal of Community Service Learning,* Fall, 13(1): 30-43.

Sotero, M. M. (2006). A conceptual model of historical trauma: implications for public health practice and research. *Journal of Health Disparities Research and Practice*, 1(1): 93–108.

Southside Health and Vitality Studies (2016). Retrieved from http://uhi-dev.uchicago.edu/what-are-south-side-health-and-vitality-studies.

United Methodist Church Global Mission: Communities of Shalom. (2015). Retrieved from http://www.umcmission.org/Give-to-Mission/Search-for-Projects/Projects/742566.

U.S. Centers for Disease Control and Prevention. (2013). *Community Health Assessment for Population Health Improvement: Resource of Most Frequently Recommended Health Outcomes and Determinants*, Atlanta, GA: Office of Surveillance, Epidemiology, and Laboratory Services.

U.S. Centers for Disease Control and Prevention. (2016). U.S. Public Health Service Syphylis Study at Tuskegee. Retrieved from http://www.cdc.gov/tuskegee/timeline.htm.

Wallerstein, N. B., & Duran, B. (2006). Using community-based participatory research to address health disparities. *Health Promotion Practice*, 7(3), 312-323.manual. Antigonish, Nova Scotia: St. Francis Xavier University, Coady International Institute.

White, J. & Gill, H. (2015). Building Integrated Communities in Winston Salem and Forsyth County, North Carolina: Demographics and Perspectives of Foreign-Born Residents. The Latino Migration Project, University of North Carolina at Chapel Hill.

ACKNOWLEDGMENTS

We wish to acknowledge Denise Koo, MD, MPH of the CDC for allowing her interview material to be included in the chapter. Additionally, we thank Michael Christensen, PhD at Drew University and Robert J. Duncan, Jr. of the Northwind Institute for their editing assistance in the section on Communities of Shalom. Likewise, we thank John Moenster and Roxanne Medina-Fulcher of Institute for People, Place and Possibility (I-P3) for reviewing and "blessing" our accuracy in describing the Community Commons model.

FULL AUTHORSHIP LISTING

Teresa Cutts, PhD, Asst. Research Professor, Wake Forest School of Medicine, Div. of Public Health Science, Dept. of Social Sciences and Health Policy, Winston Salem, NC

Ray King, PhD, MSc, Epidemiologist/Health Scientist (Informatics), Div. of Heart Disease and Stroke Prevention, Centers for Disease Control and Prevention, Atlanta, GA

Maureen Kersmarki, BA, Director, Community Benefit & Public Policy, Adventist Health System, Orlando, FL

Kirsten Peachey, MDiv, MSW, DMin, Director, Congregational Health Partnerships and Co-Director, The Center for Faith and Community Health Transformation, Advocate Health Care, Chicago, IL

Jason Hodges, PhD, Clinical Research Associate, III, Dept. of Hematology, St. Jude Children's Research Hospital, Memphis, TN

Sherrianne Kramer, PhD, Research Psychologist/Psychology Lecturer, School of Human and Community Development, University of Witwatersrand

Sandy Lazarus, PhD, Professor, University of South Africa, Medical Research Council

For more information about this chapter, contact **Teresa Cutts** at e-mail, cutts02@gmail.com or phone, (901) 643-8104.

CHAPTER 7

Integrating Care to Improve Health Outcomes: Trauma, Resilience and Mental Health

Kirsten Peachey and Teresa Cutts, with Margo DeMont, Dory Lawrence, Bryan Hatcher, Jane Berz and Lance Laurence

Researchers have consistently concluded that the factors that have the greatest impact on health arise from the environments in which we live and function in our everyday lives (see also Chapter 2 on the social determinants of health). A seminal study by McGinnis and Foege in 1993 indicated that human behaviors and interactions and the social and physical environment account for 60% of what determines health. By comparison, access to medical care only accounts for 10-15% of what contributes to the risk of premature death. Genetic pre-determination plays an important role (25-30%), but environmental factors (e.g. food consumption, toxin exposure, chronic stress) also produce epigenetic effects that

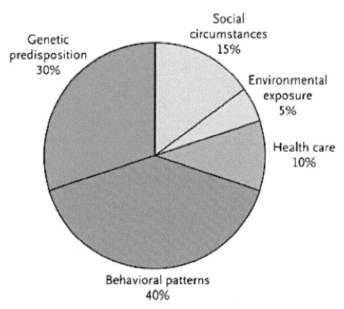

(McGinnis and Foege, 1993.)

impact health (McGinnis & Foege, 1993). In 2004, these insights were further supported by Mokdad and colleagues, who found that tobacco use, poor diet, physical inactivity, environmental factors and other health behaviors such as substance abuse continued to drive the actual causes of death for United States residents (Mokdad, Marks, Stroup, Gerberding, 2004).

Paradoxically, approximately 95% of the trillion dollars spent on health as a nation goes to medical care, with just 5% on health promotion (McGinnis & Foege, 1993; McGinnis, Williams-Ruso & Knickman, 2002). Health care systems which are built around the medical model often expend vast resources to maintain patients in their last months of life, but invest relatively little in supporting the kind of social and physical environments that would allow people in all communities to thrive and be healthy throughout their lives.

The science around how social conditions impact our bodies is rapidly developing, particularly related to the genetic and cellular implications of trauma and stress on physical and mental health, but also on possibilities for resilience and healing. Social determinants may have been dismissed in the past as soft or superfluous to the core practices of medicine, but health care systems are quickly learning to understand and engage the patient in their whole context if they are going to meet federal requirements around health outcomes and achieve the cost savings that are necessary for the survival of its organizations.

This chapter explores trauma, stress and community strength as particular factors in the social determinants of health. We start by expanding our understanding of the dynamics of trauma for individuals and at community scale. What do we mean by trauma? How does it actually affect our bodies and minds? How is resilience fostered to facilitate coping and healing? We look at the health implications and health care costs associated with unaddressed stressful childhood and community experiences, particularly around mental health, and highlight practical strategies that are being used effectively around the country to promote resilience and reduce health care costs. Finally, we focus on promising practices of integrated care that bring together what has been falsely separated—the connection between the health of our physical bodies, our mental condition, and our spiritual life at individual and community levels—what we call broadening the view of integrated health.

Defining Terms: Trauma, Resilience and Health

The social determinants of health are a broad field, but one area where headway is being made in deepening our understanding about how social conditions impact health is in the field of trauma and resilience. For decades, researchers have been able to link traumatic experience to poor health outcomes. Many studies support the role of protective factors such as positive adult-child interactions, meaningful social relationships and concrete support in times of need in mediating the effects of trauma. Public health and social scientists are zeroing in on these issues to learn more about the actual processes by which experiences we have in our social context get translated into our bodies at the cellular level.

We will explore the health and cost implications of trauma in more depth later, but first we want to define what we mean by trauma (individual, communal, and historical) and resilience. We also want to say from the outset that separating these two experiences is a false construct. In every experience of trauma, resilience is also in play. People do not have discrete experiences of trauma that are somehow devoid of efficacy, hope and strength to persevere.

INDIVIDUAL TRAUMA

Individual trauma results from an event, series of events, or set of circumstances experienced by an individual as physically or emotionally harmful or threatening and that has lasting adverse effects on

Table 1. Adverse Childhood Events and Percent Respondents Answering Positively

TYPE OF EXPERIENCE	DESCRIPTORS	PERCENT RESPONDENTS ANSWERING POSITIVELY
Abuse	Physical-Beating, Not Spanking	28%
	Physical Contact Sexual Abuse	22% Overall (28% Women, 16% Men)
	Emotional-Recurrent Threats, Humiliation	11%
Household Dysfunction	Household Member was Alcoholic or Drug User	27%
	Not Raised by Both Biological Parents	23%
	Household Member was Chronically Depressed, Suicidal, Mentally Ill, or in Psychiatric Hospital	17%
	Mother Treated Violently	13%
	Household Member was Imprisoned	6%
Neglect	Emotional	15%
	Physical	10%

the individual's functioning and physical, social, emotional, or spiritual well-being (SAMHSA, 2014). The Adverse Childhood Experiences (ACE) Study conducted by Vincent Felitti and Robert Anda from 1995 to 1997 (Felitti, Nordenberg, Williamson, Spitz, Edwards, Koss & Marks, 1998) is perhaps the most compelling explication of what individual trauma is and what effect it has on peoples' health and functioning. Felitti and Anda developed a survey with ten questions designed to indicate experiences of abuse (physical and sexual), neglect and household dysfunction. They asked over 17,000 patients in the Kaiser Permanente health system to complete a physical exam and a comprehensive confidential survey. Their questions were grouped under ten categories that were used to determine a person's ACE score. Each positive answer on the survey added a point to one's ACE score. Table 1 on the previous page summarizes the key results.

The study compared health information and ACE scores and found a stepped, dose response. The higher the ACE score, the greater the negative impact on health and social functioning. A direct link is shown between childhood trauma and adult onset of chronic disease, as well as mental illness, time in prison, and work issues such as absenteeism (Felitti et al., 1998).

This was the first study on the effects of several types of trauma rather than the consequences of just one. It found that ACEs are pervasive. About two-thirds of the adults in the study had experienced one or more types of adverse childhood experiences. Of those, 87 percent had experienced 2 or more types. People who had an alcoholic father, for example, were likely to have also experienced physical abuse or verbal abuse. In short, ACEs usually don't happen in isolation. Women are also twice as likely as men to have more than five ACEs (Felitti et al., 1998).

Adults, of course, also experience painful or highly stressful situations that impact their well-being. Post-Traumatic Stress Disorder (PTSD), a diagnosis accepted by the American Psychiatric Association, describes the symptoms that accompany severe and prolonged exposure to stressors such as abuse, assault, military service or natural disaster. PTSD is associated with greater medical service utilization for physical health problems. Depression, anger and social dysfunction are the most common symptoms, but as we have already noted, physical, mental, emotional, spiritual and relational health are all intertwined. More recent clinical studies have linked chronic stress to impairment of the nervous system, the hypothalamic–pituitary–adrenal (HPA) axis, and cardiovascular, metabolic, and immune systems which contribute to chronic diseases such as diabetes, hypertension, and cardiovascular disease (Sherin & Nemeroff, 2011). Many studies on PTSD explore the processes that cause dysfunction. Among the findings, evidence shows that not all traumas create the same risk for PTSD: traumatic injuries caused by other people are the most likely to lead to PTSD, and it may be especially severe or long lasting when the stressor is of "human design" (Charuvastra & Cloitre, 2008).

COMMUNITY TRAUMA

Community Trauma is a toxic or negative event or condition that disrupts an entire neighborhood or population. It may be caused by a natural disaster, such as Hurricane Katrina when people from the whole city and region were displaced and in need of housing, water, food, medical care, clothing. Often in natural disasters, the wider community responds with good-will. The burden and sorrow are shared. Events such as a school shooting or mass murder are shocking experiences that make everyone feel unsafe. In urban communities, trauma may come in the form of gang violence, struggle to meet daily living needs, or the stress of racial discrimination. Unlike a natural disaster where the wider community is quick to respond with assistance, communities that experience violence and crime are often isolated from the rest of society. The whole community is labeled as dangerous or unstable and those in neighboring communities may even blame the victims, assuming they are involved in gang or criminal activity. Law enforcement, normally providing a sense of safety and order, may not be responsive or trusted by the community.

The ACE scoring system was not originally designed to assess this level of stress. To begin to capture a broader conception of trauma, researchers in Philadelphia designed an Expanded ACE questionnaire (Findings from The Philadelphia Urban ACE Survey, 2013). Their 14 question survey included questions from the Conventional ACE tool, but added others that assessed community trauma, including experiencing racism, witnessing violence, living in an unsafe neighborhood, experiencing bullying, and having a history of living in foster care. It was also administered to a much more diverse sample. Whereas the majority of respondents in the original ACE study and numerous subsequent studies were White non-Hispanic, middle-class, and had more than a high school education, here the goal was to explore what ACEs look like in a more urban setting with a higher percentage of people of color.

The Philadelphia Urban ACE Survey found that the percentage of adults who experienced at least one ACE increased to 83.2% when the urban ACE survey indicators were added, compared to about 66% in the original study. Sixty three per cent of adults had a higher ACE score when including the urban ACE items. These urban ACE indicators are prevalent. During childhood, 40% of adults saw or heard violence in their community, more than a third reported feeling discrimination (for African Americans the rate is almost 50%), and almost a third didn't feel safe or that their neighbors looked out for each other (Findings from The Philadelphia Urban ACE Survey, 2013).

The Expanded ACE scores cluster around geographic areas that have the highest percentages of poverty and lowest adult educational levels. In those communities, over 45% of the population have ACE scores of four or more. Three of the five zip codes in Philadelphia with the highest percentage of Hispanic adults have a population in which 45.1% of the population has four or more ACEs (Findings from the Philadelphia Urban ACE Survey, 2013). As we will see in the next section, the connection between high ACE scores, health status and healthcare costs is staggering. The original ACE study (Felitti and Anda, 1998) showed that those with four categories of ACEs are more likely to have:

- 240% higher risk of hepatitis
- 390% higher risk of COPD (emphysema or chronic bronchitis)
- 240% higher risk of Sexually Transmitted Infections
- 200% higher risk of smoking
- 1200% higher risk of attempting suicide
- 700% higher risk to be an alcoholic.

If almost half the residents in whole zip codes experience four or more ACEs, it is no wonder that we have seemingly intractable health disparities in some communities. Clearly, expanding the way we think about Adverse Childhood Experiences to include Adverse Community Experiences is critical for health care planning around community health engagement. A few progressive hospitals, like the Community Health Enhancement Department of Memorial Hospital, South Bend in Indiana, have been incorporating ACE questions into their Community Health Needs Assessment (see sidebar on Aces Data Collection and Implementation).

HISTORICAL TRAUMA

Historical trauma is the condition in which an entire population is subjugated deliberately and systematically over an extended period of time by a dominant group or social order (See also Chapter 6). Studies crossing historical periods, global settings and types of subjugation (war, starvation, occupation, colonization, etc.) have all found an increased disease burden for those suffering the

In 2012, the Community Health Enhancement (CHE) Department of Memorial Hospital-South Bend decided to begin including eight of the ACE questions in its Community Health Needs Assessment. The subsequent data from 599 respondents, predominantly Caucasian (86%), showed that 126 (21%) had a total score of three or more on the eight items. Members of the high ACEs subgroup came from every income category. For example, 21 earned less than $10,000, but 19 earned more than $75,000.

The data also revealed similar patterns of higher associations between those with increased ACEs scores and chronic illness in the following physical health areas.

	COPD	Arthritis	Diabetes	Asthma	Heart Attack	Stroke	Kidney Disease	Obesity (BMI)
< 3 score	8.9%	34.9%	13.1%	11.4%	7.2%	6.3%	3.6%	28.9%
>3 score	16.7%	46.0%	24.8%	27.0%	10.3%	7.9%	7.9%	38.2%

In addition, the data also showed that associations between high ACE scores and mental health problems were especially troublesome.

	Anxiety	Depression
< 3 score	9.5%	15.0%
>3 score	34.9%	45.2%

Based on this data, the Community Health Enhancement Department staff decided to focus their efforts across the entire community and implement a simple three-pronged plan to impact individual experience and health, families, organizations and the community as a whole:

1. Increase community-wide awareness of ACEs and their broad effects

2. Actively support interventions to reduce trauma as well as the effect of trauma

3. Build health (cognitive, social, emotional, physical, financial).

Over time, they imagined this system-wide focus could create a culture of health where costly penal, health, educational, and social welfare interventions would be reduced and the quality of life and holistic outcomes throughout our community would increase.

To achieve these new goals, CHE has begun to implement many action steps during the past three years. Just a few examples include:

- Partnering with the public schools to teach the Mind Up resiliency training curriculum to students;

- Hosting and financially supporting training by experts in trauma-focused techniques (EMDR/A-TIP) for mental and physical health professionals;

- Participating in the building St. Joseph County Cares (SJC CARES), a community-wide trauma-focused task force. SJC CARES ensures that wherever a child or youth goes, they are greeted and treated in a way that is consistent with a trauma informed approach. Soccer coaches, pastors, after-school providers, and theatre directors are all educated to know about the impact of trauma on developing brains, identify the ways in which trauma can show up as behaviors in children and youth, recognize that they can play a role in mitigating the impact of trauma, and avoid re-traumatization;

- Funding a part-time non-medical Trauma Intervention Specialist to work with gunshot, assault, and stabbing victims and their families.

Memorial Hospital-South Bend included the ACE questions again in their 2015 Community Health Needs Assessment and noted similar results. They are continuing to make a long-term commitment to reducing trauma and its effects in their community, especially in the area of mental health.

immediate experience, but also for their children and even their grandchildren (Sotero, 2006). This transgenerational transmission of health consequences is one of the most concerning features of historical trauma in terms of its implications for managing health outcomes for our most socially complex patients. We will explore the genetic pathways that support this intergenerational effect later in the chapter.

Much of the framing of the field of study around "historical trauma" comes from the work of Maria Brave Heart and the American Indian/Native Alaskan (AINA) context. However, studies have spanned populations as diverse as those forced into labor camps during the Stalinist purges in the 1930, the renowned Dutch Famine Birth Cohort Study on the Nazi enforced Dutch "hunger winter" of 1944-5 (www.dutchfamine.nl/index.htm) and the experience of Palestinians under Israeli occupation (Danieli, 1998). In our own history as a nation, over 200 years of slavery laid the groundwork for a legacy of discrimination and institutional racism which continue to shape the daily experience and opportunities of African Americans today.

Studies also show that Native Americans are seven times more likely than the U.S. average to die from alcoholism, four times more likely to die from diabetes, twice as likely to complete suicide, and 50% more likely to die from influenza or pneumonia. In the Western Hemisphere, only Haiti has a lower life expectancy than Native American populations (Sotero, 2006). These statistics mirror health disparities experienced in the African American and Hispanic communities. While it seems overwhelming, we cannot ignore the salience of historical trauma as a contributing factor when we tend to the health of our patients, families and communities.

RESILIENCE

One of the most exciting things about the work around trauma is the finding that trauma is not destiny. When Adverse Childhood Experiences are addressed, healing can occur and health outcomes do improve. When communities have what they need and people can function in a trusting and supportive community environment, the health of the population improves. As the Children's Resilience Initiative says, "Resilience trumps trauma."

The American Psychological Association (2015) defines resilience as "the process of adapting well in the face of adversity, trauma, tragedy, threats or significant sources of stress—such as family and relationship problems, serious health problems or workplace and financial stressors. It means 'bouncing back' from difficult experiences." A very different organization, The Maine Resiliency Building Network (2015), defines resilience as "the ability to work with adversity in such a way that one comes through it unharmed or even better for the experience." This hopeful approach to resilience is central to trauma informed practices—the idea that we can thrive in spite of or even because of difficulty.

Resilience is basically our ability to modulate the stress response. Whether a person perseveres or gives up in the face of difficulty depends on many factors. These can be environmental or biological, but the strongest influence on our response to stress and ability to be resilient are psychological factors—the way we think—and relational factors—connections we have with others. The way we think about the cause of negative events, whether we feel we have the ability to exert control in most situations, and our overall outlook on life is a mindset. It is teachable, and it is one we can help others develop. Still, it is not only up to a person to foster their own resilience. It is also our responsibility to surround individuals with a supportive and positive environment while lessening the presence of risk factors. Protective factors are positive qualities located within the cognitive, emotional, environmental, social, and spiritual experience of the person that are associated with resilience and, when combined, facilitate resilience. These modifiable factors work cumulatively to empower and support a person or a child in avoiding or successfully working through negative outcomes associated with ACEs. Developing resilience is important to healthcare because research shows that people who are able to bounce back live longer, have better health, happier relationships and greater success (Reivich & Shatte, 2002).

Because trauma is fundamentally a phenomenon of dysfunctional or toxic relationships, one of the most critical protective and healing factors for both individuals and communities is strong social relationships. Many studies support the function of social support in buffering or protecting against the effects of stress. Across studies, it is clear that the quality of the relationship is more important than the quantity of relationships. For example, Liebenberg, Ungar and LeBlanc (as quoted in Ungar, 2013) showed that it was not the quantity of services that were provided, but the quality of relationships between an adult service provider and youth that was most predictive of how well a child was able to make use of the services. When adults heard and empowered children in the adult-child relationship, children functioned better.

These benefits are observed across diverse populations, from children to veterans to unemployed workers to mothers of children with serious illnesses. Strong social support helps people with depression function better and increases their likelihood of recovery. Vietnam veterans who had high levels of social support were 180% less likely to develop PTSD than counterparts who did not have strong social connections (Ozbay, Johnson, Dimoulas, Morgan, Charney & Southwick, 2007). A positive relationship with a caring adult is one of the most effective strategies for mediating the impact of ACEs. One program found that a compassionate response to students' trauma histories reduced out of school suspensions by 80% (Resilience Trumps ACEs, n.d.).

HOW DO TRAUMA AND RESILIENCE WORK?

Intuitively we can understand how toxic stress can impact a person's emotional or mental health or a community's sense of well-being and we can imagine how this would impact their physical health. We can see how stress can trigger coping mechanisms such as overeating, substance abuse, risky behaviors, multiple sexual partners and social isolation which feed poor health outcomes. Researchers are now also exploring how traumatic experience actually creates brain impairment and how this gets translated into behavior. While more needs to be learned, scientists already have a good idea how these pathways function. The diagram below shows the progression of impacts from the initial experience of trauma to poor health and social outcomes and early death.

Science is now demonstrating that, in addition to the social consequences of toxic stress, the unregulated and ongoing release of stress hormones such as cortisol and adrenaline, can activate the Hypothalamic–Pituitary–Adrenal (HPA) Axis. HPA are three endocrine glands that regulate many body processes, including digestion, the immune system, mood and emotions and how we store and expend energy. An activated HPA

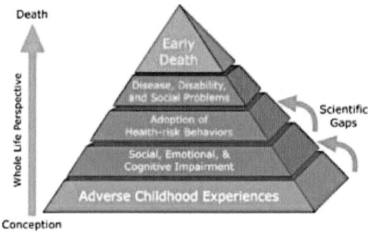

(CDC. Injury Prevention & Control: Division of Violence Prevention, 2014)

Axis can weaken body defenses and compromise the immune system's ability to protect from infection, cancer or autoimmune diseases and can also raise blood pressure, promote plaque formation in arteries and lead to neurological changes that create depressive and post-traumatic stress illnesses (Shonkoff, Garner, Siegel, Dobbins, Earls, Garner, McGuinn, Pascoe & Wood, 2012).

Trauma also causes changes to brain structure and functioning. Survivors of trauma have shown smaller brain volumes and alterations in the functioning of the neocortex and the visual and auditory cortex. These findings strongly suggest that childhood trauma may have profound negative effects on executive function, attention, memory, and visual spatial function (Danese, DeBellis & Teicher, 2015).

In addition, the field of epigenetics is exploring how trauma changes the expression of our genetic structure. While our actual DNA remains the same, our life experiences and the physical environment in which we live can turn certain features of our genes on and off or change the way they function. As noted above, these genetic shifts can be passed down through generations. For example, a study (Dias & Ressler, 2014) conducted on mice found that when a pleasant smell was associated with an electric shock, the mice began to cower and show signs of fear whenever that smell was introduced. The mice's babies also cowered when encountering the smell despite never having been shocked, and their babies also had the same reaction when they smelled the aroma. These researchers believe that the shock created an intergenerational epigenetic shift in the mice's olfactory system that connected the smell with danger (Dias & Ressler, 2014).

In Switzerland, a team of behavioral geneticists found a clue to the generational transition of aggression and violence. Their research links two observable phenomena: "the higher rate of aggression in those experiencing early-life stress and the blunted activation of a brain region known as the orbitofrontal cortex among people with pathological aggression" (Blue, 2013, p. 4). Another study (Márquez, Cordero, Larsen, Groner, Marquis, Magistretti, Trono & Sandi, 2013) showed that stressed lab animals had higher levels of testosterone, and showed more activity in the amygdala, the brain segment responsible for emotions, including fear and anxiety. There was also an altered connectivity between the seat of emotions and the prefrontal cortex, where executive functions such as decision-making, learning math, and making judgment calls are located. One of the most interesting aspects of the study was evidence that the brain alterations were correlated with enhanced expression of the gene for the monoamine oxidase A (MAOA) enzyme (Márquez et al., 2013).

In support of the claim that "resilience trumps trauma," this same study found that when an MAOA inhibitor was introduced, normal social behaviors returned and aggression was reduced (Márquez et al., 2013). It is important to remember that neuroscience research has taught us that changing our behavior over time can create changes in our brains. This is called neuroplasticity. Our brains change throughout our lifetime in response to our experiences, choices and repeated thoughts. This is the brain's way of fine-tuning itself to meet our needs. For example, if a person is exposed to ongoing trauma, the brain will respond with a heightened stress response as a survival mechanism. The opposite is also true. Ongoing exposure to supportive and caring environments will trigger resilience and healing. Any action or thought that is repeated often, whether positive or negative, becomes "hard-wired," nearly an automatic response in our brains. If traumatic experiences shift the way that our genome functions, restorative experiences can correct or redirect genetic functioning.

This is great news for teaching the skills of resilience. Practicing a positive mindset and developing resilient coping skills over time will help to make that response style more automatic. It can serve to replace the negative, reactive response style that survivors of trauma develop, normalize the HPA Axis response and rewire genetic and brain pathways. Trauma and adversity do not have to be destiny.

Communities can also foster resilience by supporting practices that enable a rapid and comprehensive response to crisis, fostering community connections through events, parks and other public spaces, and effectively connecting residents to a wide-range of social services. Resilient communities seek solutions to problems by engaging people within the community and building interventions around local customs and cultural norms. These communities are better able to bounce back from crisis and disruptions, maintain a good quality of life for the residents, prepare for uncertainties, and adapt to change.

Skills that can help us develop a less negative mindset about adversity include: optimism, gratitude, empathy, and altruism. Physiological interventions such as exercise, mindfulness, deep breathing and meditation help modulate the body's stress response. Finally, as already noted social support and connection to others are important factors in resilience. In fact, the presence of a caring adult can help to mitigate the impact of trauma in the life of a child and significantly increase that child's resilience (Hodas, 2006).

All of these elements can be learned and taught in settings as diverse as hospital workplaces, schools and even prisons. Further down or in side-bars we highlight specific modalities for fostering resilience currently used in clinical settings (see sidebars on Resilience for work done in Oncology at Advocate Children's Hospital in Chicago, and Mind Up Resiliency Building for work done in South Bend, Indiana in public schools.)

The Health Impact and Costs of Trauma

It should be the goal of every institution of human caring to ensure that no one in our society is hurt or has to endure harmful life experiences. As faith-based and/or mission driven health care providers, our traditions and values call us to create loving and just communities where all people can be healthy and whole. That is enough reason to try to reduce trauma and foster social caring and support. It turns out that attending to the environments in which our patients and families live, work, play or attend school is not only a critical part of their health journey; it promotes the financial health of our organizations, as well. Trauma, toxic stress and unstable social conditions have an astonishing impact on health outcomes. The effects of trauma reduce life expectancy and quality of life and cost health care systems millions of dollars in readmissions, noncompliance with treatment plans and unnecessary chronic disease conditions.

The health impact of traumatic experience is well documented. Studies based on the original 17,000 Kaiser Permanente patients that participated in the study showed a dose response, graded relationship between ACE scores (the number of categories of childhood experiences of trauma) and each of the adult health risk behaviors and diseases that were studied (Brown, Anda, Tiemeier, Felitti, Edwards, Croft & Giles, 2009). For instance, persons who had experienced four or more categories of childhood exposure were 4 to 12 times more likely to have increased health risks for alcoholism, drug abuse, depression, and suicide attempt. They were twice as likely to

FOSTERING STAFF RESILIENCE

Because young cancer patients and their families are involved in care over many years, our pediatric caregivers at Advocate Children's Hospital in metropolitan Chicago often witness many life changes and develop meaningful bonds with families. While strong attachments facilitate healing, they also amplify the magnitude of loss when a patient dies. Staff experience grief as well as physical and emotional stress that translate into disrupted sleep, loss of appetite, pain, and mental health issues.

Recognizing the need for staff support, leaders from Oncology and Mission & Spiritual Care divisions came together in 2013 to consider how to overcome generalized feelings of helplessness and hopelessness that result from these profound losses. New interventions, from scheduled debriefings to group prayer, have already proven important to staff morale and resiliency. The Vice President of Mission and Spiritual Care worked with nursing leadership and other hospital managers to seek funding from the LiveStrong Foundation to conduct three, three-day resiliency trainings for members of the interdisciplinary teams at the two main campuses of the children's hospital.

The grant funded the implementation of a train-the-trainer program with VitalHearts, a non-profit organization from Colorado, led by psychologist, Henry Tobey. The Resiliency Training Initiative's mission is caring for cancer treatment providers who suffer from secondary or vicarious trauma, which is a significant, although hidden problem. Secondary Traumatic Stress includes such reactions as: depression, anxiety, persistent trauma imagery, sleep disturbances, mistrust of their organization, isolating from family/friends, frequent illness and loss of mission optimism, among other symptoms, due to the deep exposure to suffering that care providers experience. VitalHearts' program, the Secondary Trauma Resiliency Training (STRT), revitalizes care providers, often saving careers of those who work with cancer patient and survivors by making them more resilient. This allows institutions to better retain their staff expertise, which gives crucial value to patients.

To date sixty members of the interdisciplinary team have participated in the training and with the grant ending in 2015, the Mission and Spiritual Care Department has received budget approval to conduct three more trainings in 2016. Participants in the first three trainings have overwhelmingly recommended that more members of Advocate Children's Hospital team have the opportunity to take part in the training. This training and recent efforts from staff chaplains to provide regular staff support sessions, including weekly resiliency rounds, have begun to transform the culture of the hospital to be one where health care professionals are reflecting and living out of a place of resiliency.

be smokers, 12 times more likely to have attempted suicide, 7 times more likely to be alcoholic, and 10 times more likely to have injected street drugs. People with high ACE scores had a 2 to 4-fold increase in smoking, poor self-rated health, multiple sexual partners, and sexually transmitted disease and were 1.5 times more likely to be physically inactive or severely obese. Adult diseases including ischemic heart disease, cancer, chronic lung disease, skeletal fractures, and liver disease were all associated with the presence of ACEs. Compared with people with zero ACEs, those with four categories of ACEs had a 240 % greater risk of hepatitis, were 390% more likely to have chronic obstructive pulmonary disease (emphysema or chronic bronchitis), and a 240% higher risk of a sexually-transmitted disease. Persons with two or more ACEs were found to have a 70% increased risk for hospitalization for autoimmune disease compared with people with no ACEs and 100% increased risk for rheumatic diseases. They also had more social problems—more absences from work, more injuries, more marriages, etc. People with six or more adverse experiences died on average 20 years sooner than those with no ACEs (Felitti & Anda, 2009).

MIND UP RESILIENCY BUILDING

Community Health Enhancement of Memorial Hospital-South Bend is offering resiliency building classes at Rise-up Academy, South Bend public schools' alternative school for youth 16–21 wanting a second chance. The facilitator is utilizing a curriculum entitled Mind Up. Developed by the Hawn Foundation, this curriculum uses research to teach basic neuroscience and build resilience at the same time. Students learn how to self-regulate by practicing controlled breathing and mindfulness as they learn about the associated brain processes. In addition, lessons in optimism, empathy, gratitude and altruism help students develop a positive mind-set. Each lesson features classroom activities as well as a link to specific neuroscience research around resilience. Students also learn strategies to improve focus and attention as well as manage stress. Concepts in the curriculum meet health and science standards. Both teachers and students are fascinated by the neuroscience lessons and report that the activities increase coping skills. Outcomes are measured with pre/post testing that includes knowledge acquisition and behavioral change. In addition, the Resiliency Scales for Children & Adolescents™—A Profile of Personal Strengths (RSCA) is also administered pre and post training to measure growth in three areas: Sense of Mastery, Sense of Relatedness, and Emotional Reactivity.

Overview and Impact/Cost of Mental Illness and Substance Abuse

We now review the cost of mental health conditions to the health care system and discuss treatment models for integrating mental health and physical health. Although we address those experiencing severe and persistent chronic mental illnesses, we will focus more on those in the lower segments of the population health management pyramid, those described by our colleague, Steve Tierney, MD, of South Central Foundation, as having the (imagined) Diagnostic and Statistical Manual-V type diagnosis: "My Life is a Mess, Not Otherwise Specified." In short, we refer to vulnerable persons who have ongoing life stressors, often tied to their status as under-served, unemployed and/or working multiple low-paying jobs, living in poverty and/or unsafe environments, replete with more susceptibility to abuse or neglect, toxins, violence and in poor living conditions.

We recognize that many such people have likely experienced trauma, making them more susceptible to developing clinical depression, anxiety and/or substance abuse, in a cyclical toxic interaction. The embodiment of those stressors can lead to a host of stress-related illnesses (see "How stress gets under our skin", HSLG, 2013, p. 41). Dube, Felitti, Dong, Chapman, Giles and Anda (2003) found that ACEs seem to account for one half to two thirds of serious problems with drug use. In a study of over 8000 patients in a primary care clinic, each ACE increased the likelihood for early initiation of drug use two to four times. As the ACE score increased, the initiation of drug use and drug addiction increased. Compared with people with zero ACEs, people with more than five ACEs were seven to ten times more likely to report illicit drug use problems, addiction to illicit drugs, and IV drug use.

Adverse Childhood Experiences have real health care costs in financial terms, health outcomes, quality of life and community stability. Those with four categories of ACEs are more likely to have:

- 240% higher risk of hepatitis
- 390% higher risk of COPD (emphysema or chronic bronchitis)
- 240% higher risk of STDs
- 200% more likely to smoke
- 1200% more likely to have attempted suicide
- 700% higher risk to be an alcoholic (Felitti and Anda, 1998).

A recent CDC study looked at confirmed child maltreatment cases. The total lifetime estimated financial costs associated with just one year of confirmed cases of child maltreatment (physical abuse, sexual abuse, psychological abuse and neglect) is approximately $124 billion. That breaks down to a lifetime cost of $210,012 for each victim of child maltreatment who lived, which is comparable to other costly health conditions. The costs of each death due to child maltreatment are even higher. The researchers based their calculations on only confirmed cases of physical, sexual and verbal abuse and neglect, which child maltreatment experts say is a small percentage of what actually occurs.

The breakdown per child is:

- $32,648 in childhood health care costs
- $10,530 in adult medical costs
- $144,360 in productivity losses
- $7,728 in child welfare costs
- $6,747 in criminal justice costs
- $7,999 in special education costs.

The estimated average lifetime cost per death includes:

- $14,100 in medical costs
- $1,258,800 in productivity losses (CDC, 2014).

COSTS OF MENTAL HEALTH

Estimates in 2007-08 were that severe mental illness costs in the US were approximately $308 billion, due to 60.8% lost earnings, 31.5% direct health care costs and 7.7% disability benefits (Insel et al., 2008; Marks, 2007).

In a 2004 study, 10 health conditions were assessed via large medical/absence data bank across many major corporations (Soni, 2009). Overall economic burden of illness: #1 hypertension ($392 per eligible employee per year), #2 heart disease ($368) and #3 depression and other mental conditions. In a more recent estimate, the Agency for Healthcare Research and Quality, cites a cost of $57.5 billion in 2006 for mental health care in the U.S. (AHRQ, 2010).

This graded relationship persists across all populations and age groups dating back to 1900, which suggests that this association is true despite changes in the availability of drugs and social attitudes toward drugs over the years (Dube et al, 2003). When we look at just male children, we find that those with an ACE score of 6 or more have a shocking 4,600% increased likelihood of becoming an injection drug user, compared to a male with an ACE score of 0 (Felitti, 2002). This strongly suggests that medical practice and addiction treatment programs should become "trauma informed" and integrate methods to address the experiential sources of substance abuse and addiction.

The relationship between stress, poverty, trauma and mental illness and substance abuse problems has also been well-documented. Essentially, common mental disorders occur at over twice the rate for those experiencing poverty than those who are rich (WHO, 2007). Depression is also strongly associated with trauma even fifty to sixty years after ACEs occurred. One study shows that 54% of current depression and 58% of suicide attempts in women can be attributed to adverse childhood experiences (Felitti & Anda, 2009). Whatever later factors might trigger suicide, childhood experiences cannot be left out of the equation. A similar relationship exists between ACE Score and later hallucinations (Felitti & Anda, 2009.) Also, depression is 1.5 to 2 times more prevalent for under-served parts of populations (WHO, 2007). From an epidemiological standpoint, these researchers defined "under-served parts of the population" as those living in poverty, with low socioeconomic status (measured by social or income class), unemployment and low levels of education (Saraceno & Barbui, 1997).

Likewise, those experiencing food insecurity or debt are more likely to manifest mental disorders, as well as those experiencing overcrowding and sub-standard housing. The

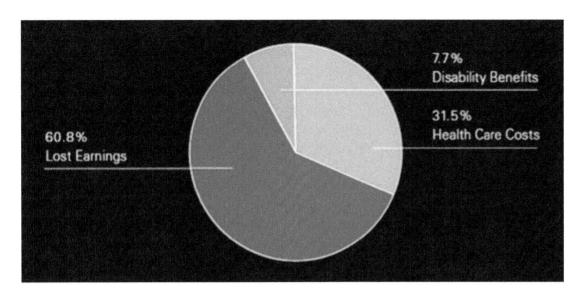

Costs of Mental Illness in the U.S.: 2007-2008. Data derived from Insel, 2008 and Mark et al., 2007"

WHO and others argue that breaking the cyclical nature of poverty is a key consideration for preventing more mental illness and note the lack of adequate funding devoted at national and international levels to both prevention of mental illness and poverty reduction efforts. Substance abuse has a similar relationship to poverty and stress in under-served populations. A recent SAMSHA report (2014) found that among the 43.8 million adults aged 18 or older in 2013 with any mental illness in the past year, 17.5 percent (7.7 million adults) met criteria for a substance use disorder (i.e., illicit drug or alcohol dependence or abuse). Among the 10 million adults with severe mental illness in the past year, 23.1 percent also had past year substance dependence or abuse. In comparison, 6.5 percent of adults who did not have mental illness in the past year met criteria for a substance use disorder.

What is the cost and impact of mental illness and substance abuse to our society? Estimates in 2007-08 were that severe mental illness costs in the U.S. were approximately $308 billion, owing to 60.8% lost earnings, 31.5% direct health care costs and 7.7% disability benefits (Insel, 2008; Mark et al., 2007; slide above reproduced courtesy of Dr. Thom Bornemman of the Carter Center's Mental Health Program).

Psychiatrically disabled persons (those with severe mental illness) in Massachusetts with co-occurring substance abuse disorders manifested 60% higher costs than those with only substance abuse issues, mostly due to inpatient psychiatric admissions (Dickey & Azeni, 1996). However these costs do not even begin to account for the quality of life lost due to mental illness, for both the persons experiencing these illnesses and their family members.

Collectively, claims for depression, anxiety and stress cost U.S. employers an estimated $344 billion each year due to lost productivity, accidents, disability claims and medical fees (Insel, 2008). Estimates range from 18% to 81% of current lost productivity costs associated with presenteeism ("at the job but not performing well"). Of course, these illnesses co-occur with many chronic medical conditions. In a 2004 study, ten health conditions were assessed via a large medical/absence data bank across many major corporations (Soni, 2009). In this study, depression and other mental conditions ranked number three in terms of cost per eligible employee per year in terms of economic burden of illness (see Medical Cost Offsets of Behavioral Health Treatment (Laurence, 2013) for details).

Costs in hospital emergency rooms are also significant. Dealing with mental illness/substance abuse prevention and front line treatment is critically important, especially in our health systems, where those inappropriately using emergency room services often have both medical and psychiatric or stress-related illnesses. Total annual visits to emergency rooms in the United States from 1997-2007 increased by 23% (Tang, Stein, Hsia, Maselli & Gonzales, 2010), yet during part of that timeframe (1992-2003) mental health-related ER visits increased 75% (Salinksky & Loftis, 2007). Compared to patients without psychiatric disorders, those with psychiatric disorders are more likely to use the ER on multiple occasions and to have multiple hospitalizations (Baillargeon, Thomas, Williams et al., 2008). Almost 12 million ER visits in the U.S. in 2007, roughly 1 in 8, were due to mental health and/or substance use problems in adults (AHRQ, 2010). Of these 12 million visits, 63.7% were related to mental health problems, 24.4% involved substance use disorders and 11.9% involved co-occurring psychiatric and substance use disorders (AHRQ, 2010).

Specific to health systems, we know at local and state levels that many super-utilizers or over-utilizers of emergency services have co-occurring medical and mental illness/substance abuse issues. For instance, CDC analyzed ED visits occurring in North Carolina during the period 2008–2010 captured by the North Carolina Disease Event Tracking and Epidemiologic Collection Tool (NC DETECT). This report indicated that nearly 10% of ED visits had one or more mental health diagnoses assigned to the visit and the rate of mental health related ED visits increased seven times as much as the overall rate of ED visits in North Carolina during the study period. Those with a mental health diagnoses were admitted to the hospital from the ED more than twice as often as those without such diagnoses. Stress, anxiety, and depression were diagnosed in 61% of mental health-related ED visits. The annual rate of mental health-related ED visits for those aged ≥65 years was nearly twice the rate of those aged 25–64 years; half of those aged ≥65 years with mental health diagnoses were admitted to the hospital from the ED (CDC, 2013). Looking at these numbers can cause even the most optimistic among us to feel despair about making a difference in persons with these issues.

Although these cost figures are staggering, there is good news. Numerous experiments in care for persons covered under Medicaid and other programs for the under-served exist to show that incorporating any level of mental health screening, care and treatment can save money for health plans, hospital, individuals and other stakeholders, and, more importantly, improve the quality of life for both individuals and families (see Medical Cost Offsets of Behavioral Health Treatment sidebar for details).

Additionally, there is hope for prevention of mental illness and substance abuse through evidence-based practices that could be implemented at the community level. For example, the Institute of Medicine (2009; 2012) reports that these practices exist for both youth and those in later life. Muñoz et al. (2012) report estimates from meta-analyses that suggest that 22-38% of initial major depressive episodes could be prevented with available methods. These include strength-based and resiliency training, cognitive behavioral programs, web-based programs, public health efforts, taking a developmental perspective, targeting high risk populations (post-partum, elderly, college students, etc.) and testing evidence-based interventions with the widest reach. Other prevention efforts center on dealing with poverty and adverse events in youth and children (Yoshikawa, Aber & Beardslee, 2012; Blair & Raver, 2012). Actively engaging these programs or knowledge at community scale may help prevent unnecessary suffering. Stakeholder Health believes that offering resiliency training, mindfulness and other strategies proactively to all children and youth would decrease the stigma of designating persons as traumatized and could

Excerpted from 2013 Presentation by Lance Laurence

Numerous natural experiments, in care for persons covered under Medicaid and other programs for under-served, exist to show that incorporating any level of mental health screening, care and treatment can save money for health plans, hospital, individuals and other stakeholders.

In 1990, the Hawaii Medicaid Program dropped MH/SA services in Medicaid due to costs. As a result, Medicaid costs escalated as those with mental health problems sought help from PCPs at twice the rate of those without such issues and visited the ED more frequently. In 1991, the Hawaii Medicaid Program reinstituted a full array of mental health services, including no utilization review, a process often required in advance to justify reimbursement for therapy visits. Costs in the Medicaid Program decreased. One aspect of the Hawaii Medicaid Study focused on high users with targeted mental health care. Cost reductions in medical care for those receiving services were 38% for those not chronically ill, 18% for those chronically ill, 15% who had substance abuse diagnoses. These high users sought medical help 200-250% more frequently than those not seeking mental health intervention.

In a follow up of the same study cohort, high users (80% of costs used by 20% of the patients) were randomly assigned to receiving mental health care or not. After 18 months, those getting mental health care showed a 44% reduction in general medical costs. Likewise, in a 2008 study, high users receiving psychotherapy showed a 38% reduction in office visits, 56% reduction in laboratory/x-ray visits, and 78% reduction for urgent care visits.

Biodyne Institute's 4-year study of 16,000 lives in the Hawaii Medicaid population and 30,000 federal employees showed that patients who received targeted, focused mental health care experienced a 35-38% drop in medical costs after receiving treatment. Those who got no focused mental health care saw medical cost increases from 0-25%, depending on the patient.

Likewise, Kaiser Permanente's HMO found that those who received psychotherapy showed a 77.9% decrease in average length of stay in the hospital, a 66.7% decrease in the frequency of hospitalizations, a 48.6% decrease in the number of prescriptions written, 47.1% decrease in physician office visits, 45.3% decrease in emergency room visits, and 31.2% decrease in telephone contacts. One million patient contacts were reviewed. Sixty-eight per cent of these persons were on medication at the onset of the study. Mental health interventions provided a 13% reduction in those on medication at the end of the study.

While early medical cost offset studies focused on high utilizers of medical services, later work also expanded to look at those who were on the low end of the utilization spectrum. Again, the use of some level of mental health care demonstrated improvements. A study with 8,100 enrollees at Boston Clinic demonstrated that those receiving psychotherapy for non-chronic condition (i.e., not bipolar, etc.) reduced their non-psychiatric medical services by 7.2%; similarly diagnosed patients who did not receive mental health care increased 9.5%—effects lasted over a two year period. In a BCBS Federal Plan, those who received psychotherapy along with treatment of their medical conditions used 56% less medical services than those with similar medical conditions and no psychotherapy.

Finally, meta-analysis of 91 peer reviewed cost-offset studies of those without severe and persistent mental illness showed that 90% of the studies reported a 20-30% medical cost offset savings when compared to those who did not receive psychological services (Chiles, Lambert & Hatch, 1999).

prevent untold pain and suffering and violence against self and others. Our question to ourselves as health system staff interacting with the community is, "Why are we not using these strategies to improve the mental health, resiliency and well-being of all persons?"

We now attempt to answer that question by first, broadening the view of what constitutes all facets of integrated health, particularly in terms of future training in health systems, and then sharing select, potential solutions and interventions for addressing ACEs, mental health and substance abuse problems at both individual and community-scale, highlighting exemplary practices and organizations.

Moving Toward a New Model of Integrated Medicine or Health

BROADENING THE VIEW OF INTEGRATED HEALTH

While most health systems have barely adopted the now dated "bio-psycho-social" model (Engel, 1977) of care delivery, SH and others suggest that the current iteration of the full spectrum of Integrated Health should be expanded beyond this model to include, as delineated by many including the World Council of Churches Reference Group on Mental Health and Faith Communities (WCC, 2007), the dimension of faith or spirituality, broadly defined—a bio-psycho-social-spiritual model. The World Health Organization has also advocated adding a spiritual component to their definition of health: "Health is a dynamic state of complete physical, mental, spiritual and social well-being and not merely the absence of disease or infirmity" (WHO, 2001).

We go even further in seeing Integrated Health not only in terms of the individual but also at community level. This view incorporates, within a health systems framework, current models of population health metrics and interventions now capturing the attention of both public health and clinical practitioners. An example is the Institute for Healthcare Improvement's ambitious Triple Aim to improve quality of care or patient experience and health outcomes while decreasing costs at community scale (Bisognano & Kenney, 2012). We advocate an even more expansive view, however, adding health equity to a "Quadruple Aim" (see our earlier work, Health Systems Learning Group, 2013, p. 12) to insure justice in healthcare and elsewhere. We now explore how integrated care is being adopted by health systems, and early returns on investment that can result.

INTEGRATED CARE IN HEALTH SYSTEMS

In the light of federal regulations requiring not-for-profit health systems to demonstrate community benefit and ensure high quality patient outcomes, health care systems are seeing the benefit of addressing the social determinants of health and providing care that brings in wisdom from other disciplines. Though a move to integrated, patient centered medical homes gained ground in the '60s and early '70s, the managed care decade of the 80s successfully re-siloed the healthcare disciplines and, instead, valued services on volume. The more tonsillectomies performed or broken bones cast, the more money earned or saved—a business model that invited payment for sick care and less for health and prevention.

The idea of multi-disciplinary care, coordination, collaboration, and integration of services is resurfacing at a time when the business model is beginning to shift from fee-for-service to outcomes (or values) based payment models, such as per member per month incentives (actually penalties) to reduce readmissions and for ED diversions. This alters the model of care delivery and brings medical providers (broadly defined) to consider public health and population health models that look at "big data" and aim at the overall minimization of symptoms and diagnoses in large groups and communities. Behavioral health, similarly, is finding a new home in primary and specialty outpatient and inpatient care delivery. Touted as the response to lack of follow through for referrals for behavioral health treatment in other settings, medical treatment noncompliance, management of "difficult" patients, and real-time consultation for patients exhibiting depression, anxiety, suicidality or other complex symptomology, behavioral health (psychiatric and non-medical) is finding its way into these clinics.

The Health Research Services Agency (HRSA) suggests that the integration of primary medical care, behavioral health, public health, oral health, weight management (an option for impacting metabolic syndromes), and pharmacy should be the norm in all clinics, and, depending on the patients served and community needs, other services (physical therapy, nutrition, etc.) might also be appropriate to the mix. We would add spiritual care as another discipline that needs to be at the table, as well as those who help improve social and economic well-being (such as financial or life skills counselors).

Limiting most of these models is an approach that generally involves medicine "integrating" other "ancillary" services into their practice. Workflows might shift, thorough screenings might invite the clinic to treat some depression, anxiety or addiction that might have otherwise been missed, services can be enhanced, but the basic limit is still there—treat what is broken, ill, or diseased, and follow the known best protocol. The focus stays on the biological aspects of the person. This contrasts with the holistic model of assessment, treatment, prevention and wellness, particularly as the key to managing chronic health conditions, that many promote, including the World Council of Churches, National Institutes of Health, Doctors Without Borders, Association of Clinical Pastoral Education, American Association of Pastoral Counselors, and American Psychiatric Association.

While the rigid view of integrated care refers to a behavioral health provider embedded in a medical clinic sharing outcomes through patient registry data and population health management, we suggest a broader view of Integrated Health that (more and more) encompasses care in the community. Increasingly, no longer is it simply the expectation that the patient come to the provider for care. Rather, providers (physicians, social workers, psychologists, nutritionists, etc.) are leaving the clinic and basing their efforts in the heart of community programs and locations where those who need the help the most might receive better access to quality care. For example, free dental clinics are becoming commonplace and low cost or free medical clinics (integrated with behavioral health) are being housed in houses of worship when those buildings would otherwise be empty. Likewise, community members are inviting behavioral health providers to screen for depression and anxiety and provide referral resources at local health fairs.

INTEGRATED CARE: RETURN ON INVESTMENT

Almost every integration effort with a true patient-centered philosophy and practice is providing positive results in their practice. Well known for successes are Intermountain Health Care in Utah, and Cherokee Health Systems in Tennessee. A "Becker's Hospital Review" article from May 2013 (Rodak, 2013) lists 100 integrated health systems across the country. SAMHSA's Primary and Behavioral Health Care Integration program names these benefits from current integrated care settings:

• Improved access to primary care services;

• Improved prevention, early identification, and intervention to reduce the incidence of serious physical illnesses, including chronic disease;

• Increased availability of integrated, holistic care for physical and behavioral disorders; and

• Improved overall health status of clients.

Models that work around policy and funding barriers include Federally Qualified Health Centers and Rural Health Centers that provide services through large blocks of funding rather than reimbursement in the fee-for-service paradigm. These Centers screen all patients for anxiety, depression, and substance use behaviors, embedding behavioral health consultants and co-locating counselors for onsite psychotherapy.

As noted (Medical Cost Offsets sidebar, above), outcomes related to the integration of clinical and community services are very positive. Consistently, integrated primary care clinics are showing improved general health for patients, reduced length of illness for acute patients, reduced hospital admissions and readmissions, and increased treatment compliance metrics in their patient groups. Unexpectedly, clinicians and non-clinicians alike receiving training in integrated modalities, behavioral health interventions, and educational programs are seeing improved mental health themselves—such as improved coping techniques and qualities of resiliency, self-differentiation, and increased emotional intelligence.

Training for integrated care practices also invites a shift in our educational structures. Siloed training based on disciplines is counter to the idea of integrated practice and to the collaborative approach of many programs of inter-professional training. Likewise, developing integrated practice in medical clinics is less about staffing all the necessary disciplines and more about creating a culture of collaboration with flat structures to the fullest degree possible.

The Emotional Fitness Center is an exemplary, individual and community-based practice that integrates behavioral health care through the African-American churches in Tennessee. The Emotional Fitness Center was born out of a crisis in The Healing Center church in Memphis, Tennessee. Early Monday morning, after a wonderful Easter service in 2002, a member of the congregation came to the grounds of the church, got under the cross and took her life. This tragedy shook the congregation to its core in light of the fact that its leader, Bishop and Dr. William M. Young, was a counselor and therapist. How could this suicide happen on his watch? After colleagues came in to help the congregation recover from this loss, a fire was lit in the hearts of the Bishop Young and his wife, Minister Dianne Young, to sound the alarm that suicide was a growing phenomenon in the African American community that could no longer be ignored. From this tragedy, the Youngs formulated the First National Suicide and the Black Church Conference in June, 2003. The conferences continue bi-annually and draw 350 attendees from across the country. The Youngs were also supported by Methodist Le Bonheur Health System, who helped with crafting their first grant to the state and helped sponsor their bi-annual conferences.

The Youngs, now realizing the power of faith and community, with knowledge and hunger to help those with mental, emotional and behavioral health challenges, presented a concept to the State of Tennessee, Department of Mental Health and Substance Abuse in 2007, to develop the Emotional Fitness Centers of Tennessee. The program has been funded by the Tennessee Department of Mental Health and Substance Abuse since 2008. The use of the term "Emotional Fitness" removes the stigma in itself because "Mental Health" to most African Americans sends a negative message culturally. The church removes much of the stigma by giving individuals permission to seek care for their mental health, offering church sites as places where individuals in the community can go and be screened for emotional distress or trauma. After being screened, those dealing with these challenges would be triaged to support groups, counselors, mental health facilities or hospitals to receive the needed care.

Currently, The Emotional Fitness Center utilizes over 20 Peer Advocate Liaisons (PALS) to screen and navigate persons with behavioral health needs to appropriate mental health care, The PALS are based at 7 African American churches, offering multiple entry points through which persons can come into their system. Persons screened by the PALS are then triaged by Bishop Young (also a licensed professional counselor and family and marital therapist by the State of Tennessee) to local psychiatrists, psychologists, social workers and/or to a series of support groups at the Center, ranging from care for family survivors of suicide, anger management, those dealing with violence in their lives and more. The program serves an essential feature in decreasing stigma of mental health care, providing a strong safety net in the community and building strong ties between the African-American church and traditional mental health services.

Over 50 PALS in total have been trained since 2007, with up to 13 churches in Memphis and West Tennessee participating since 2008. Over 3,500 persons have been served in this program since 2008 and most of these individuals would never have received services had they not been made available utilizing the church as the hub for navigation of care. The Youngs, through the Emotional Fitness Centers of Tennessee, have proven the combination of faith and mental health is a best practice for getting individuals into care. Though the funding is not adequate to roll out the program throughout the state, it is definitely a proven best practice, especially since over half of the residents in the State of Tennessee identify themselves as having a faith home.

Resilience Solutions

Mindfulness is derived from centuries-old meditative traditions. It is simply the cultivation of inner resilience and well-being through attention and awareness. Although it can be taught in a secular way, it is a component of many faith traditions and allows each person to bring their own perspective and approach to finding meaning, purpose, and well-being in their lives. It can be as simple as learning how to breathe deeply and purposefully when feeling anxious. The Psalmist in the 23rd Psalm reminds us that it is beside still waters that the soul is restored. It is a powerful tool whether one is looking to find a healthy way to reduce stress and become more self-aware, a child who needs to calm down and focus, a veteran battling post-traumatic stress disorder, a cancer patient seeking strength and perspective for the journey ahead, and more.

The secular practice of mindfulness entered the mainstream in large part due to the groundbreaking work of Jon Kabat-Zinn and his Mindfulness-Based Stress Reduction (MBSR) program at the University of Massachusetts Medical School. Kabat-Zinn describes mindfulness, at its core universal and not particular to any culture, tradition or belief system, as quieting the mind and paying attention in the present moment, on purpose, and without judgment, staying curious instead of reacting (Kabat-Zinn, 1994). The physical and mental health benefits of mindfulness have been so well documented that they have inspired countless programs to adapt the MBSR model for schools, prisons, hospitals, veterans' centers, and more.

World-renowned neuroscientist Dr. Richard J. Davidson at The Center for Investigating Healthy Minds at The Waisman Center, University of Wisconsin-Madison, has been leading rigorous scientific studies for decades on the psychological and neurological evidence for the benefits of mindfulness training. Mindfulness has been linked to heightened activation in brain regions responsible for regulating attention, or focus, and positive affective states such as compassion, kindness and empathy (Davidson, Kabat-Zinn, Suchmacher, Rosenkranz, Muller, Santorelli et al., 2003; Lutz, Greischar, Rawlings, Ricard & Davidson, 2004; Lutz, Slagter, Dunne & Davidson, 2008). Researchers have discovered that the neuroplasticity of the brain, its ability to change structure and function, comes not only from external experiences but also internally through thoughts and intentions. Their evidence-based studies suggest that one can develop concrete skills of inner preparedness to face stress, shock and trauma through meditation and other cognitive behavior training.

Studies also reveal that emotions, attention, and introspection are ongoing and changing processes that may be understood and mastered as skills similar to sports, math, and music (Davidson & McEwen, 2012). A Kindness Curriculum for pre-kindergarten students using Kabat-Zinn's adult-based MBSR curriculum as a model is being used in a research study in the Madison Metropolitan School District with positive results to be published soon. Mindfulness in Schools, a project at the University of Exeter, UK, has created a mindfulness curriculum for middle school students with the goal of teaching skills that cultivate well-being and promotion of mental health. Results reported in the British Journal of Psychiatry (Kuyken, Weare, Ukoumunne et al., 2013) show evidence of its benefit in reducing stress and enhancing well-being and reducing depressive symptoms in students.

The UCLA Mindful Awareness Research Center and The Cousins Center for Psychoneuroimmunology has ongoing studies using mindfulness to lower blood pressure and boost the immune system, increase attention and focus and help with anxiety and depression, foster well-being and create less emotional reactivity, and change the brain in areas in charge of decision making, emotional flexibility, and empathy. Their affiliate program, Inner Kids, provides a mindfulness curriculum for K-12 education with the goal of cultivating more thoughtful, resilient, and empathetic children. Also, Emory University has created the Emory-Tibet Partnership and developed Cognitively Based Compassion Training (CBCT), a program that intentionally and systematically works to cultivate compassion for self and others. A recent study from researchers at Emory focused on foster kids (Reddy, Negi, Dodson-Lavelle et al., 2013) showing promising results in using CBCT in at risk populations.

In Chattanooga, Tennessee, people from various backgrounds including medicine, nursing, theology, social work, psychology, business, education, healing arts, and other professional and religious traditions created the Center for Mindful Living. This non-sectarian, non-profit organization serves the community through teaching mindfulness as a tool for living. Classes are offered in Kabat-Zinn's MBSR, Emory-Tibet's CBCT, Mindfulness in Schools, Mindful Eating, Meditation, Tai Ji, Yoga, Centering Prayer, and many other workshops and classes. The center has created programs for public schools in underserved areas of the community, offers mindfulness camp for kids, and works with local hospitals to create programs for cancer patients to learn to breathe during treatment. Outreach classes are also offered in the corporate/business setting (including some hospitals) as well to provide onsite meditation and yoga sessions with positive results.

Mindfulness can no longer be considered "fluff' or strictly a Buddhist practice. It has entered the mainstream based on rigorous scientific research and positive outcomes and should not be ignored by the traditional medical model of healthcare. Mindfulness is a tool for reducing the effects of trauma and, more importantly, teaching resilience at the earliest age as a prevention strategy for building healthy, mindful communities.

TRAUMA INFORMED OR FOCUSED COGNITIVE BEHAVIORAL THERAPY

Trauma-Focused Cognitive Behavioral Therapy (TF-CBT) is a model of psychotherapy that effectively combines trauma-sensitive interventions with cognitive behavioral therapy (Child Sexual Abuse Task Force and Research & Practice Core, 2004). Cognitive Behavior Therapy (CBT) was initially developed by Aaron Beck and others in the 1970's and has been shown to be a strong evidence-based modality to treat anxiety, depression (Beck, Rush, Shaw & Emery, 1979; Butler, Chapman, Forman & Beck, 2006; Wolitzky-Taylor, Zimmerman, Arch, De Guzman & Lagomasino, 2015), various personality disorders (Linehan, 1993), as well as Post Traumatic Stress Disorder (PTSD), especially when combined with other interventions (Mueser, Rosenberg, Xie et al., 2008; Foa, Keane, Friedman & Cohen, 2008).

CBT contends that specific exercises changing thinking and behavior can dramatically improve mood, personality and help persons better process trauma. For example, TF-CBT is designed to address the needs of children with Post Traumatic Stress Disorder (PTSD) or other significant behavioral problems related to traumatic life experiences (Child Sexual Abuse Task Force and Research & Practice Core, 2004). Core elements of effective TF-CBT for children include trauma assessment, utilizing cultural strengths, addressing safety, engagement, attachment and positive focus on the child-caregiver relationship, attention to the social context, trauma processing, consolidation and post-traumatic growth syndrome, therapist self-care and common core interventions (Strand, Hansen & Courtney, 2013). These common core interventions include psycho-education, parent training and developmental guidance, feeling identification, problem solving and social skills cognitive interventions, relaxation and stress reduction, and affective interventions along with creation and processing of the child's trauma narrative (Strand, Hansen & Courtney, 2013).

This treatment results in improvements in PTSD symptoms such as depression, anxiety, behavior problems, sexualized behaviors, trauma-related shame, interpersonal trust and social competence. It has been recognized by SAMHSA nationally (Elliott, Bjelajac, Fallot, Markoff & Reed, 2005) and by many state level behavioral health initiatives (e.g., Minnesota) as a useful intervention to be implemented at community scale. Likewise, trauma informed CBT has been used successfully in quasi-experimental trials to treat adults with co-occurring substance abuse issues (Morrissey, Ellis, Gatz, Amaro, Reed, Savage, Finkelstein, Mazelis, Brown, Jackson & Banks, 2005). Health systems (such as Memorial Hospital in South Bend, as described above) are increasingly interested in use of trauma informed CBT as a model that can be adopted to address issues resulting from ACEs, and prevent the impact of ACEs as described above.

EYE MOVEMENT DESENSITIZATION AND REPROCESSING (EMDR)

Eye Movement Desensitization and Reprocessing (EMDR) is a well-known, but often controversial, therapeutic modality that has been used in both outpatient and inpatient settings to treat Post-Traumatic Stress Disorder or PTSD. EMDR was developed by Francine Shapiro to reduce the effects of distressing memories by a multi-stage approach designed to help a patient more effectively process such memories and associated stimuli (Shapiro & Laliotis, 2010). Essentially, a patient is asked to recall distressing memories while receiving one of several types of bilateral sensory input from a practitioner, such as side-to-side eye movements (Feske, 1998). EMDR has been shown to be more beneficial than no treatment and is similar to trauma-informed cognitive behavior therapy (CBT) in helping persons with chronic PTSD (Bisson, Roberts, Andrew, Cooper & Lewis, 2013; Watts, Schnurr, Mayo, Young-Xu, Weeks & Friedman, 2013). EMDR requires extensive training of clinical professionals, but similar models to the intervention have been developed (e.g., Acute Trauma Incident Processing or A-TIP; Community Resiliency Model; Emotional Freedom Technique or EFT) that have been shown efficacious in clinical trials (Feinstein, 2012) and can be implemented at community scale by laypersons (see the EMDR and Other Hospital-Based Approaches for Mediating Adverse Childhood Experiences sidebar for more details).

COMMUNITY-BASED TRAININGS

In addition to traditional healthcare providers, we are also seeing more and more laypersons being pulled into the larger integrated care networks, as their skills in health literacy, cultural competency and holding implicit trust in community renders them essential players on the broader care team. SH also advocates that health systems provide wholesale and free training of community members/volunteers to build capacity for early recognition, screening, prevention, triage to traditional treatment, as well as enhanced self-management of behavioral health issues. The following trainings are available at community scale.

BETTER BRAINS FOR BABIES/BRAIN HEALTH THROUGH THE AGES

Better Brains for Babies is a community-based training designed to teach parents and other caregivers four strategies for stimulating and nurturing early brain development: touch, talk, read and play, as well as addressing how early neglect and trauma impacts brain development and physical and emotional well-being as children develop. Better Brains for Babies was developed by University of Georgia researchers (Bales, 2005) and further refined in work with the churches in Memphis, through The Urban Childhood Institute (TUCI). In collaboration with the Congregational Health Network, the training was further expanded to include healthy strategies for brain protection and enhancement through the lifespan, focusing on healthy exercise, nutrition, minimizing use of alcohol and abstaining from drugs, as well as other behavioral strategies for preventing dementia and tips for caregiving those with dementia. This training has been taught to over 100 persons in the Memphis area and has been well-received by younger persons, as well as the older generation, in terms of both early brain development and good brain health promotion strategies throughout the lifespan.

MENTAL HEALTH FIRST AID

In terms of Integrated Health at community scale, educational programs for lay persons, such as Mental Health First Aid are aimed at building community capacity to promote wellness and prevention, stigma reduction, skill development for helping managing acute episodes toward stability and appropriate professional or community support. Mental Health First Aid (MHFA) is a training designed to help lay persons navigate peers to traditional mental health services and resources. This eight-hour course teaches participants how to help someone who is developing a mental health problem or experiencing a mental health crisis, by identifying, understanding and responding to signs of mental illness or substance abuse problems (Kitchener & Jorm, 2008).

MHFA was created in 2001 by Betty Kitchener, a nurse specializing in health education, and Anthony Jorm, a mental health literacy professor. Kitchener and Jorm run Mental Health First Aid™ Australia, a national non-profit health promotion charity focused on training and research. This has now expanded to the US and 22 other countries under MHFA International (Mental Health First Aid website, 2015). ALGEE is the core training technique and mnemonic device that aids in retaining the information learned in MHFA.

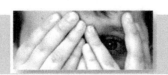

In 2012, with the completion of the mandated Community Health Needs Assessment, the Community Health Enhancement team of Memorial Hospital of South Bend became keenly aware of the community's concerns regarding the seemingly out-of-control Violence and Safety in the neighborhoods, as well as domestic and relationship violence.

The team began to seriously investigate the correlation between childhood adverse experiences (ACE) and the startling variety of mental and physical health diseases in adulthood. They took heart with the multiple professional sources that were consistent in stating childhood trauma need not plant and nourish the horrible projected destiny. They avidly consumed studies which developed a forecast of the potential for mediation and prevention. Two evidence-based interventions came to their attention, Resiliency and Eye Movement Desensitization and Reprocessing (EMDR); EMDR, developed by Frances Shapiro, is a psychotherapeutic approach to help cliental process traumatic experiences.

An informal poll of St. Joseph and Elkhart Counties, the two locations served by both Beacon Health System and the area's community mental health center, Oaklawn, suggested there were fewer than a half-dozen therapists trained in EMDR. The first initiative was pretty obvious: they needed EMDR trained therapists. Connecting with a therapist and EMDR trainer, to-date, they have provided training to more than 100 therapists, making this evidenced-based program widely available to their community.

Building upon the training for licensed therapists, they have also offered Acute Trauma Incident Processing (A-TIP) training which would include first responders, teachers, justice officers, adult Parks and Recreation program leaders, etc. With awareness comes a strong internal entreaty to make a difference, to intervene, to assist their children to succeed academically and socially; to increase the odds for a healthy future for themselves and their children. South Bend has found many opportunities to use the knowledge and training that is available, many of which are embedded in best practices. Among their first partners in preventing and treating the trauma was Youth Services Bureau, a safe shelter for homeless teens, the St. Joseph County Juvenile Justice Center; Memorial Hospital's regional, level II Trauma Center providing immediate intervention to stabilize the patient emotionally and subsequently physiologically. The Trauma Center also employs a well-respected gentleman from the community as the Community Trauma Liaison, providing a link for healing victims, families and the community. The South Bend Police Department has been a critical partner as they work to ameliorate violence in our neighborhoods.

Elkhart's law enforcement officers were trained in a communications/brain based program, "Policing the Teen Brain"; South Bend's Police Department will be immersed in the train-the-trainer model after the first of the year. They have presented the impact of ACE on children's brain development to parents at two urban parochial schools; in addition, the school counselor was trained in EMDR. Immediately, parents besieged the team asking for training for them to assist their children in dealing with trauma. They are researching possibilities and in conversation with professionals. A presentation to an alternative school's teachers and principal evolved into a seven-week course for the students, ages 16 to 21.

From February 2016, Memorial partnered with local agencies and organizations to host the PBS series on childhood in America, including "Healing the Wounds." Another colleague is investigating funding opportunities to bring "Paper Tigers," a documentary about ACEs, to the area. Memorial was part of a research study being conducted at the University of Notre Dame, measuring the impact of the 400 subject/mothers trauma experiences on the birth outcome and the first six-months of the infants' life development. Accrual and intervention has been completed; this cutting-edge research is in the analysis stage before submission for publication.

Two additional expansions for next year include the train-the-trainer workshops, "ACE Interface," with Dr. Rob Anda and Laura Porter. This training is currently scheduled for South Bend; however, a grant submission is being prepared to replicate the training in Elkhart. The community health team will also be developing a series of programs which will be geared toward different audiences, from an intention of raising awareness, to becoming a change agent for children, parents and organizations providing services to our vulnerable children.

An indicator of success might be when other groups begin to own the concept and bring it to children and parents in the agencies from which they serve. Key service agencies in Elkhart and St. Joseph County have coalesced to transform shared interests into a community-wide organization based upon trauma-informed-care. The University of Notre Dame invited Dr. Bruce Perry, pediatric psychiatrist and author *The Boy Who Was Raised As A Dog* and *Born to Love*, to play a key role in an academic symposia on child development. They have been blessed by the early work of many pioneers who began the research and continue to validate the implications of trauma and health. South Bend, St. Joseph County, Elkhart, Elkhart County are opening their eyes and hearts to serve their beloved communities.

Assess for risk of suicide or harm

Listen nonjudgmentally

Give reassurance and information

Encourage appropriate professional help

Encourage self-help and other support strategies

Mental Health First Aid USA is listed in the Substance Abuse and Mental Health Services Administration (SAMHSA)'s National Registry of Evidence-based Programs and Practices. The SAMHSA Intervention Summary for MHFA suggests that the training (intervention) was useful in building knowledge and confidence in interacting with and providing help to, persons with mental illness and substance abuse problems and decreasing sense of social distance from those with such illnesses (SAMHSA National Register of Evidence-based Programs and Practices, 2015). Several states and groups have adopted large scale MHFA training to improve community capacity to respond to and help persons with mental illness and substance abuse problems, building a stronger safety net. For example, North Carolina's Dept. of Health and Human Services along with SAMHSA funding, has trained almost 12,000 persons in MHFA since 2008.

FAITH COMMUNITY EFFORTS

Increasingly faith communities are providing support groups and educational programs for grief and other life transitions. Likewise, faith leaders often serve as front line responders for behavioral health issues. Many people will go to their pastor, priest, rabbi, cleric, shaman, or lay leader for help in understanding and managing distress (chronic and acute) in their lives before seeking other professional resources. Programs to train and support faith leaders in this role are evolving rapidly, although seminaries, divinity schools and other theological training programs have included pastoral care or counseling techniques in the curriculum for decades. In 2016 the American Psychiatric Association published *Mental Health: A Guide for Faith Leaders*, a booklet and quick reference guide for understanding, managing, and referral sources for mental health issues.

Additionally, laypersons are now being seen and trained as critical parts of this Integrated Health system. For example, Stephens Ministries, a program designed to equip and empower lay caregivers, has trained over 600,000 Stephens Ministers since 1975, who provide high-quality, confidential care to people who are hurting, from the Christian perspective (Stephens Ministries website, 2015).

Community Scale Screening and Assessment: Population Health Management Tools

In terms of solutions to behavioral health issues, Stakeholder Health holds a core belief that communities can partner more intentionally with health systems to improve overall health and well-being within the broad integrated health view described above. One mechanism to achieve this is to train and engage laypersons in the use of screening and assessment tools now being used in population health management efforts across health systems and in community mental health settings. Just as Mental Health First Aid training expands the broader knowledge of how to deal more appropriately with mental illness and substance abuse, these screening tools help to better integrate the work of community-based peers and laypersons working in their churches and organizations with that of traditional mental health practitioners and organizations. The more familiarity the public has with these tools, the more they can partner to help detect problems in peers and family members and thus broaden the community safety net to prevent intra-personal and inter-personal harm and violence at all levels. Below we describe briefly some commonly used tools, with links to their access. All of the tools discussed in this section are available in Appendix 2.

TAKE AN ACE HISTORY: NOTICE AND ASK ABOUT TRAUMA

A critical first step in moving toward resilience may be as simple as asking people about their experience. Following up from the ACE study, Kaiser Permanente began taking an ACE history for each of their patients in their outpatient clinics. When respondents answered "yes" to one of the questions on the ACE tool, the provider simply said, "I see that you have experienced …. Tell me how that has affected you later in your life." Simply asking the question, taking it seriously and responding in a compassionate way had a measurable impact on use of health care resources. Over a two-year period with 100,000 patients, when practitioners used this approach, an independent study showed a 35% reduction in doctor office visits (DOVs) in the year subsequent to evaluation, compared to the year before. Additionally, analysis showed an 11% reduction in Emergency Department (ED) visits and a 3% reduction in hospitalizations. Even though the question was asked and recorded in the medical record, practitioners did not usually continue to address the issues in subsequent visits. Just asking the question and recognizing that it had an impact on the person seemed to have a positive impact. Interestingly, however, these benefits did not last beyond the first year, so additional follow up and treatment is certainly also necessary (Felitti & Anda, 2009).

SBIRT AND AUDIT

Trauma and substance abuse scales can be used by trained laypersons to determine what kind of extra support a person might need. For example, *SBIRT – Screening, Brief Intervention, Referral to Treatment –* is a comprehensive, public health approach to the delivery of early intervention and treatment services for persons with substance use disorders, as well as those at risk of developing these disorders." As indicated by the acronym, there are three distinct phases to SBIRT:

• Screening can assess the severity of substance use, dependence and abuse at hopefully early stages of the game, identifying appropriate levels of treatment.

• Brief intervention offers the possibility of behavior change by raising awareness of personal practices and their consequences. In addition to psycho-education, Motivational Interviewing is a primary tool utilized in this phase to invite behavior change as indicated.

• Referral to treatment is the methodology offered to those with more severe addiction (or potential addiction) issues, again with a goal of intervening as early in the process as possible with the appropriate level of care.

Tools used in SBIRT include the AUDIT and NIAAA Low Risk Drinking Guidelines. The AUDIT (*Alcohol Use Disorders Identification Test*), developed by the World Health Organization in 1982, is a brief 10-question addendum to SBIRT used in many primary care settings to identify those who are at risk of excessive alcohol use. It is available in English, Japanese, Spanish, and Slovenian (www.who.int/substance_abuse/ activities/sbi/en). The AUDIT-C is a modified version of the 10-question AUDIT instrument that can reliably identify patients who are hazardous drinkers or who have active alcohol use disorders. A score of 4 for males or 3 for females is considered positive, indicating need for further conversation or possible intervention. Similarly, the National Institute on Alcohol Abuse and Alcoholism (NIAAA) Low Risk Drinking Guidelines are short questions designed to determine if a person's drinking patterns put them at risk in terms of health.

Two scales for assessing depression and anxiety at population levels, the Personal Health Questionnaire-9 (PHQ-9) and Generalized Anxiety Disorder-7 (GAD-7), were developed by Spitzer and colleagues as part of the PRIME-MD study, for assessment efforts in primary care and other settings (Spitzer, Williams, Kroenke, Linzer, deGruy, Hahn, Brody & Johnson, 1994; Spitzer, Williams & Kroenke 2000; Kroenke, Spitzer & Williams, 2001; Kroeneke & Spitzer, 2002).

The PHQ-9 is now widely emerging as a gold standard tool for screening for depression and has been embedded in many health system electronic medical records. It starts with items 1 and 2 (PHQ-2) which, if scored above 3 points, suggests a need for use of the whole 9 item scale (free at the website noted for AUDIT above, along with an instruction manual). Scores and actions appropriate to depression levels suggested by scores are found in the instruction manual in Table 1, and all tools and scoring are public domain, courtesy of Pfizer.

PHQ-9 Scores and Proposed Treatment Actions suggest that a score of 0-4 indicates None-minimal action; a score of 5-9 indicates Mild Watchful waiting and repeat PHQ-9 at follow-up; a score of 10-14 indicates a Moderate Treatment plan, considering counseling, follow-up and/or pharmacotherapy; a score of 15-19 suggests Moderately Severe Active treatment with pharmacotherapy and/or psychotherapy; while a score of 20-27 suggests Severe levels, with Immediate initiation of pharmacotherapy and, if severe impairment or poor response to therapy, expedited referral to a mental health specialist for psychotherapy and/or collaborative management (Kroenke & Spitzer, 2002).

GENERALIZED ANXIETY DISORDER-7

The Generalized Anxiety Disorder-7 is a similar brief screening tool that can also be administered by lay persons to discern whether more follow up is needed. As with the PHQ-9, scores above 3 suggest the need to administer the full seven items and take further action to prevent more problems secondary to anxiety symptoms.

Conclusion

At The Center for Faith and Community Health Transformation, an initiative in Chicago that works with faith communities to advance health equity by drawing on the unique spiritual power that resides in the practices and commitments of their faith, one of the core organizing principles is the interplay between hurt and hope. The idea is that we find our resilience both when fully engaged with trauma (or challenge) and when exercising our capacities to find meaning and purpose, experience kindness and loving relationships, and heal and be healthy. Our experience as individuals and as communities is that we are always living at the intersection of challenge and hope. The power for transformational change comes when we are aware of both and integrate both perspectives into our identity.

For example, many in the African-American community experience the deep and enduring impact of historical trauma, yet in countless African American churches across the nation, hope and love nevertheless prevail. This reality has been a constant for centuries, all the way back to the origins of African American spirituals—songs of hope sung during times of persecution and despair. The message was enlarged in 1956 by Dr. Martin Luther King who said on the night his home was bombed, "We must love our white brothers no matter what they do to us. We must make them know that we love them. Jesus still cries out in words that echo across the centuries: 'Love your enemies; Bless them that curse you; pray for them that despitefully use you.' ... We must meet hate with love." This speech inspired the non-violent approach to Civil Rights protests in the South. This model of resilience is seen today in the response by the members of the Emanuel African Methodist Episcopal Church in Charleston to the horrible shootings that took place there in June of 2015. As CNN reported in an online news story, the Reverend Norvel Goff told the congregation, "Lots of folks expected us to do something strange and break out in a riot. Well, they just don't know us. God shows how to love our neighbors as we love ourselves." Many of the family members of the victims offered forgiveness directly to the shooter in court, and the son of Sharonda Coleman-Singleton, one of the victims said, "Love is always stronger than hate," echoing Dr. King's message almost 60 years later (Capelouto, Shoichet & Savidge, 2015).

This example may seem distant from the medical concerns of health care systems, but it is not. People in our hospitals and clinics are experiencing this kind of reality every day—crisis, abuse, discrimination, violence, life-threatening illness, social isolation—and meeting it with hope that comes out of deep faith commitment, personal values, fearless love and a capacity for unimaginable grace. Our patients and families come to us with experiences of trauma and stress—personal, community and historical. But they also come with the capacity to be resilient in the face of difficulty. We know that these realities impact the physical, mental and spiritual health of the people we serve. One of the most important things we can do as health care providers is simply to notice this larger context and, with the patient or with the community, recognize how it is functioning in their lives. Science is with us on this, ready to make a difference for our patients and for our communities, and helping our health care ministries and/ or mission driven initiatives thrive as well.

REFERENCES

Agency for Healthcare Research and Quality (AHRQ). (2010). Mental Disorders and/or Substance Abuse Related to One of Every Eight Emergency Department Cases. *AHRQ News and Numbers*, July 8. Rockville, MD. Retrieved from http://www.ahrq.gov/news/nn/nn070810.htm.

Anda, R. F. & Brown, D. W. (2010). *Adverse Childhood Experiences & Population Health in Washington: The Face of a Chronic Public Health Disaster.* Prepared for the Washington State Family Policy Council.

American Psychological Association. The road to resilience. (2015). Retrieved from http://www.apa.org/helpcenter/road-resilience.aspx.

Baillargeon, J., Thomas, C.R., Williams, B. et al. (2008). Emergency department utilization patterns among uninsured patients with psychiatric disorders. *Psychiatric Services.* 59: 808–811.

Bales, D. W. (2005). Sharing the message about early brain development: Georgia's Better Brains for Babies collaboration. *Forum for Family and Consumer Issues*, 10. Retrieved from http://www.ces.ncsu.edu/depts/fcs/pub/10_2/pa3.html.

Beck A., Rush A.J., Shaw, B.F. & Emery, G. (1979). *Cognitive Behavior Therapy.* New York: The Guilford Press.

Bisognano, M., Kenney, C. (2012) *Pursuing the Triple Aim: Seven Innovators Show the Way to Better Care, Better Health, and Lower Costs.* San Francisco: Jossey-Bass Publishers.

Bisson, J., Roberts, N.P., Andrew M., Cooper R. & Lewis C. (2013). Psychological therapies for chronic post-traumatic stress disorder (PTSD) in adults. *Cochrane Database of Systematic Reviews. 12: CD003388.*

Blair, C. & Raver, C.C. (2012). Child development in the context of adversity: Experiential canalization of brain and behavior. *American Psychologist.* 67: 309-318.

Blue, B. (2013) Childhood Trauma Leaves Legacy of Brain Changes: Painful experiences early in life can alter the brain in lasting ways. *TIME.* January 16.

Brown, D.W., Anda, R.F., Tiemeier, H., Felitti, V.J., Edwards, V.J., Croft, J.B. & Giles, W.H. (2009). Adverse childhood experiences and the risk of premature mortality. *Am J Prev Med.* Nov. 37(5):389-96.

Butler, A.C., Chapman, J.E., Forman, E.M. & Beck, A.T. (2006). The empirical status of cognitive-behavioral therapy: A review of meta-analyses. *Clinical Psychology Review*, 26 (1): 17-31.

Capelouto, S.; Shoichet, C. & Savidge, M. (June 21, 2015) Charleston Minister: "No evildoer, no demon" can close the church. *CNN.* Retrieved from http://www.cnn.com/2015/06/21/us/charleston-church-shooting-main/.

Centers for Disease Control and Prevention. Morbidity and Mortality Weekly. (2013). Emergency Department Visits by Patients with Mental Health Disorders—North Carolina, 2008–2010, 62 (23): 469-472.

Centers for Disease Control and Prevention. Injury Prevention & Control: Division of Violence Prevention. (2014) Retrieved from http://www.cdc.gov/violenceprevention/acestudy/.

Charuvastra, A. & Cloitre, M. (2008). Social Bonds and Posttraumatic Stress Disorder. *Annual Review of Psychology.* 59: 301–328.

Child Sexual Abuse Task Force and Research & Practice Core, National Child Traumatic Stress Network. (2004). *How to Implement Trauma-Focused Cognitive Behavioral Therapy. Durham, NC and Los Angeles, CA: National Center for Child Traumatic Stress.*

Chiles, J. A., Lambert, M. J. & Hatch, A. L. (1999). The Impact of Psychological Interventions on Medical Cost Offset: A Meta-analytic Review. *Clinical Psychology: Science and Practice*, 6: 204–220.

Collins C., Hewson D.L., Munger R. & Wade T. (2010). Evolving Models of Behavioral Health Integration in Primary Care, Milbank Memorial Fund, http://www.milbank.org/reports/10430EvolvingCare/EvolvingCare.pdf.

Danese, A., DeBellis, M.D., & Teicher, A. (2015). Biological Effects of ACEs. *Academy on Violence and Abuse (AVA)*. Retrieved from http://www.avahealth.org/aces_best_practices/biological-impacts.html.

Danieli, Y. (Ed.) (1998). *International Handbook of Multigenerational Legacies of Trauma*. New York: Plenum Press.

Davidson, R. J., Kabat-Zinn, J., Schumacher, J., Rosenkranz, M. A., Muller, D., Santorelli, S. F., Urbanowski, F., Harrington, A., Bonus, K., & Sheridan, J. F. (2003). Alterations in brain and immune function produced by mindfulness meditation. *Psychosomatic Medicine*, 65: 564-570.

Davidson, R. J. & McEwen, B. S. (2012). Social influences on neuroplasticity: Stress and interventions to promote well-being. *Nature Neuroscience*, 15(5): 689-95.

Dias, B.G. & Ressler, K.J. (2014). Parental olfactory experience influences behavior and neural structure in subsequent generations, *Nature Neuroscience*. 17: 89–96.

Dickey, B. & Azeni, H. (1996). Persons with Dual Diagnoses of Substance Abuse and Major Mental Illness: Their Excess Costs of Psychiatric Care. *American Journal of Public Health*, 86(7): 973-77.

Dube, S., Felitti, V., Dong, M., Chapman, D., Giles, W. & Anda, R. (2003). Childhood Abuse, Neglect, and Household Dysfunction and the Risk of Illicit Drug Use: The Adverse Childhood Experiences Study. *Pediatrics,* 111 (3), March.

Elliott, D. E., Bjelajac, P., Fallot, R. D., Markoff, L. S. & Reed, B. G. (2005). Trauma-informed or trauma-denied: Principles and implementation of trauma-informed services for women. *Journal of Community Psychology*, 33:461–477.

Engel, G. (1977). The Need for a New Medical Model: A Challenge for Biomedicine. *Science* 196(4286): 129-36.

Fanga, X., Brown, D.S., Florencea, C.S., & Mercy, J.A. (2012). The economic burden of child maltreatment in the United States and implications for prevention. *Child Abuse & Neglect,* 36(2): 156–165.

Feinstein, D. (2012). Acupoint stimulation in treating psychological disorders: Evidence of efficacy. *Review of General Psychology*, 16(4), 364-380.

Felitti, V., Anda, R., Nordenberg, D., Williamson, D., Spitz, A., Edwards, V., Koss, M., & Marks, J. (1998). Relationship of Childhood Abuse and Household Dysfunction to Many of the Leading Causes of Death in Adults The Adverse Childhood Experiences (ACE) Study. *American Journal of Preventive Medicine*. 14(4): 245-258.

Felitti, V. (2002). The Relationship of Adverse Childhood Experiences to Adult Health: Turning gold into lead. *Z Psychsom Med Psychother*. 48(4): 359-369.

Felitti, V. & Anda, R. (2009). The Relationship of Adverse Childhood Experiences to Adult Medical Disease, Psychiatric Disorders, and Sexual Behavior: Implications for Healthcare in *The Hidden Epidemic: The Impact of Early Life Trauma on Health and Disease*. Lanius R & Vermetten E, editors. Cambridge University Press.

Feske, U. (1998). "Eye movement desensitization and reprocessing treatment for posttraumatic stress disorder. *Clinical Psychology: Science and Practice 5 (2): 171–181.*

Findings from the Philadelphia Urban ACE Survey. (2013). Prepared for Institute for Safe Families by The Research and Evaluation Group at Public Health Management Corporation, 260 S. Broad St., Philadelphia, PA. September 18.

Foa, E.B., Keane, T.M., Friedman, M.J. & Cohen, J.A. (2008). *Effective Treatments for PTSD, Second Edition: Practice Guidelines from the International Society for Traumatic Stress Studies*. New York: The Guilford Press.

Hodas, G.R. (2006). *Responding to childhood trauma: The promise and practice of trauma informed care*. Pennsylvania Office of Mental Health and Substance Abuse Services. February.

Insel, T.R. (2008). Assessing the economic costs of serious mental illness. *American Journal of Psychiatry*. 165(6):703-711. PMID: 18519528.

Institute of Medicine (IOM) (2009). *Preventing Mental, Emotional, Behavioral Disorders Among Young People: Progress and Possibilities*. Rockville, MD.

Institute of Medicine (IOM) (2012). *The Mental-Health and Substance Use Workforce for Older Adults*. Rockville, MD.

Kabat-Zinn, J. (1994). *Wherever you go, there you are*. New York: Hyperion.

King, M.L., Jr. (1958). *Stride Toward Freedom: The Montgomery Story*, New York: Harper and Brothers.

Kitchener, B.A. & Jorm, A.F. (2008). Mental health first aid: An international programme for early intervention. *Early Intervention in Psychiatry,* 2:55-61.

Kroenke, K., Spitzer, R.L., Williams, J.B.W. (2001). The PHQ-9: Validity of a brief depression severity measure. *Journal of General Internal Medicine*, 16:606-613.

Kroenke, K. & Spitzer, R.L. (2002*).* The PHQ-9: A New Depression Diagnostic and Severity Measure. *Psychiatric Annals*, 32:509-521.

Kuyken, W., Weare, K., Ukoumunne, O.C., Vicary, R., Motton, N.,Burnett, C., Hennelly, S., & Huppert, F. (2013). Effectiveness of the Mindfulness in Schools Programme: non-randomised controlled feasibility Study. *The British Journal of Psychiatry*, 1-6.

Laurence, L. (2013). Improving Patient Outcomes: The Medical Cost-Onset Effect & Value of Psychological Services. Keynote presentation at the Tennessee Psychological Association annual conference, November, Nashville, TN.

Liebenberg, L., Ungar, M., & LeBlanc, J. C. (2013). The CYRM-12: A brief measure of resilience. Canadian Journal of Public Health, 104(2): 131-135.

Linehan, M. (1993). *Cognitive-Behavioral Treatment of Borderline Personality Disorder*. New York: The Guilford Press.

Lutz, A., Greischar, L., Rawlings, N. B., Ricard, M., & Davidson, R. J. (2004). Long-term meditators self-induce high-amplitude synchrony during mental practice. *Proceedings of the National Academy of Sciences*, 101: 16369-16373.

Lutz, A., Slagter, H. A., Dunne, J., & Davidson, R. J. (2008). Attention regulation and monitoring in meditation. *Trends in Cognitive Sciences*. 12(4): 163-169.

Maine Resiliency Building Network. (2015). Retrieved from http://www.maineaces.org.

Mark, T., Levit, K., Coffey, R., McKusick, D., Harwood, H., King, E., Bouchery, E., Genuardi, J., Vandivort-Warren, R., Buck, J., & Ryan, K. (2007). National Expenditures for Mental Health Services and Substance Abuse Treatment, 1993–2003, *SAMHSA publication number SMA 07-4227*. Rockville, MD: Substance Abuse and Mental Health Services Administration.

Márquez C, Poirier GL, Cordero MI, Larsen MH, Groner A, Marquis J, Magistretti PJ, Trono D, and Sandi C. (2013). Peripuberty stress leads to abnormal aggression, altered amygdala and orbitofrontal reactivity and increased prefrontal MAOA gene expression. *Translational Psychiatry*. Jan. 3(1): e216.

Mayo Clinic. (n.d.). Resilience: Build Skills to Endure Hardship. Retrived from http://www.mayoclinic.org/tests-procedures/resilience-training/in-depth/resilience/art-20046311.

McGinnis, J.M. and Foege, W.H. (1993). Actual causes of death in the United States. *JAMA*. 270:2207-2212

Mokdad, A., Marks, J., Stroup, D., Gerberding, J. (2004). Actual Causes of Death in the United States--2000. *JAMA*. 291(10):1238-1245.

Morrissey, J.P., Ellis, A.R., Gatz, M., Amaro, H., Reed, B.G., Savage, A., Finkelstein, N., Mazelis, R., Brown, V., Jackson, E.W. & Banks, S. (2005). *Journal of Substance Abuse Treatment. 28(2):121-33.*

McGinnis J.M., Williams-Ruso P., Knickman J.R. (2002). The case for more active policy attention to health promotion. *Health Affairs*, 21(2):78-93.

Mueser, K. T., Rosenberg, S. D., Xie, H., Jankowski, M. K., Bolton, E. E., Lu, W., & Wolfe, R. (2008). A Randomized Controlled Trial of Cognitive-Behavioral Treatment of Posttraumatic Stress Disorder in Severe Mental Illness. *Journal of Consulting and Clinical Psychology*, 76(2): 259–271.

Muñoz, R. F., Beardslee, W. R., & Leykin, Y. (2012). Major Depression Can Be Prevented. *The American Psychologist*, 67(4): 285–295.

Ozbay F, Johnson DC, Dimoulas E, Morgan CA, Charney D, Southwick S. (2007). Social support and resilience to stress: from neurobiology to clinical practice. *Psychiatry (Edgmont).* May 4(5):35-40.

Rodak, S. (2013). 100 Integrated Health Systems to Know. Becker's Hospital Review, May 15, 2013; retrieved from http://www.beckershospitalreview.com/lists/100-integrated-health-systems-to-know.html.

Reddy, S.D., Negi, L. T., Dodson-Lavelle, B., Ozawa-de Silva, B., Pace, T.W.W, Cole, S.P., Raison, C.L., & Craighead, L.W. (2013). Cognitive-Based Compassion Training: A Promising Prevention Strategy for At-Risk Adolescents. *Journal of Child and Family Studies.* 22: 219–230.

Reivich K., & Shatté A. (2002). *The Resilience Factor*. New York: Broadway Books.

Resilience Trumps ACEs. (2015). Children's Resilience Initiative. Retrieved from www.resiliencetrumpsaces.org.

Saraceno B. & Barbui, C. (1997). Poverty and Mental Illness. *Canadian Journal of Psychiatry*, 42(3): 285-290.

Salinsky, E., & Loftis, C. (2007). Shrinking Inpatient Psychiatric Capacity: Cause for Celebration or Concern? *National Health Policy Forum, Issues Brief 823: 1-21*, George Washington University, Washington, DC.

Shapiro, F. & Laliotis, D. (2010). "EMDR and the adaptive information processing model: Integrative treatment and case conceptualization." *Clinical Social Work Journal* 39 (2): 191–200.

Sherin, J. & Nemeroff, C. (2011). Post-traumatic stress disorder: the neurobiological impact of psychological trauma. *Dialogues in Clinical NeuroSciences*. September; 13(3): 263–278.

Shonkoff, J.P., Garner, A.S., Siegel, B.S., Dobbins, M.I., Earls, M.F., Garner, A.S., McGuinn, L., Pascoe, J., & Wood, D.L. (2012). The Lifelong Effects of Early Childhood Adversity and Toxic Stress. *Pediatrics*. Jan; 129(1): e232-e246.

Soni, Anita. (2009). *The Five Most Costly Conditions, 1996 and 2006: Estimates for the U.S. Civilian Noninstitutionalized Population*. Statistical Brief #248. Agency for Healthcare Research and Quality, Rockville, MD. http://www.meps.ahrq.gov/mepsweb/data_files/publications/st248/stat248.pdf .

Sotero, M. (2006). A Conceptual Model of Historical Trauma: Implications for Public Health Practice and Research. *Journal of Health Disparities Research and Practice*, Fall 1 (1): 93–108.

Spitzer, R.L., Williams, J.B.W., Kroenke, K., Linzer, M., deGruy, F.V., Hahn, S.R., Brody, D., Johnson, J.G. (1994). Utility of a new procedure for diagnosing mental disorders in primary care: The PRIME-MD 1000 study. *JAMA*, 272:1749-1756.

Spitzer R.L., Kroenke K., Williams J.B.W. and the Patient Health Questionnaire Primary Care Study Group. (1999). Validation and utility of a self-report version of PRIME-MD: the PHQ Primary Care Study. *JAMA*, 282 (3):1737-1744.

Spitzer R.L., Williams J.B.W. & Kroenke K. (2000). Validity and utility of the Patient Health Questionnaire in assessment of 3000 obstetrics-gynecologic patients. *Am J Obstet Gynecol*, 183(4):759-769.

Stephen Ministries. (2015). Stephen Ministry by the Numbers. Retrieved from Stephen's Ministries website, at https://www.stephenministries.org/stephenministry/default.cfm/917.

Strand, V., Hansen. S. & Courtney, D. (2013). Common Elements Across Evidence-Based Trauma Treatment: Discovery and Implications. *Advances in Social Work*, Fall 14(2): 334-354.

SAMHSA Primary Care and Behavioral Care Integration (PBHCI) Program. Retrieved from http://www.integration.samhsa.gov/about-us/pbhci.

SAMHSA National Register of Evidence-based Programs and Practices. (2015). Retrieved from http://nrepp.samhsa.gov/ViewIntervention.aspx?id=321.

Substance Abuse and Mental Health Services Administration. SAMHSA's Concept of Trauma and Guidance for a Trauma-Informed Approach. (2014). *HHS Publication No. (SMA) 14-4884*. Rockville, MD: Substance Abuse and Mental Health Services Administration.

Substance Abuse and Mental Health Services Administration, (2014). Results from the 2013 National Survey on Drug Use and Health: Mental Health Findings, NSDUH Series H-49. *HHS Publication No. (SMA) 14-4887*. Rockville, MD: Substance Abuse and Mental Health Services Administration.

Tang, N., Stein, J., Hsia, R.Y., Maselli, J.H., & Gonzales, R. (2010). Trends and characteristics of US emergency department visits, 1997-2007. *JAMA*, 304(6): 664-70.

The Philadelphia Urban ACE Study. (2013). Retrieved from http://www.instituteforsafefamilies.org/philadelphia-urban-ace-study .

Ungar, M. (2013). Family Resilience and At-Risk Youth. In D. Becvar (Ed.), *Handbook of Family Resilience.* New York, NY: Springer.

Watts, B.V., Schnurr, P.P., Mayo, L., Young-Xu, Y., Weeks, W.B., & Friedman, M.J. (2013). "Meta-analysis of the efficacy of treatments for posttraumatic stress disorder". *Journal of Clinical Psychiatry 4 (6): e541–550.*

Wolitzky-Taylor K., Zimmermann M., Arch J.J., De Guzman E., & Lagomasino, I. (2015). Has evidence-based psychosocial treatment for anxiety disorders permeated usual care in community mental health settings? *Behaviour Research and Therapy*, 72: 9-17.

World Council of Churches. (2007). Consultation on Mental Health and Faith Communities, Vellore, India: Christian Medical College. Available at www.arhap.uct.za.

World Health Organization. (2001). *World Health Report —WHO Mental Health: New Understanding*, New Hope, Geneva.

World Health Organization (2007). Breaking the Vicious Cycle between Mental Ill-Health and Poverty. Geneva. Retrieved from (http://www.who.int/mental_health/policy/development/en/index.html.)

Yoshikawa, H., Aber, J.L., & Beardslee, W.R. (2012). Poverty and the mental, emotional and behavioral health of children and youth: Implications for prevention science. American Psychologist, 67: 272-284.

ACKNOWLEDGMENTS

We wish to thank Minister Dianne Young for vetting the sidebar written about The Emotional Fitness Center, as well as Dr. Thom Bornemann of the Carter Center Mental Health Program, for use of his PowerPoint presentation slides.

FULL AUTHORSHIP LISTING

Kirsten Peachey, MDiv, MSW, DMin, Director, Congregational Health Partnerships and Co-Director, The Center for Faith and Community Health Transformation, Advocate Health Care, Chicago, IL

Teresa Cutts, PhD, Asst. Research Professor, Wake Forest School of Medicine, Div. of Public Health Science, Dept. of Social Sciences and Health Policy, Winston Salem, NC

Margo DeMont, Ph.D., M.Ed., L.C.S.W., Executive Director of Community Health Enhancement, Community Hospital, South Bend, Indiana

Dory Lawrence, M.A., Brain Health Educator, Memorial BrainWorks, Beacon Health System, South Bend and Elkhart, Indiana

Bryan Hatcher, LCSW, MDiv, Chief Operating Officer, CareNet, Wake Forest Baptist Medical Cener, Winston Salem, NC

Jane Berz, MSN, Breast Center Consultations, Catholic Health Initiatives, Chattanooga, TN

Lance Laurence, PhD, Adjunct Professor, University of Tennessee, Knoxville, Knoxville, TN

For more information about this chapter, contact **Kirsten Peachey** at e-mail, kirsten.peachey@advocatehealth.com or phone, (630) 929-6107.

CHAPTER 8

Financial Accounting that Produces Health

Kevin Barnett with Teresa Cutts and Jeremy Moseley

Overview

In 1948, the United Nations approved the Universal Declaration of Human Rights, Article 25 that states "Everyone has the right to a standard of living adequate for the health and well-being of himself and of his family, including food, clothing, housing, medical care, and necessary social services" (United Nations, 1948). The establishment of health as a basic human right would appear to position it beyond economic considerations, but the practical reality is that governments and others make daily decisions about systems of taxation, economic incentives, and allocation of resources that directly impact the health and well-being of individuals, families, and populations.

As the wealthiest nation on the planet, one committed to the idea of minimally regulated capitalism, we are engaged in a perpetual struggle between two versions of reality. On one hand, we see ourselves through a lens of what some would refer to as a delusion of rugged individualism, where we are the masters of our own destiny, and all who work hard and play by the rules will succeed. A more sober analysis leads us to recognize that there are winners and losers in our capitalist enterprise, and there is a need for investment of resources to provide support and/or create opportunities for those who may be less fortunate or capable of providing for themselves. While providing this support may be viewed as essential in an advanced society, determining what forms, how much, and when to provide it calls for an assessment of costs and the associated returns on these investments.

What we are learning, and will discuss in this chapter, is the fact that inadequate investment in addressing the social determinants of health often results in more costly negative outcomes. This is so whether we are talking about a lack of investment in disease prevention that then yields high acuity and costly inpatient care for preventable chronic conditions, or about a lack of investment in early childhood education which contributes to higher costs for special education in the medium term and higher rates of incarceration over the long term. In this context, the driving motivation may be a commitment to make better business investments at the societal level.

At present, the U.S. ranks last among 11 peer countries on dimensions of access, efficiency, and health care equity (David, Stremikis & Shoen, 2014). Whereas Organization for Economic Cooperation and Development countries (OECD) spend an average of $2 on social services for every $1 spent on health care, the United States spends 60 cents (Bradley & Taylor, 2013). Table I highlights the disparity, which is driven at least in part by higher per capita costs for health care. For example, while the U.S. has shorter lengths of stay in hospitals and fewer discharges per 1000 people, spending per discharge in 2009 was $18,142, compared to $11,112 in Denmark, $5,204 in France, and $5,072 in Germany. In addition, prices for drugs in the U.S. are one third higher than in Canada and Germany, and double what is spent in Australia, France, and the U.K. (Squires, 2012).

There are multiple factors driving the disparity in health care and social service expenditures between the U.S. and other developed nations. In some cases, we have chosen to charge more on a per capita basis for the same goods and services than other countries; in others, we have decided that regardless of our assets, we do not focus on providing affordable childcare, education, housing, and transportation at the level that matches other economically advanced countries. It is unavoidable that these decisions made in the public and private sector impact health and well-being at the family, community, and societal level.

In this chapter, we'll first summarize current dynamics and emerging trends in the context of health reform with a focus on implications in the shift from fee-for-service to value-based reimbursement. Next we'll discuss how the history and legacy of discrimination has created pockets of extreme poverty, social dysfunction, and persistent health problems in communities across the country. These geographic concentrations of economic, social, and health inequities highlight the need for focused attention and investment not just by health care organizations but by a broad spectrum of stakeholders across sectors in order to produce meaningful and sustainable improvement. This may be one of the most significant challenges we face in building a healthy society in the coming years.

We will then review the emerging focus on comprehensive approaches to health improvement that leverage the resources of the health and community development sectors. We'll also explore the emerging roles of employers as potential partners in health production, touching on some of the most innovative practices and outcomes to date. Finally, we close the chapter by sharing sample innovative practices of Stakeholder Health members that build systems to support and reinforce an ethic of shared ownership for health with the broader community.

Health vs. Social Services Expenditures in Industrialized Countries: U.S. Priorities Are the Outlier

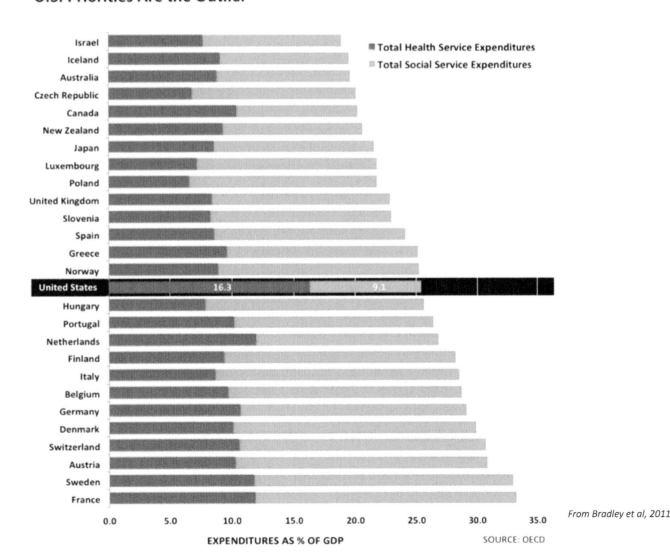

From Bradley et al, 2011

SOURCE: OECD

Health Care Financing in Context: Considering the Challenges

Fee-for-service (FFS) reimbursement has been the predominant form of payment for health care in the 20th and the 21st Centuries. This form of payment rewards the producers of increasingly costly procedures, equipment, pharmaceuticals, and facilities for treatment of illnesses (many of which are preventable). Not only has the capital necessary to finance this medical care juggernaut been allocated at the expense of investments in the leading causes of life, but it has also contributed to an erosion in the profitability of other economic sectors.

In the face of the continued escalation of costs in recent decades, health care leaders increasingly recognize that the FFS model is unsustainable. The passage of the Affordable Care Act (ACA) has put into play an incremental series of changes that are gradually but inexorably moving us towards what is currently referred to as "pay for value," a generalized term that is intended to communicate a shift in financial incentives away from conducting procedures and filling beds and towards keeping people healthy and out of clinical care settings. We used to call this form of payment capitation, until that term became associated with the practices of some insurers in the 1990s when care "gatekeepers" focused more on limiting access to specialty services than proactively managing care (i.e., with an emphasis on prevention).

Examples of incremental steps in the evolution to a "pay for value" system have included, but are not limited to, "bundling" payments for sets of procedures for a particular diagnosis, establishing shared savings for achievement of established quality metrics and associated utilization patterns for population groups, and limiting reimbursement for readmissions for particular procedures, as CMS has done in recent years. A growing number of providers and payers have made a more complete shift to full-risk capitation, or what is most often referred to as global budgeting.

The ACA has significantly expanded coverage, despite the fact that only 30 of 50 states have participated in the Medicaid expansion to date. Medicaid coverage has increased by 14 million since October 2013, and reports indicate that this expansion has not resulted in a reduction in employer-based coverage (Lyons, 2015). Most new enrollees are low-to-moderate income individuals that receive some form of subsidies. While there were concerns about the risk pool of new enrollees, approximately half are under 35, and it appears that the newly insured are in better health than those who remain uninsured.

Uninsured rates were 10.5% in the second quarter of 2015, down from 16.6% in 2013. States that participated in the Medicaid expansion experienced reductions in the percentage of uninsured from 14.9% in 2013 to 8.5% in 2015 (Kaiser Family Foundation, 2015). Gaps in coverage still exist for approximately 3 million adults who are low-wage workers who don't meet income thresholds, live in states that are not expanding Medicaid, or are undocumented immigrants. Most of those individuals live in states like Texas, Florida, Georgia, and North Carolina.

The combined impact of an expansion in coverage to low-to-moderate income individuals (who live in communities where social determinants serve as obstacles to desired health behaviors) and the assumption of financial risk presents an immense challenge to providers in the years ahead. A current CMS program that ties Medicare reimbursement to improved performance will reduce payments by 1% for the lowest performing quartile of hospitals in 2016, with a net estimated reduction of $364 million in spending for those 700-800 hospitals (Evans, 2015).

Some have made the case that it will be difficult for low performers to improve because the CMS risk adjustment measure fails to adequately reflect that poor and sicker patients with more complex conditions will continue to experience disproportionate adverse events. CMS recently acknowledged that Medicare underpays for dual eligible patients (i.e., those who are both poor and either elderly or disabled), and has launched a retrospective analysis of 2014 data. Preliminary indications are that CMS overpays for beneficiaries with low medical costs, and underpays for those with high costs. CMS plans to publish final changes in February 2016 (Dickson, 2015).

On the positive side, states that have implemented the Medicaid expansion have reported savings in behavioral health, criminal justice, and uncompensated care as well as increased revenue (Cunningham et al., 2015). Federal officials have calculated that charity care has dropped by $3.9 billion in states that expanded Medicaid. At the same time, Medicaid shortfalls have expanded. Medicaid shortfalls accounted for 48% of what hospitals reported as community benefit in 2013, a figure that is approximately twice as large as was reported for charity care (24%). As part of a strategy to better target resources, health systems like Dignity Health have indicated that they are directing an increasing share of their community benefit dollars to increase access to primary care for Medicaid patients (Evans, 2015).

The imperative for a more comprehensive approach to improving health and reversing the prevalence in diabetes, heart disease, and other chronic diseases is becoming clearer with each passing day. Non-communicable Diseases (NCDs) account for 7 of the top 10 causes of death in the U.S., and heart disease and cancer account for 48% of all deaths (Heron, 2013). NCDs account for more than 80% of U.S. health care costs, estimated at $2.9 trillion, or 17.4% of the GDP in 2013 (CMS, 2015). While deaths due to lung cancer and heart disease have declined over the last two decades due to decrease in tobacco use and improved care management, deaths from diabetes and mental illness are continuing to trend upward (Lancet, 2015). Between 1990 and 2013, the prevalence of obesity in the U.S. increased 153%, from 11.6 to 29.4% of U.S. adults (UnitedHealth Foundation, 2014).

Likewise, the growth in the proportion of seniors in the population also presents our health care system with significant challenges in the coming years. Americans aged 65 years or older are expected to represent approximately 19% of the total population by 2030, nearly one in five people (U.S. Department of Health and Human Services, Administration for Community Living, Administration on Aging, Aging Statistics, 2015). Among the challenges of managing the care for a growing senior population with higher rates of NCDs is coming to grips with the limits of doing so in traditional long term care institutions, and the increasing demand for supportive services in community-based settings.

The challenges faced in the transformation of health care in the U.S. are myriad, but they are centered on moving from a fragmented and reactive system of resource allocations for treatment for often preventable conditions in acute care settings to the financing of a health producing enterprise at the institutional, community, and societal level. In this new world, acute medical care services are essential elements of a larger system of primary care, preventive services, and strategic investments in social and physical infrastructure that together comprise the leading causes of life. The accounting for this system will view health systems as "nestled" enterprises that thrive when services, activities and investments are optimally aligned to foster life, liberty, and the pursuit of happiness.

We must seek an alternative to the historical frame that looks at health care expenditures in isolation, with only the providers, payers, equipment manufacturers, and pharmaceutical companies setting the terms of transactions. The net result has been a steady upward spiral of costs, driven in part by economic mechanisms (e.g., barriers to market entry, imperfect information, high complexity, societal view of medical care as essential services) that contribute to the unfettered escalation of costs. It is time for a dialogue that looks beyond who should pay for goods and services that are unhinged from basic market mediators, and considers the relative value of medical care delivery in the context of a broader set of societal investment options.

Health Inequities and Community: How Did We Get Here?

THE SOCIAL DETERMINANTS OF HEALTH

A search for improved health outcomes naturally leads us to a complex array of social, economic, and environmental factors that play a fundamental role in influencing our ability to meet our basic needs and feel a sense of stability, hope, purpose, and connectedness to the world around us. As reviewed in Chapter Two of this volume, these social determinants of health impact health in ways that far outweigh traditional medical care.

A central consideration in an examination of the social determinants of health (SDH) is the degree to which investment in primary prevention produces impacts on health status, costs, and other outcomes of interest to diverse stakeholders. Woolf and Braveman (2011) describe four elements of complexity, including:

- Different determinants, or *factors that influence* health
- Different *dimensions impacted* by determinants, including morbidity, mortality, function, and well-being
- Different *causal pathways* in which SDH exert their influence, depending on differential configurations, intensity, temporality, etc.
- Different *levels of influence,* at the individual, cultural group, neighborhood, societal.

All four elements play out differentially in complex ways in which individuals respond according to different times in their lives, the unique circumstances of the moment, what kinds of support systems may be in place, and reasons they may be more or less receptive, responsive, or resistant to particular factors in place.

Social and physical environmental factors include income and wealth, family and household structure, social support, education, occupation, neighborhood, social institutions, and it is important to consider how their influence is exerted and what is reinforced or ameliorated in the life course and across generations. All this makes it very difficult to parse out and attribute relative contributions to individual factors. Appropriate attention is being given to the impact of SDH at the earliest ages, including a more substantial impact on cognitive and non-cognitive development (e.g., executive function), which in turn affect behavioral tendencies (e.g., deferred gratification) and, hence, increases in risk behaviors. Growing attention to epigenetics points to the ways in which exposures to traumatic experiences in vivo and in the earliest years of life can also serve as genetic triggers that contribute to the development of chronic diseases later in life (see Chapter 7).

In consideration of the substantial contributions of the social determinants to health or illness, we would naturally want to know the relative cost of ensuring access to things such as quality education, and compare those costs to the downstream costs for failing to ensure quality. In the educational arena, one study reported that interventions that increase high school graduation rates produce an average of $166,000 in savings of government expenditures associated with higher tax revenues, reduced crime, and lower public health costs (Levin, Belfield, Meunnig & Rouse, 2007).

The growing focus on walkability is supported by findings that increased walking and decreased driving contribute to reduced stress, increased social capital, improved public safety, and reduced rates of traffic fatalities and violent crime (Furie & Desai, 2010; Litman, 2010).

Historical factors that have contributed greatly to the persistent and profound health inequities are concentrated in specific communities across the country. As noted in the introduction to this chapter, these "facts on the ground" are driven in part by a series of decisions made in the public and private sectors that have contributed to the flight of capital and the concentration of poverty and poor health in particular neighborhoods across the country.

While the pattern of discriminatory public policies can be traced back much further in our history as a nation, we'll start with efforts to reduce poverty and create opportunities during the Great Depression. One element of Franklin D. Roosevelt's New Deal involved the establishment of the Home Owner's Loan Corporation in 1933. One of the early actions of this federal agency was to draft maps of communities to determine which were worthy of mortgage lending. Neighborhoods were ranked and color-coded, and the D-rated ones—with "inharmonious" racial groups—were outlined in red. This strategy was quickly adopted by private banks, and "redlined" communities were effectively cut off from essential capital.

This policy was implemented during a time when millions of African Americans were fleeing oppression during the Jim Crow era in the South in search for job opportunities and stability for their families. The expansion of industrial production during and in the wake of World War II provided substantial impetus and hope for these families. In their search for housing, African Americans and other ethnic minorities quickly discovered that their options were often limited to these "redlined" communities. Given the high demand and limited availability, landlords were able to charge exorbitant prices for often dilapidated housing, with "contract mortgages" (Satter, 2010) that enabled them to evict families without equity payouts after years of making payments.

One of the numerous actions taken by the federal government that impeded the accumulation of capital among low-income communities was the passage of the Housing Act of 1949 with the stated purpose to provide "a decent home and a suitable living environment for every American family." In order to secure the votes for this law, low income housing advocates had to agree to the parallel clearing of "blighted" areas from the urban core. The Housing Act provided a subsidy to municipalities covering two thirds of the costs of clearing, and language covering the use of the land indicated that development would be "predominantly residential" (50% of construction had to be residential) allowing for inclusion of commercial properties as part of renewal initiatives (Biles, 2000). The net effect, in many cities, was the displacement of large numbers of residents of color.

In 1956, the Federal Aid Highway Act shifted control over highway development, so decisions were made to route highways directly through what had been economically vibrant urban neighborhoods in the interest of expediting traffic in and out of the city core. The resulting deterioration of commercial activity in turn degraded the tax base of cities, and the only housing options for many people of color who were displaced were highly concentrated public housing projects.

Further amendments to the Housing Act in 1954 and 1959 included the addition of Section 112, which made universities eligible for funds without requirements for links to residential housing. This was extended to hospitals in 1961 at the request of the American Hospital Association. In addition, Section 112 permitted cities to claim expenditures by universities or hospitals as part of their 2:1 Federal-local match. If the expenditures surpassed the match, cities were given credits towards further urban renewal projects, which created an incentive for cities to expand their urban renewal efforts. By 1964, 154 projects involving 120 universities and 75 hospitals had taken advantage of Section 112. Examples include Detroit Medical Center, which is currently a for-profit facility, and Johns Hopkins University Medical Center.

Redlining was technically outlawed by the passage of the Fair Housing Act of 1968, but more subtle forms of discrimination continue to this day (see sidebar on Banks Assessed Penalties for Redlining).

These longstanding patterns of discrimination have had a profound intergenerational impact upon the ability of African American and Latino populations to accumulate capital. Harmful public policies, lending practices, and capital flight have all conspired to limit the wealth that parents in each successive generation can pass on to their children.

Given this history, it is not surprising that the residents of urban inner city neighborhoods continue to struggle with limited capital, poor housing quality, dysfunctional schools, and a lack of access to healthy food, banking services, retail goods, transportation, and employment opportunities. While there have been an array of initiatives launched by private foundations, going back as far as the Gray Areas program led by the Ford Foundation in the 1940s and by the federal government (the War on Poverty in the 1960s, Model Cities in the 1970s, and the Empowerment Zones initiative in the 1990s), none of these efforts have brought a sufficient concentration of resources and support services to overcome the deeply established structural inequities that were put in place in the early to mid-20th century.

Setting aside for a moment the geographic concentrations of inequities, a 2009 study found that the average wealth of white heads of households in the U.S. was 20 times higher than black heads of households (Taylor et al., 2011). A recent report cited an estimate that the U.S. economy loses approximately $309 billion per year due to the direct and indirect impact of disparities (Norris & Howard, 2015).

As noted in the beginning, the scope and scale of these challenges is daunting, yet there are emerging signs of understanding and commitment in both the public and private sector that offer hope for the future. The next section will provide an overview of recent actions being taken by public sector agencies to implement financial innovations that encourage work across sectors, with a central focus in communities and with populations where health inequities are concentrated.

BANKS ASSESSED PENALTIES FOR REDLINING

At least six banks have been assessed penalties in the last five years for discriminatory lending practices, including:

- **Hudson City Savings Bank** (CT, NJ, NY)
  Paid a $33 million fine to the Consumer Financial Protection Bureau and the Justice Department after review of data indicated that only 25 of 1,886 approved mortgages in 2014 (.013%) went to black borrowers. Of 54 branches opened between 2004 and 2010, only 3 were in predominantly Black or Latino neighborhoods. While these neighborhoods accounted for more than a third of the market in NY and NJ, Hudson deployed only 12 of their 162 brokers in those communities (Swarns, 2015).

- **Associated Bank** (WI)
  Agreement to pay $10 million in mortgage assistance and finance $200 million in loans in selected census tracts in response to documented patterns of discriminatory lending.

- **Evans Bancorp** (NY)
  Agreed to pay a $1M fine and $200k in advertising in low income African American neighborhoods after investigators discovered a map that defined trade areas that excluded Buffalo's east side.

- **Santander Bank** (RI - Providence)
  In a settlement with the City of Providence, Santander agreed to give $350,000 to the Providence Community Library for programs on financial literacy and homeownership; $450,000 to a nonprofit community arts center to support a mixed-use project; and $500,000 to the Rhode Island Local Initiatives Support Corp to help pay mortgage down payments and closing costs for low- and moderate-income Providence residents. (Providence Journal, 2014).

- **Five Star Bank** (NY - Rochester)
  Investigators discovered a map that excluded downtown and suburban census tracts with majority minority populations. In the settlement, Five Star will drop their mortgage minimum (75,000) and will open branches and offer $750,000 in discounts and loan subsidies in minority neighborhoods. (Daneman, 2015).

Financial Innovations: A Review of Emerging Models

Since the passage of the ACA, the Center for Medicare and Medicaid Services, the Centers for Disease Control and Prevention, and other federal agencies are working with states, providers, and payers to launch initiatives that encourage work across sectors—with a central goal to "bend the cost curve." The following is a sampling of state level strategies documented in a recent report (Spencer et al, 2015):

- **OREGON**

  Has established Coordinated Care Organizations (CCOs) under the 1115 waiver, with a global budget and a fixed trend rate, with incentive payments to meet performance objectives. CCOs develop payment methodologies for providers that tailor services to meet specific community needs. Parameters used in determining the scope of services include that they a) are "health-related," b) lack billing codes, and c) have the potential to be cost-effective alternatives to covered benefits and produce cost savings. Examples of services include but are not limited to transportation, gyms, cooking classes, athletic shoes, farmers markets, referrals to job training, and housing repairs.

  Early reports indicate that the integration of these kinds of non-traditional services has been a gradual process which, because the scope of services ranges beyond billable codes, has required considerable deliberation in the development of clear policies to provide guidance. A key factor in the expansion of the scope of services was diversity in the competencies and experience of CCO board members.

- **UTAH**

  Engaged four managed care organizations (MCOs) to develop full-risk capitated ACOs as part of their 1115 waiver. The ACOs are charged by the state legislature with "delivering the most appropriate services at the lowest costs" (Lundquist, 2014). No specific scope of services is defined, and ACOs can pay for self-help activities, housing supports, and living improvements.

- **VERMONT**

  The Blueprint for Health Initiative is a multi-payer, patient-centered medical home program delivered by diverse Community Health Teams (CHTs). The Blueprint includes elements such as the Support and Services at Home (SASH) initiative, which links seniors and persons with disabilities with support services and affordable housing. In this initiative, regional housing authorities link with home health, mental health agencies, and agencies on aging to establish care teams that provide a broad array of services. In addition to State funding, SASH now also receives funding through Medicare's Multi-Payer Advanced Primary Care Practice (MAPCP) demonstration program. The configuration of team members is based upon identified community needs.

  Providers that have established Primary Care Medical Homes (PCMHs) receive a per-member-per-month (PMPM) payment (referred to as a capacity payment) tied to their performance against NQCA ratings, and payers share in the cost at $1.50 a month per beneficiary. Integration of data systems was identified as one of the most significant near term challenges. For the next phase of systems redesign, Vermont is negotiating the establishment of an all payer, full risk capitated system for all providers to be launched in early 2017.

- **NEW YORK**

  A Medicaid Redesign Team (MRT) was established in 2011, and includes supportive housing, with a focus on dual eligible beneficiaries. An affordable housing work group was established with over 40 stakeholders, with a charge to identify barriers to housing and to propose solutions. The outcome was the launch of the two-year, $10 million MRT Supportive Housing Olmstead Housing Subsidy Program in October 2015. The program will establish supportive housing for Medicaid recipients who need nursing home level care, and will use non-Medicaid state funds to provide rental subsidies and coordination with community support services. Health care providers are required to coordinate with non-health service providers, including supportive housing organizations.

  MRT is linked with the DSRIP (Delivery System Reform Incentive Payment) program, which has allocated $9 million over two years for rental subsidies. Since Medicaid does not pay for rental subsidies or capital funding, it is paid for by NY's state-share Medicaid dollars. In 2015, NY allocated $47 million in state-share Medicaid funding to expand supportive housing units for high cost Medicaid patients, another $38 million in rental subsidies and related supportive services, $24 million in supportive housing pilot programs, and $2.5 million for monitoring and evaluation.

- **MASSACHUSETTS**

  The state has established a program that focuses on supportive services for treatment of high-risk pediatric asthma patients to cover things such as bed covers, filters, and housing remediation for pests. It is a single bundled payment arrangement for a defined period for an episode of care. This, the Children's High Risk Asthma Bundled Payment (CHABP) program, was initially authorized by the state legislature in 2010. CMS provided an 1115 waiver in 2011 for a pilot, and approved a protocol for formal implementation in 2014. The first phase of the program included a $50 per patient per month (PMPM) payment for high risk patients 2-18 years of age.

  Providers are required to use community health workers (CHWs), do monthly monitoring of patients, and could use funding for home assessments and provision of filters, bed covers, and pest management supplies. CHWs were also authorized to support advocacy for landlord improvements. Unfortunately, the program did not proceed beyond the first phase, given other dynamics around health care financing. CMS provided guidance on June 26, 2015, with the release of an Informational Bulletin that outlined the kinds of services and activities that could be integrated into reimbursement strategies.

In recent years, CMS launched two programs that give particular attention to Medicaid coverage of housing-related activities and services, with a "goal of promoting community integration for individuals with disabilities, older adults needing long term care services and supports (LTSS), and those experiencing chronic homelessness" (DHHS, 2015). These services do not include funding for room and board, but a variety of other essential housing-related services and activities.

Two programs in particular, the Money Follows the Person (MFP) rebalancing demonstration program and the Real Choice Systems Change (RCSC) grants, provide excellent models for health care organizations and partners that seek support from Medicaid to cover housing-related activities and services. Participants in MFP have shown that engaging housing specialists, assisting with searches, and paying for moving expenses have reduced health care costs by transitioning individuals out of high cost nursing homes and into community living (Lipson et al, 2011). There are three categories of housing related activities and services, including:

INDIVIDUAL HOUSING TRANSITION SERVICES

Services include:

- Tenant screening and housing assessment
- Individualized housing support plan
- Assistance with housing application process
- ID resources to cover security deposit, moving costs
- Ensure safety in living environment
- Arrange and manage move
- Develop housing support crisis plan.

INDIVIDUAL HOUSING & TENANCY SUSTAINING SERVICES

Services include:

- Early ID and intervention for behaviors that may jeopardize tenancy
- ED and training on tenant responsibilities
- Coaching on relationships with landlords
- Assistance in resolving disputes
- Advocacy and links with community resources
- Assistance with housing recertification
- Review and update of plan.

STATE LEVEL HOUSING RELATED COLLABORATIVE ACTIVITIES

Services include:

- Develop agreements and working relationships with state and local housing and Community Development Corporations (CDCs)
- Participating in state and local housing and CDCs
- Create and ID opportunities for additional housing options.

There are also a number of federal waivers that states can use to cover many of these kinds of expenditures. The 1915(c) HCBS (Housing and Community Based Services) Waivers can be used by states to cover some housing transition, tenancy sustaining activities and environmental modifications. The 1915 (i) HCBS State Plan Optional Benefit helps those transitioning out of Medicaid-funded institutions to a private residence, and Medicaid can provide reimbursements for security deposits, set up fees for utilities and phone, essential household furnishings, moving expenses, and cleaning prior to occupancy. The 1915 (k) Community First Choice (CFC) State Plan Optional Benefit permits reimbursement for person-centered home and community-based attendant services and supports.

The 1915 (b) Waivers permit states to use savings from services covered through 1915 (b) waiver to provide additional services. Examples include a behavioral health waiver in Iowa, specialty inpatient health plans for children with serious emotional disturbances in Michigan, a family care waiver in Wisconsin, and an integrated care delivery system waiver in Ohio. Finally, there are Section 1115 Research and Demonstration Programs, which are approved for a five-year period and can be renewed, typically for three years. The core condition is that they have to be budget neutral for the federal government. Examples include the Road to Community Living Program in Washington State, which uses funds to support housing-related transition and sustaining services, and to support collaboration across agencies, while Texas uses administrative funding to support collaboration between state housing and local agencies.

The most recent national initiative launched by the Center for Medicare and Medicaid Innovation (CMMI) is Accountable Health Communities (AHC). Successful applicants for this initiative will receive between $1-4.5 million in funding to support the establishment of an "integrator" function that facilitates the alignment of population health management strategies with a broad array of non-health care services and activities in communities, ranging from food to housing support.

HEALTH AND SCHOOL FUNDING

Regarding areas for targeted investment to improve health, it is important to consider public expenditures associated with K-12 schools, and financial losses associated with absenteeism, truancy, suspensions, and dropouts. Since schools are paid through a formula based upon daily attendance, each of these problems directly impacts their bottom line. In 2013, California schools lost over $1 billion in funding due to truancy alone (Office of the CA Attorney General, 2014).

Absenteeism is highest in the earliest years of elementary school, when the foundation for learning is being established with a focus on reading skills. In California, over 250,000 students were absent 18 or more days per year. Forty thousand (40,000) of those missed more than 36 days per year (Office of the CA Attorney General, 2014).

The figures on dropouts are even more alarming. Each year, approximately 120,000 California residents reach the age of 20 without a high school diploma. A 2007 study estimated the annual cost to the state of California at $46 billion per year in lost tax revenues, medical costs, welfare, and criminal justice expenditures. Conversely, the economic benefit of each additional graduate would be $392,000 (Rumberger, 2007).

Strategies that focus on creating the conditions that support increased attendance and improved performance, particularly at the early years, offer considerable potential to contribute to increases in funding for local schools, improved health, increased life expectancy, and increased economic vitality.

One of the most exciting financial innovations in recent years is the pay for success (PFS) model. At the most basic level, the PFS model looks to investors to make financial bets that an intervention will yield financial returns beyond the initial investment. Most of the PFS models tested to date focus in areas such as early childhood education to reduce the demand for special education, and life and job skills training and placement for incarcerated youth to reduce recidivism. Successful implementation of these models offers the promise to both improve health and well-being and reduce financial burden in the public sector. For health care providers and payers, PFS investments offer the potential to prospectively finance strategies to reduce the demand for treatment of preventable health problems, ranging from chronic diseases such as asthma and diabetes to behavioral health issues. Examples of PFS models include:

- **Early childhood intervention (Chicago)**—A $16.9 million social impact bond (SIB) deal was secured in 2013 in Chicago to provide early childhood educational services (pre-K) to up to 2,620 children over four years. The intervention is a half-day Child-Parent Center (CPC) model, funded by the Goldman Sachs' Social Impact Fund and Northern Trust and the J.B. and M.K. Pritzker Family Foundation. The intervention goals are to increase kindergarten readiness, improve third-grade literacy, and reduce the need for special education. The program is intended to serve 4 year old children who qualify for the federal free and reduced lunch program, but do not attend at least a half-day of pre-kindergarten. If successful, Chicago public schools will receive approximately one third of the savings generated, with the rest going to pay back investors. The loans and repayments will be managed by IFF, a nonprofit community development financial institution (CDFI). The program covered 374 children in the first year, up to 782 in the next two years and at least 680 in the fourth year. This covers more than half of the roughly 1,500 eligible low-income children who currently do not receive pre-K services. The remaining half will start getting pre-K education in the 2015-16 school year through $9.4 million in additional funding from the city and Chicago Public Schools, plus a $4.5 million state grant.

- **Reducing asthma (Fresno, CA)**—In 2012 a pilot program was launched in Fresno, California, with a goal to reduce asthma acuity and incidence. Approximately 20% of the population in Fresno has asthma, compared to an 8% rate at the national level (Badawy, 2012). This is the first PFS model to be implemented in the health care arena, and is being coordinated by Collective Health and Social Finance. Payers hoping to reduce costs include Anthem Blue Cross and Health Net, and care is being coordinated by Clinica Sierra Vista, a federally qualified health center serving low-income residents in the region. The development of the PFS and piloting phase is being supported through a grant from The California Endowment. The average baseline costs of care for targeted patients is approximately $15,000 per year. A total of 200 patients are being served during the pilot phase, with a plan to expand to 3,500 patients with investments from banks, individuals and foundations. In addition to care coordination services, the intervention includes home cleaning services, weatherizing, bed covers, and pest extermination.

- **Reducing recidivism (New York City)**—In 2012, New York launched the first social impact bond in the country. Program funding was provided through a $9.6 million loan from the Urban Investment Group of Goldman Sachs, and Bloomberg Philanthropies covered most of that investment with a $7.4 million loan guarantee. If the program intervention produced a reduction in recidivism beyond a target of 10%, Goldman Sachs would secure a substantial profit. MDRC served as an intermediary, working with partners to negotiate the financial elements, and oversaw the implementation of the intervention at New York City's

Rikers Island. The Adolescent Behavioral Learning Experience (ABLE) program, a cognitive behavioral therapy program for 16- to 18-year-olds was carried out by the Osborne Association and Friends of Island Academy. The program focused on personal responsibility education, training, and counseling. An independent evaluation of the program was conducted by the Vera Institute of Justice. In August of 2015, shortly after the release of a preliminary report (Vera Institute of Justice, 2015), the decision was made to terminate the program based upon findings that the program did not meet the target established in order for the City of New York to repay investors.

Each of these three early experiments offers invaluable insights in consideration of similar strategies going forward. The use of social impact bonds (SIBs) to fund these types of interventions is a new concept, with the earliest testing in Great Britain in 2010. As such, assessing the relative effectiveness of specific programs and understanding the implications for similar efforts is still in its infancy. On one hand, New York taxpayers avoided paying the costs for the failure to meet the objectives of the Riker's Island program. Some would posit that while narrowly focused programs provide the basis for clear-cut evaluation of relative effectiveness, a failure to produce a measurable impact reflects the reality that producing measurable outcomes will require more comprehensive strategies. A related concern is that these PFS models are limited by a demand for near term results, leading to a bias towards approaches that contribute to overly simplistic public discourse about solving complex problems. Complexity also works against the design of mechanisms for financial returns. In Fresno, considerable time and effort has been devoted to sorting through how savings from reduced preventable utilization will be secured by providers and repaid to investors, given the complexity of financial mechanisms in health care financing.

Some concern exists that SIBs are not viable for the long-term, but are simply the latest "fad" for philanthropy. On the positive side, program-related investments (PRIs) or below-market rate investments that are primarily made to achieve programmatic rather than financial objectives by foundations, have served as a mechanism to move beyond annual grant financial targets. The potential downside is that increased expectations for foundations to "smooth the path" for investors may divert attention and program support for other innovative programs.

INTERMEDIARIES AS THE "GLUE" FOR COLLABORATION

At the same time that many are looking to philanthropy to direct funds towards social impact bonds (SIBs), there is a parallel (and somewhat related) emphasis on support for local/regional intermediaries, or "backbone" entities which can serve as objective brokers of diverse stakeholders for "collective impact" approaches to solving complex social, economic, and health-related problems. These terms have been popularized by FSG, a consulting firm based in Boston and San Francisco, through a series of articles published in the Stanford Innovation Review over the last five years. The initial article (Kania & Kramer, 2011) profiled the Strive initiative in Cincinnati, an effort to align the broader educational community on an organized set of strategies to improve academic performance among youth.

The Collective Impact model identifies five conditions for success: 1) a common agenda, 2) shared measurement systems, 3) mutually reinforcing activities, 4) continuous communication, and 5) a backbone organization. The backbone organization is intended to be an independent organization (separate from organizations charged with roles in interventions) with standing among diverse stakeholders which can serve as a convener, facilitator, manager, administrator, and monitor of progress.

There is growing recognition among philanthropic organizations that demands for communities to "collaborate" without an infrastructure to facilitate the kind of deeper engagement and mutual accountability envisioned in the collective impact model has been unrealistic at best. With this in mind, there are calls not only for national foundations, but particularly for local and regional foundations to step definitively into this role. In many communities (particularly in urban settings), there are a plethora of public and private sector organizations delivering an array of most often individually-focused services in an inefficient, and often duplicative manner. Achievement of the Collective Impact objective of mutually reinforcing activities will often require a substantial re-design process. Options can include, but are not limited to co-location of activities, consolidation of program elements and administration, and co-investments in new program areas of focus. While larger organizations such as hospitals and local public health agencies may view themselves as appropriate entities to serve as "backbones," the need for an independent organization viewed as an objective broker may lead local stakeholders in different directions (see Chapter 3 on leading complex health structures).

There is much to learn about these new areas of partnership, investment, and alignment of programs, services, and activities across sectors. In such an environment, philanthropy can play a key role, and it is important to preserve a focus on relatively untested innovations that help to solve complex problems. Chapter 9 offers more details on how philanthropy can be leveraged to best impact broader community health.

THE LEADERSHIP ROLE OF MISSION-DRIVEN HEALTH SYSTEMS: HOW DO WE FINANCE SHARED OWNERSHIP?

Giving more focus to the social determinants of health and to geographic areas where health inequities are concentrated represents a shift for health care organizations from the question "**Who** is at greater risk for disease?" to the question "**Why** are some people at greater risk of preventable illness, injury and death than others?" The next, even more critical question, however, is "**What** are we going to do about it?" This section outlines the unique responsibility of mission-driven health systems to provide leadership in bringing health care costs under control and into the broader context of a "leading causes of life" investment strategy.

In consideration of what forms of leadership to provide in mission-driven health systems, it is essential to consider how best to establish and reinforce an ethic of shared ownership for health. As noted in Chapter 3, this approach requires hospitals and health systems to reconsider a more traditional "command and control" approach to engagement and explore a more generative model that seeks to optimize participation and encouragement of distributed leadership among diverse stakeholders. Key framing here is how best to align a spectrum of internal and external "assets" that offer the greatest potential to leverage the important, but limited resources of health care organizations.

Within the broader responsibility to provide leadership, this work will continue to evolve in different demographic, regional, and regulatory environments (e.g., states where the Medicaid expansion is not occurring, different payer mixes and reimbursement rates, federal, state, and local resource allocations for essential services and infrastructure, etc.).

INVESTMENTS IN DATA INFRASTRUCTURE

In order to effectively monitor progress in comprehensive approaches to health improvement, it is essential for hospitals to build the data capacity that will allow for a more in depth analysis of utilization patterns, and identification of pathways to health and illness in the geographic community context.

This is not only essential for individual organizations; systems are needed that support interoperability across provider organizations as an essential path to timely assessment of costs, quality, and outcomes. The configuration of stakeholders, their relative capacity, local/regional demographics, and the larger regulatory environment differs widely across the country—as such, there is no single rule of thumb, beyond a commitment to shared ownership for health.

In the development of these more comprehensive data systems, there is growing recognition (Morrissey, 2015) that electronic health records (EHRs) that are designed for a FFS system are not sufficient for fee-for-value systems. As noted in Chapter Four, a more evolved system requires accommodation of a more complex array of care settings, providers, and so on who are assuming risk and can contribute to improved outcomes through different modalities of treatments, procedures, input, and health improvement strategies.

As coverage continues to expand, hospitals and health systems will see a drop in the demand for charity care, and while some of those resources will be directed towards a growing population of Medicaid patients, hospitals are beginning to increase their allocation of charitable resources towards more proactive community health improvement strategies. Stakeholder Health partner Ascension Health System reported a 9.3% drop in traditional charity care in FY15. Some of these funds were shifted to Medicaid shortfalls, but they also increased their allocations for community health initiatives by 6.2%, or $37 million. In states that have not implemented the Medicaid expansion, bad debt reporting in hospitals in Medicaid expansion states increased 8.9%, compared to only 2.5% in states that expanded Medicaid coverage (Kutscher, 2015).

Scrutiny of tax-exempt hospitals can be expected to increase in the coming years, with growing pressure by advocacy groups to eliminate the group exemption that allows health systems to provide only aggregate totals in their 990H, and begin to require facility-specific reporting of community benefit contributions. Challenges such as the most recent tax settlement by Morristown Medical Center (NJ) to pay $26 million in property taxes are expected to continue. A growing number of hospitals are coming to the conclusion that access to care is not the most important public health issue in their community. In communities like the Tenderloin District of San Francisco, Saint Francis Memorial Hospital, part of the Dignity Health System, is giving focus to issues such as crime reduction, toxic stress, and substance abuse, and homelessness. In order to monitor progress in addressing these complex issues, and to partner effectively with diverse stakeholders, data systems are needed that connect these dots.

HEALTH AND COMMUNITY DEVELOPMENT: ROLES FOR HOSPITALS AND HEALTH SYSTEMS

Approximately four years ago, with support from the Robert Wood Johnson Foundation, the Federal Reserve Bank of San Francisco began to convene a series of regional meetings across the country that brought together financial institutions and the public health community. These meetings focused on the fact that many of the kinds of investments made by financial institutions in fulfillment of their Community Reinvestment Act (CRA) responsibilities had important health implications. The focus of these investments ranged from affordable housing and childcare centers to job training programs, grocery stores, charter schools, and federally qualified health centers. Much of the early dialogue focused on how to move towards more of a health frame in the selection of investments, and on developing metrics that better capture health impacts and reinforce a more integrated approach across the health and community development sectors.

In consideration of this important new development, it was suggested (Barnett, 2012) that these conversations would benefit from bringing a key stakeholder to the table with a shared interest in a more comprehensive approach to community health improvement, i.e., hospitals. Like financial institutions, tax-exempt hospitals have a legal obligation—and increasingly a strategic imperative—to target their resources in communities where health inequities are concentrated, and to leverage those resources through alignment with those of diverse community stakeholders. With this in mind, there is growing attention among hospitals and health systems across the country in the formation of partnerships with CDFIs, community development corporations, and other stakeholders in the community development arena. Many of these partnerships focus on real estate investments linked explicitly to better management of chronic diseases such as diabetes, cardiovascular disease, asthma, as well as mental and behavioral health issues.

As part of these health-community development partnerships, a number of Stakeholder Health systems are directing a portion of their investment portfolios to support linked development strategies. Dignity Health, Trinity Health, Bon Secours, and Henry Ford Health System all have well established track records, often making strategic investments at the pre-development phase that provide a critically important bridge and stability as local developers and CDFIs seek loans for construction. Other health systems are beginning to step into this arena as well, in recognition of the need for alignment across sectors.

Engagement of hospitals and health systems in these targeted investment strategies address a critical need among CDFIs and other community development stakeholders to secure early capital that creates a glide path for CRA-related investments by financial institutions. At the same time, these strategic-minded health systems are optimally leveraging their resource allocations in health improvement activities by linking them to the kinds of physical infrastructure investments that are critically needed to reverse the negative health impacts associated with decades of redlining and disinvestment.

This expanding arena of strategic investment and alignment of the health and community development sectors is reinforced by the recent framing of hospitals, academic institutions, and other large employers with a mission focus as "anchor institutions" (Kelly & McKinley, 2015). This framing strengthens a focus on "place" in local economic development. It also emphasizes the need to bring a "third player" beyond cities and businesses, where historical dynamics have led to a process where a city's ability to deliver value to its residents is undermined by a bidding war in which revenues are sacrificed in the form of tax abatements to influence corporate location decisions. The "third player" is the combined force of anchor institutions, community groups, community-based organizations, philanthropy, and local small businesses.

Whereas a recent focus has been on pressuring larger businesses, there is a growing movement towards a more proactive form of systems level planning and economic development. A key dimension is developing, expanding, and building the capacity of under-utilized local assets. Examples include social networks, physical infrastructure, arts and cultural communities, and so on. In one recent example, spending resources at locally owned firms created a feedback loop where wealth recirculated at least three times as much in the local economy (Chevas, 2013).

The framing of tax-exempt hospitals and universities as potential anchor institutions involves over $1 trillion in economic activity, representing approximately 7% of GDP (Institute of Education Sciences, 2013; CMS, 2014). Hospitals and health systems alone account for more than $780 billion in total annual expenditures, $340 billion in purchasing of goods and services, and more than $500 billion in investment portfolios (Norris & Howard, 2015). Examples of an anchor institution approach is reflected in the following examples:

- A plan to spend $1.2 billion for facility development between 2005 and 2010 by University Hospitals (UHS) in Cleveland. UHS partnered with the Mayor's office and local building trade unions to establish the Vision 2010 program with a goal of procuring 80% of the $1.2 billion from local and regional firms. Over the next five years, they created over 5,000 jobs, and procured 92% from local and regional firms. More recently, UHS developed a Step Up to UH program that includes training and wrap around support services in a pipeline to hire residents of proximal low-income African American communities (Serang, Thompson, & Howard, 2013). In another example, the Mayo Clinic in Rochester, MN helped to finance a community land trust to ensure long term affordable housing for employees and the larger community (Zuckerman, 2013).

- The Fifth Season Cooperative, a multi-stakeholder food hub established in 2010 in La Crosse, WI, was launched with the support of the Gunderson Lutheran Health system, the University of Wisconsin-La Crosse, and three local public school systems. The cooperative provides ongoing technical assistance to members to support the scaling of the operation. Early support came from the Vernon County Economic Development Association through a local state grant, as well as from fundraising through the sale of stocks to local residents.

- New Orleans Works (NOW) is a workforce initiative with support from the National Fund for Workforce Solutions, and is a partnership with local health care sector stakeholders, including the Ochsner Health System, the Southeast Louisiana Veterans Healthcare System, and Delgado Community College. A current focus is on the training and deployment of Medical Assistants (Greater New Orleans Foundation, 2014).

The anchor institution perspective involves a more global consideration of potential contributions of hospitals, moving beyond the compliance-constrained idea of community benefit to "be accountable for all of their impacts on community health, and leveraging all of their assets to ensure the well-being of the community in which they are based" (Norris & Howard, 2015; Page 5).

Moving in this direction also calls for colleagues in the community development arena to expand their thinking beyond building physical structures (and on a single transaction) without consideration of the neighborhood context. This historical, decontextualized approach to development closely parallels a similar focus on individuals or groups of patients in the health care sector—both must be remedied if we are to address the persistent and profound social, economic, and health inequities that are prevalent in the most affluent society on the planet. Super Church (2013) cites as an example one of the first Whole Foods stores (located in Dedham, MA) to achieve Green Globe certification, but it is located in a strip mall area that is "virtually unreachable on foot from nearby neighborhoods."

A more contextual approach to community development brings attention to a broader array of factors in planning and decision-making. For example, a recent study in Washington, DC observed that more walkable neighborhoods with proximity to transit have higher rents, retail revenues, and housing values than less walkable neighborhoods. Whereas the cause and effect dynamic suggests that investments in walkability are hand-in-glove with the gentrification process that often displaces low income residents, it is appropriate to consider walkability as an important part of neighborhood revitalization that contributes substantially to improvements in health status and quality of life (Leinberger & Alfonso, 2012). Housing prices in walkable neighborhoods fell substantially less than the national average between 2006 and 2011, and the U.S. Conference Board estimated that they will rise much faster than the national average between 2014 and 2017 (Urban Land Institute, 2011).

Super Church (2013) notes that new financial tools are needed to support more comprehensive approaches to community development, pointing to substantial financing gaps for both moderate-income housing and retail/commercial and industrial development: "The available subsidies are very limited and highly competitive, and most developers do not have sufficient equity to self-fund projects of this scale." An additional complicating factor is the impact of the Supreme Court ruling in June 2015 on the Fair Housing Act, which has resulted in the lack of Low Income Housing Tax Credits in neighborhoods where there is a concentration of poverty.

Many project underwriters have been unwilling to finance larger scale efforts, since project costs are high, rents are limited, and there is insufficient evidence that rents would increase at a level that would overcome near term concerns. Increased investments are needed by private equity funds established through contributions from philanthropy (program-related investments) and impact investors, including hospitals and health systems.

A recent Health Affairs blog (Somers & McGinnis, 2014) expanded on the concept of the ACO model to reflect a trend towards the assumption of responsibility under global budgeting for a broader array of services beyond medical care delivery (e.g., mental health, substance abuse treatment, housing support services). These entities are referred to as "totally accountable care organizations," or TACOs. While such an integrated role is largely an aspiration at this juncture in the national health reform process, a growing number of organizations have taken important steps in this direction.

The development of a Medicaid ACO at Hennepin County Medical Center (HCMC) represents an early model worth examining. HCMC works with homeless shelters, supportive housing providers, the criminal justice system, and the public health department. Because HCMC already operates under a global budget system, incentives have driven investments in areas such as a sobering center, a far more humanistic and cost-effective option than care in ED settings and county incarceration facilities. As a county facility (but with operation as a 501c3 nonprofit), HCMC is in a good position to explore opportunities with local public sector agencies for a more cost-effective allocation of resources. State agencies across the country are in an optimal position to signal to localities that similar approaches may be rewarded.

A CATALYZING ROLE FOR EMPLOYERS

U.S. employers have a major stake in the achievement of the goals of national reform given the fact that they provide coverage for approximately 54% of the population (Smith & Medalia, 2014). In 2012, they spent $578 billion on group health coverage, a 72% increase over the $336 billion spent in 2000 (CMS, 2014).

Steady increases in obesity in the U.S. have taken their toll on employers, with some industries more impacted by others. One study found, for example, that obese women with a BMI of 40 or greater miss 8.2 days/year, 141% or nearly 1 week more than normal weight women (Finkelstein et al, 2005). Overall, it is estimated that obesity produces an additional $1,152 in medical expenditures per year for males and $3,613 for females in the U.S. Lost productivity is estimated at $3,792 for males, and $3,037 for females (The Week, 2012). Over a decade ago, productivity losses due to absenteeism were estimated to cost employers approximately $226 billion per year (Stewart et al, 2003). Trends suggest that current costs are likely to be significantly higher.

Nearly 80% of U.S. employers offer workplace wellness programs, given considerable evidence of substantial returns on their investment. A review of 36 peer reviewed studies of workplace wellness programs found an average reduction in medical care costs of $3.27 for every dollar invested (Baicker, 2010).

The next frontier for employers in efforts to supporting wellness and reducing health care costs involves expanding their engagement beyond employees to their families and surrounding communities. Approximately 90% of larger firms offer some form of wellness programs for employees, but only 63% offer them to spouses or dependents, and only a fraction of those to surrounding communities (Kaiser Family Foundation, 2013).

A growing number of larger firms are moving beyond the more narrow interpretation of corporate responsibility articulated by Milton Friedman (1970), and thinking about their roles in fostering health in the communities in which their employees and families reside. For example, Friedman's narrow view is frequently illustrated by this quote: "There is one and only one responsibility of business—to use its resources and engage in activities designed to increase its profits, so long as it stays within the rules of the game, which is to say, engages in open and free competition without deception or fraud." (Friedman, 1962). The concept of corporate social responsibility emerged in the 1970s, and led a number of companies to begin to direct resources towards investing in local economic development and in some cases, social policy development (Carroll, 1999). Consideration of the roles of firms in this regard has continued to evolve towards a more integrated approach framed as "Shared Value," where competitiveness in the marketplace is directly tied to advancing the economic and social vitality of communities in which they operate (Porter et al, 2011). A recent report (Oziransky et al, 2015) commissioned by the Robert Wood Johnson Foundation offers a number of excellent examples, including:

- A $10 million, 10 year corporate investment by Campbell's Soup in a Collective Impact approach to reducing obesity and hunger by 50% in Camden, NJ.

- A partnership between General Dynamics Bath Iron Works and L.L. Bean to fund diabetes prevention programs for their workforce, their dependents, and the local community near both corporate headquarters.

- A multi-stakeholder health system initiative in Cincinnati, Ohio, supported by General Electric to improve quality of care, reduce costs, and improve health outcomes for its employees and the larger community.

In short, the corporate community increasingly recognizes the practical reality that their long term vitality is inextricably tied to the health and well-being of their employees, which in turn is inextricably tied to the communities in which they reside. This placed-based, integrated view of the health enhancement process is essential if we are to begin to address the profound and persistent economic, social, and health inequities that are concentrated in urban and rural communities across the country.

We'll close this chapter with sidebar profiles of internal and external systems development by two Stakeholder Health member organizations to build a framework for shared ownership for health with local community stakeholders.

Summary

In summary, health systems must begin to explore new means of financial accounting that expands beyond their walls and incorporates partnerships with other entities, as well as allowing them to be better positioned and resourced to help address the social determinants of health. While these efforts are at a rudimentary stage, promising practices from many SH partners offer hope for a new way of doing business that can result in improved health and healthcare outcomes for all.

To date, few health systems have actually created financial metrics to show ROI, much less SROI. Basic financial accounting finds both the scope and the ability to assign "causation" in a broad model that includes numerous internal health systems, as well as community partners to be a difficult task. However, in our work with faith-based and community partners and networks in both Memphis, TN (with the Congregational Health Network or CHN) and Wake Forest (with Supporters of Health—hybrid community health workers), we have created very granular accounting and data dashboard strategies for outlining system costs and share these beginning models here.

CONGREGATIONAL HEALTH NETWORK OF METHODIST LE BONHEUR HEALTHCARE, MEMPHIS, TN

The work of the Memphis Model or Congregational Health Network (CHN) was highlighted extensively in the first HSLG monograph. Now over 600 congregations, with mostly African-American members, the CHN members showed decreased healthcare utilization for Methodist Le Bonheur Healthcare (MLH). For example, using predictive modeling, we showed that CHN members vs. non-members (matched on 8 variables) had significantly longer times (69 days) to readmissions (Barnes et al., 2014). Place-based efforts in zip code 38109 and the smaller neighborhood of Riverview Kansas began in 2010, anticipating the ACA and readmission non-payment. Focus groups with clergy, community coalitions and lay persons in this violent and decimated neighborhood revealed a need for increased access to health care. CEO Gary Shorb took a community tour with Rev. Drs. Chris Bounds and Bobby Baker (Director of Faith and Community Partnerships) and then brought his leadership team to Rev. James Kendrick's church, Oak Grove, since Rev. Kendrick had been working with the disenfranchised young men of color on the streets in his Health Watch ministry for many years. The CHN's first place-based navigator, Joy Crawford Sharp, was hired in 2011 and hit the ground running. The Wellness without Walls initiative began with bi-monthly events at the local community center and careful follow up of every need by Joy. By 2012, aggregate charity care charges had dropped overall for MLH, particularly in the target zip code of 38109. See table 1 below.

	Year	Visits	Full Costs	Variable Costs	Average per Capita Charity Costs	Net (Percent) Charity Care Change from Prior Year
38109	2010	5,566	$6,269,769	$4,737,311	$1126.44	NA
	2011	6,772	$9,055,808	$6,732,605	$1337.24	$2,786,039 increase (↑30.8 %)
	2012	6,568	$8,249,922	$6,404,569	$1256.08	$-805,866 decrease (↓8.9 %)

The Chief Financial Officer then suggested that a cost to charge ratio be calculated, versus looking only at encounters, so we began tracking cost associated with the write-off amount, based on transaction, not discharge date, which increased the numbers evaluated. Those data are presented below, but still represented a decrease in charity care costs.

CHARITY CARE 38109 - NEW METHODOLOGY		
Year	Write-Off Cost*	Volume
2010	$6,505,332.19	6,905
2011	$6,826,729.90	7,104
2012	$6,676,539.42	7,595
July YTD 2013	$3,012,650.18	4,930

*Cost of Write-off = cost to charge ratio applied to transaction amount

Cost to charge ratio 2010 = 25%

Cost to charge ratio 2011 =23.5%

Cost to charge ratio 2012 =23.15%

Cost to charge ratio 2013 = 23.15%

WAKE FOREST BAPTIST MEDICAL CENTER (WFBMC):
SUPPORTERS OF HEALTH COHORT AND AGGREGATE SELF-PAY DATA

As reported in the HSLG monograph (2013, p. 60) and related in a blog by IHI's Kathy Luther (http://www.ihi.org/communities/blogs/_layouts/ihi/community/blog/itemview.aspx?List=7d1126ec-8f63-4a3b-9926-c44ea3036813&ID=111), in 2012, soon after starting work, VP Gary Gunderson stepped up to save the jobs of 267 environmental service workers who were under threat of outsourcing. He managed this by promising to cross-train some of these workers as community health workers, as part of the FaithHealth divisional work. The Supporters of Health model of hybrid community health workers/community care triagers was born and now WFBMC has 5 FTE Supporters, or what we term the "Fab Five." Supporters of Health efforts, along with our full FaithHealth division, Transitional Care staff, Patient Financial Services and more, are responsible for the aggregate and cohort data seen below.

Supporters of Health Cohort: Financial Data: Six Months Prior and After Enrollment

	6 MONTHS PRIOR TO ENROLLMENT	6 MONTHS AFTER ENROLLMENT
Total Encounters	875	877
Patients	132	130
Average Encounters Per Patient	6.6	6.7
Average Cost Per Encounter	$2,208	$1,846 (16%↓)
Average Cost Per Patient	$14,634	$12,451 (15%↓)
Charges	$5,514,374	$4,624,047 (16%↓)
Charges Per Inpatient Encounter	$19,293	$18,794 (3%↓)
Charges Per Outpatient Encounter	$1,927	$1,741 (10%↓)

Early Supporters of Health cohort data have been very promising. See above financial data from the first six months of work of the Supporters (1.2 FTEs, as the program was started) with 132 patients. The average cost per patient decreased by 16% from pre- and post-enrollment and there was a significant move toward ambulatory vs. inpatient treatment.

One of Gary's promises to the WFBMC Board when he started employment at Wake Forest in 2012 was that FaithHealth efforts would show a decrease in charity care costs overall and in five target zip codes by Year Three efforts. In order to show that FaithHealth was impacting charity care, a very granular aggregate self-pay data dashboard was developed in conjunction with Financial Services staff. Inpatient and outpatient ratios were calculated, along with direct variable costs per encounter, which we believe are key parts of costs to the health system that can be decreased (versus indirects).

Gary's predictions for WFBMC have been realized since 2012. In aggregate, overall total self-pay costs to the system have dropped by 4% from FY12 to FY15, resulting in decreased costs to the system of $2,508,460.

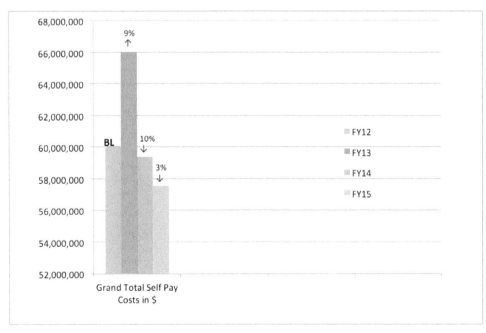

Additionally, charity care costs in our 5 target under-served zip codes have decreased by $1,040,459, with a decrease in direct variable cost per encounter from $202 to $200.

FISCAL YEAR	UNIQUE PATIENTS (N)	TOTAL COST ($)*	TOTAL COST PER ENCOUNTER ($)	DIRECT VARIABLE COST PER ENCOUNTER ($)	MEDIAN INCOME ($)
FY12	11,661	18,552,721	490	**202**	36,386
FY13	13,500	19,899,214	488	**200**	36,011
FY14	12,316	18,622,795	483	**201**	35,636
FY15	12,218	17,512,262	489	**200**	35,636

REFERENCES

Alliance for Advancing Nonprofit Healthcare, "Basic Facts & Figures: Nonprofit Community Hospitals," The Alliance, http://www.nonprofithealthcare.org/resources/BasicFacts-NonprofitHospitals.pdf.

Badawy, M. (2012). "California City Seeks to Cut Asthma Rate Via Bond Issue." Reuters, October 19, 2012.

Baicker, K., Cutler, D., & Song, Z. (2010). "Workplace Wellness Programs Can Generate Savings." *Health Affairs* 29, no. 2 (2010): 304-11, February.

Barnes P.B., Cutts T.F., Dickinson S.B., Hao G., Bowman S. & Gunderson G. (2014). "Methods for Managing and Analyzing Electronic Medical Records: A Formative Examination of a Hospital-Congregation Based Intervention." *Population Health Management*, October 17(5): 279-286.

Barnett, K. (2012). Meeting with David Erickson and Ian Galloway, Federal Reserve Bank of San Francisco, September.

Biles, R. (2000). "Public Housing and the Postwar Urban Renaissance, 1949-1973." In From *Tenements to the Taylor Homes: In Search of an Urban Housing Policy in Twentieth Century America*, Ed. John F. Bauman, Roger Biles, and Kristin S. Szylvian (University Park: Pennsylvania State University Press).

Bradley, E.H. & Taylor, L.A. (2013). "The American Health Care Paradox: Why Spending More is Getting Us Less." New York, New York: Public Affairs.

Bradley, E. H., Elkins, B. R., Herrin, J. & Elbel, B. (2011). Health and Social Services Expenditures: Associations with Health Outcomes. *BMJ Qual Saf*, 20, 826-831.

Braveman P.A., Cubbin C., Egerter S, Williams, D.R., and Pamuk E. (2010). "Socioeconomic disparities in health in the U.S.: What the patterns tell us." *Am. J. Public Health*,100 (Suppl. 1), S186-96.

Carroll A.B. (1999). "Corporate social responsibility: evolution of a definitional construction." *Bus Soc.*, 38:268-295.

Chevas, D. (2013). "Buy Local: Celebrate Local Business-All Year Long." *Tucson Sentinel*, June 24.

CMS. (2014). National Health Expenditure Data. Available at http://www.cms.gov/Research -Statistics-Data-and-Systems/Statistics-Trends-and-Reports/NationahealthExpendData/NationalhealthAccountsHistorial.html.

CMS. (2014). National Health Expenditure Data. Available at http://www.cms.gov/Research -Statistics-Data-and-Systems/Statistics-Trends-and-Reports/NationahealthExpendData/NationalhealthAccountsHistorial.html.)(Employee Benefit Research Institute. BBRI Databook on Employee Benefits. Updated July 2014. http://www.ebri.org/pdf/publications/books/databook/db.chapter%2002.pdf.

CMS. (2014). https://www.cms.gov/research-statistics-data-and-systems/statistics-trends-and-reports/nationalhealthexpenddata/downloads/highlights.pdf.

Cunningham, P., Garfield, R. & Rudowitz, R. (2015). "How are Hospitals Faring under the Affordable Care Act? Early Experiences from Ascension Health." Kaiser Commission in Medicaid and the Uninsured, April.

Daneman, M. (2015). "NY Settles with Five Star Over Mortgages." *Democrat and Chronicle* (Rochester), January 15.

Davis K., Stremikis K., Shoen C., and Squires D. (2014). "Mirror, Mirror, on the Wall 2014 Update: How the U.S. Health Care System Compares Internationally." The Commonwealth Fund, June. Available at http://www.commonwealthfund.org/publications/fund-reports/2014/jun/mirror-mirror)

DHHS. (2015). Center for Medicare & Medicaid Services, CMCS Informational Bulletin, Coverage of Housing-Related Activities and Services for Individuals with Disabilities. June 26, Vikki Wachino.

Dickson, V. (2015). "CMS admits bad dual-eligible math." *Modern Healthcare*, November 9.

Evans, M. (2015). "Providers Struggle on CMS Measures." *Modern Healthcare*, December 14.

Evans, M. (2015). "Medicaid Losses Lead the Pack." *Modern Healthcare*, November 2.

Federal Housing Act of 1949, Title V of P.L. 81-171.

Federal Highway Act of 1956, Public Law 84-627.

Finkelstein E.A., Fiebelkorn L.C., & Wang G. (2005). "The costs of obesity among full time employees." *Am J Health Promotion*, 20(1), 45-51.

Friedman, M. (1962). *Capitalism and Freedom*. USA: University of Chicago Press.

Friedman, M. (1970). "The Social Responsibility of Business is to Increase Its Profits," *New York Times Magazine*. September 13 issue.

Furie, G., & Desai, M. (2012). "Active Transportation and Cardiovascular Disease Risk Factors in U.S. Adults." *American Journal of Preventive Medicine*, 43: 621-28.

Greater New Orleans Foundation. (2014). "New Orleans Works (NOW)." Greater New Orleans Foundation, May.

The Lancet. (2015). "Global, regional, and national age–sex specific all-cause and cause-specific mortality for 240 causes of death, 1990–2013: a systematic analysis for the Global Burden of Disease Study 2013." Volume 385, Issue 9963, 117-171.

Health System Learning Group. (2013). *Health System Learning Group (HSLG) Monograph, Prepared from shared learning for use at Strategic Investment in Shared Outcomes: Transformative Partnerships between Health Systems and Communities*, April 4, Washington, DC.

Heron, M. (2013). "Deaths: Leading causes for 2010." National Vital Statistics Report 2013:62(8). Available at http://www.cdc.gov/nchs/data/nvsr62/nvsr62_06 pdf.

Institute of Education Sciences. (2013). "Digest of Education Statistics." U.S. Department of Education, , https://nces.ed.gov/programs/digest/2014menu_tables.asp.Centers for Medicare and Medicaid Services, National Health Expenditures 2013 Highlights," CMS, 2014, https://www.cms.gov/research-statistics-data-and-systems/statistics-trends-and-reports/nationalhealthexpenddata/downloads/highlights.pdf.

Kaiser Family Foundation and Health Research and Educational Trust. (2013). "Employer Health Benefits. 2013 Annual Survey." Available at http://kaiserfamilyfoundation.files.wordpress.com/2013/08/8465-employer-health-benefits-20131.pdf

Kaiser Family Foundation and Health Research and Charitable Trust. (2015) "Key Facts about the Uninsured Population. Available at http://kff.org/uninsured/fact-sheet/key-facts-about-the-uninsured-population/

Kania, J, & Kramer, M. (2011). "Collective Impact." *Stanford Social Innovation Review*, Winter. http://ssir.org/articles/entry/collective_impact.

Kelly, M., & McKinley, S. (2015). "Cities Building Community Wealth," Democracy Collaborative, November.

Kutscher, B. (2015). "Taking a broader view of health." *Modern Healthcare*, November 23, pp. 14—18.

Leinberger, C., & Alfonso, M. (2012). "Walk this Way: The Economic Promise of Walkable Neighborhoods in Metropolitan Washington, DC." Washington DC: Brookings Institution, Metropolitan Policy Program, May 9-12.

Levin, H.M., Belfield, C., Muennig P. & Rouse C. (2007). "The public returns to public educational investments in African American males." Econ Educ. Rev. 26(6): 699-708.

Lipson, D.J., Valenzano, C.S. & Williams, S.R. (2011)."What Determines Success in State MFP Transition Programs?" National Evaluation of the Money Follows the Person (MFP) Demonstration Grant Program, Report from the Field, No. 8, Washington, DC: Mathematica Policy Research, October.

Litman, T. (2010). Evaluating Public Health Transportation Benefits." Victoria BC: Victoria Transport Policy Institute, June, 8-9.

Lundquist, D. (2014). "Utah's Medicaid Reform has been a Quiet Success." *The Desert News*, April 14.

Lyons, B. (2015). "The ACA Coverage Expansions: Where are We, and What's Ahead?" Boardroom Press, The Governance Institute, December.

Morrissey, J. (2015). "The Cost of Value-Based Care," *Trustee*, September.

Nelson, K., Rafalski, E. Bailey, S. & Marinescu, R. (2015). Managing Rising-Risk Patients in a Value-Based World. 2015 Congress on Healthcare Leadership.

Norris, T., & Howard, T. (2015). "Can Hospitals Heal America's Communities? All in for Mission is the Emerging Model for Impact," Democracy Collaborative.

Office of the Attorney General. (2014). "In School + On Track, 2014," AG's 2014 report on California's Elementary School Truancy and Absenteeism Crisis.

Oziransky, V., Yach, D., Tsu-Yu, T., Luterek, A., & Stevens, D. (2015). "Beyond the Four Walls: Why Community is Critical to Workforce Health." The Vitality Institute, commissioned by the Robert Wood Johnson Foundation, July.

Porter M., & Kramer, M. (2011). "Creating Shared Value." *Harvard Business Review*, January. Available at https://hbr.org/2011/01/the-big-idea-creating-shared-value.

Providence Journal. (2014). "Providence settles redlining lawsuit with Santander Bank." Staff reporters, November 5.

Rumberger, R. (2007). "Dropouts Cost the State $46.4 Billion," California Dropout Prevention Research Project, October 8.

Satter, B. (2009). "Family Properties: Race, Real Estate and the Exploitation of Black Urban America." Henry Holt and Company, March 17.

Serang, F., Thompson, J.P. & Howard, T. (2013). "The Anchor Mission: Leveraging the Power of Anchor Institutions to Build Community Wealth." Takoma Park, MD, The Democracy Collaborative, February.

Silver-Greenberg, J., & Corkery, M. (2015). "Evans Bank Settles 'Redlining" Lawsuit." New York Times, September 10.

Smith, J. & Medalia, D. (2014). "Health Insurance Coverage in the U.S.: 2013." United States Department of Commerce, U.S. Census Bureau, September.

Somers, S. & McGinnis, T. (2014). "Broadening the ACA Story: A Totally Accountable Care Organization." Health Affairs Blog, January 23, (http://healthaffairs.org/blog/2014/01/23/broadening-the-ACA-story-a-totally-accountable-care-organization/

Spencer, A., Lloyd, J., & McGinnis, T. (2015). "Using Medicaid Resources to Pay for Health-Related Supportive Services: Early Lessons," Center for Health Care Strategies, Inc., December.

Squires, D. (2012). "Explaining High Health Care Spending in the United States: An International Comparison of Supply, Utilization, Policies, and Quality." Issues in International Health Policy, Commonwealth Fund, May.

Stewart, W.F., Ricci, J.A., Chee E. & Morganstein, D. (2003) Lost productive work time costs from health conditions in the United States; results from the American Productivity Audit. *J Occupational Environ Med*; 45(12):1234-1246.

Super Church, M. (2013). "Neighborhood Health: A New Framework for Investing in Sustainable Communities," Community Development Investment Review, Federal Reserve Bank of San Francisco.

Swarns, R. (2015). "Biased Lending Evolves, and Blacks Face Trouble Getting Mortgages, *New York Times*, October 30.

Taylor, P., Kochhar R., Fry R., Velasco G., Motel S. (2011)."Wealth gaps rise to record highs between whites, blacks, and Hispanics," Washington (DC): Pew Research Center.

The Week. (2012). "The Heavy Price of Obesity in America: by the Numbers." May 2.

UnitedHealth Foundation. (2014). "America's Health Rankings." Available at http://www.americashealthrankings.org/.

United Nations. (1948). Universal Declaration of Human Rights. Accessed at http://www.un.org/en/universal-declaration-human-rights/)

Urban Land Institute. (2011). "Emerging Trends in Real Estate." Washington, DC, Urban Land Institute, 12.

U.S. Department of Health and Human Services. Administration for Community Living. Administration on Aging. Aging Statistics. http://www.aoa.acl.gov/Aging_Statistics/index.aspx.

Woolf, S.H. & Braveman, P. (2011). "Where Health Disparities Begin: The Role of Social and Economic Determinants—And Why Current Policies May Make Matters Worse." Health Affairs, 30:11, October.

Zuckerman, D. (2013). "How Nonprofit Hospital Wealth Can Build Assets for Low Income Communities." The Democracy Collaborative, March 8.

FULL AUTHORSHIP LISTING

Kevin Barnett, DrPh, MCP, Senior Investigator, Public Health Institute, Oakland, CA

Teresa Cutts, PhD, Asst. Research Professor, Wake Forest School of Medicine, Div. of Public Health Science, Dept. of Social Sciences and Health Policy, Winston Salem, NC

Jeremy Moseley, MHA, Director of Community Engagement, Wake Forest Baptist Medical Center, Winston Salem, NC

For more information about this chapter, contact **Kevin Barnett** at e-mail, kevinpb@pacbell.net or phone, (510) 917-0820.

CHAPTER 9

Philanthropy, Health Systems and Community Health Improvement

Doug Easterling, Allen Smart and Laura McDuffee

Introduction

Our Stakeholder Health "movement" is intentionally disruptive. It calls for hospitals and health care systems to re-imagine their role in advancing health. Rather than diagnosing and treating patients one at a time, healthcare organizations are being challenged to intervene in ways that maintain and improve the health of entire populations.

This new way of doing business requires an expanded perspective—seeing the whole person full of complexities, challenges and assets, rather than honing in on a particular illness, chronic condition, injury or set of symptoms. Likewise, Stakeholder Health redirects our sight upstream—moving from the immediate proximal causes of mortality and morbidity to the more fundamental social and economic determinants that either undermine or enhance health.

By acknowledging the broad and complex range of factors that determine health, one necessarily must accept the limited scope of influence of any single institution or sector, including health care. Stakeholder Health (HSLG, 2013, p. 14) thus counsels hospitals and healthcare organizations that they "do not need to carry the freight of solving complex social issues on their own. [Instead] they can strategically align their resources and efforts with those of others who specialize in [housing, transportation, education, agriculture, public health, economic development and business]" (HSLG, 2013, p. 14). Cross-sector partnering is a core element of the "accountable communities for health" (ACH) concept, which calls for healthcare organizations to enter into coalitions with others from public health, education, business, social services, faith and the larger community (Hacker & Walker, 2013; Tipirneni, Vickery & Ehlinger, 2015).

Stakeholder Health defines a path whereby hospitals can work respectfully and synergistically with various partners who influence health, ranging from small churches and neighborhood associations to established institutions in the governmental, private and nonprofit sectors. Cross-sector partnering is similarly a core element of the "accountable communities for health" (ACH) concept, which calls for healthcare organizations to enter into coalitions with others from public health, education, business, social services, faith and the larger community (Hacker & Walker, 2013; Tipirneni, Vickery & Ehlinger, 2015).

Foundations are a natural partner for us, and in fact have a few distinct advantages over hospitals when it comes to our line of work. For example, foundations inherently seek to advance the health and well-being of populations rather than individual patients, clients or customers. Their accountability is typically linked to improving the lives of people rather than achieving targets for revenue or profit. Perhaps even more importantly for the purposes of Stakeholder Health, foundations have a broader scope of influence over the determinants of health than do health care organizations. They have close working relationships with nonprofit organizations and government agencies in many different sectors who operate on the full range of factors that influence health (e.g., public health, mental health, social services, housing, schools, child development). And they bring a wealth of assets that extend well beyond their bank accounts and investment portfolios.

Here we describe how foundations can be brought into the work of Stakeholder Health, especially in ways that go beyond providing financial support for projects and programs. Foundations have shown that they have the means and the skills to convene actors from throughout a community, to publicize issues with institutional leaders and the broader public, to advocate for policies and other systems-level remedies, to inject innovative ideas into the development of community-health strategies, and to build the capacity of the people and the organizations that need to be engaged in the work. Hospitals have much to gain and to learn through partnering with foundations. On the flip side, foundations can come closer to their goals by forging stronger and more strategic alliances with hospitals, something that many foundations have been reluctant to do. In fact, there are significant historical tensions between hospitals and foundations, a critical aspect that we will deal with later.

The Foundation Landscape

Before probing how hospitals can work productively with foundations, it is useful to present a few fundamentals on how foundations are structured and how they go about their work. At the most general level, a foundation is an organization that disburses money for activities that the Internal Revenue Service regards as "charitable."

When the topic of philanthropy arises, one typically thinks of high-profile national foundations with billions of dollars in assets, such as the Bill and Melinda Gates, Ford, the Rockefeller, Robert Wood Johnson, and William K. Kellogg Foundations. However, foundations come in all shapes and sizes. Some are highly visible (for example, those that sponsor National Public Radio) while others can be found only by searching a philanthropic database. Some foundations make grants throughout the world while others focus on a particular state or community. A typical grant in some foundations is well over $100,000 while in others it is under $10,000. Some have a large staff with specialized expertise while others have a barebones administrative structure. Some have highly defined funding interests while others are more open and responsive to ideas that come from outside.

Foundations also vary in their organizational structure and legal status. "Grantmaking foundations" disburse charitable funds to nonprofit organizations and government entities, while "operating foundations" carry out charitable work themselves. Among grantmaking foundations, some draw from an endowment (often established through a bequest or an estate), while others raise the money they give away. From the standpoint of the Internal Revenue Service, the former are "private foundations" while the latter are "public charities." Federal tax law requires that private foundations spend at least 5% of their assets each year on charitable expenses (which includes not only grants made to nonprofits but also the foundation's own administrative costs). Public charities are not subject to the same requirement but in practice most of these foundations give away at least 5% of their assets each year. However, since fundraising foundations rely more on ongoing donations than on endowments, this statistic is less meaningful.

All this to say, when imagining how foundations can support the work of Stakeholder Health, it is useful to think in terms of specific types of foundations rather than the whole sector (see sidebar, on the most prominent types of foundations, *Taxonomy of Grantmaking Foundations*, which is intended to assist in navigating an admittedly complicated landscape).

Two specific types of foundations are particularly relevant to Stakeholder Health: hospital foundations and health conversion foundations. Each has an intimate linkage to health care organizations, but they have very different lineages, purposes and lines of accountability.

- **Family foundations** are endowed by a wealthy benefactor who defines the mission and funding priorities. Typically these are private foundations (because there is a single source for the charitable funds). As such they are required to pay out at least 5% of their assets each year for charitable purposes (which include grants and qualifying administrative expenses). Most but not all family foundations are designed to operate in perpetuity, based on the premise that investments will return more than 5% each year. Sometimes the founder sets up a board structure that keeps control over the foundation within the family, while other times the board will be made up of a mix of family and non-family members. The mix often changes over time. The Ford Foundation began as largely a family affair when Henry Ford died, but it became an independent entity that actually feuded with Henry Ford II in the 1970s (MacFarquhar, 2016). Some foundations are relatively closed when selecting grantees, while others have a more transparent and inclusive process.

- By definition, private foundations derive the majority of their assets from a single source, but this source is not always a wealthy individual or family. **Corporate foundations** are private foundations that disburse charitable funds on behalf of the parent corporation. This segment of philanthropy accounts for a major portion of the charitable dollars that are given in the U.S. each year. Much of this giving is directed toward charitable purposes (especially capital campaigns and sponsorships) within the communities where the parent corporation has offices. But an even greater amount is given by the "patient assistance foundations" that provide free or reduced-cost prescriptions to those without the means to pay. These patient assistance foundations are linked with different pharmaceutical firms. Eight of the ten most "generous" foundations (of any type) fall into this category. The patient assistance foundations associated with AbbVie, Bristol-Myers Squibb, Johnson & Johnson, Merck, Genentech, Pfizer, GlaxoSmithKline, and Lilly each reported over $500 million in charitable giving in 2013 (Foundation Center, 2015).

- A foundation is classified as a "public charity" by the IRS if its funding comes from multiple contributors within the "general public," or alternatively, it is supported by a governmental unit or tax-exempt income. Most public charities spend those dollars on their own programming (i.e., the "nonprofit organizations" that we typically think of), but many of the biggest **public charities** are grantmaking organizations. The United Way organizations that raise and distribute dollars in most U.S. communities are a prominent example.

- **Community foundations** are one of the most important grantmaking organizations that fit within the public charity category. A community foundation raises funds from local donors and provides these donors with administrative, programmatic and investment services. Donors can either set up their own distinct funds, each of which has a particular funding priority, or contribute to the foundation's discretionary fund. Some of the community foundation's grantmaking is directed by individual donors, while some grants are awarded by the board of trustees taking into account the staff's recommendations. The boards of community foundations are usually comprised of community leaders representing different institutions and sectors.

- A **hospital foundation** raises funds from individuals and organizations, and then disburses those funds in support of a particular hospital. When that hospital is a nonprofit organization, the foundation if often set up as a unit of the hospital (technically referred to as "supporting organizations"). In contrast, for-profit hospitals often find it advantageous to establish a distinct organization that is recognized by the IRS as a public charity.

- **Health conversion foundations** (also called "health legacy foundations") are created when a nonprofit hospital, health care system or health plans is sold to a for-profit firm or converted into a for-profit entity. Federal tax law requires that the proceeds from the transaction remain within the nonprofit sphere and be used for comparable purposes (e.g., to improve the health status of the same population that was served by the entity that was sold or converted). Typically a new health foundation is created. It is a separate legal entity with its own mission and governance structure.

- Philanthropy also occurs through **trusts** that are managed by financial institutions. A trust is either set up by a living donor or established as a condition of the will when a donor dies. Rather than being governed by a board of trustees, the financial institution serves as the trustee and controls the disbursement of grants, investment decisions and the hiring of staff. One example of a trust that funds health projects is Kate B. Reynolds Charitable Trust in Winston-Salem, NC, which is a trust account of Wells Fargo. When the Kate B. Reynolds Charitable Trust was initially established (upon the death of Mrs. Reynolds), the will stipulated that there would be three trustees, two of Mrs. Reynolds' relatives and Wachovia Bank (which was then based in Winston-Salem), and that Wachovia would become the sole trustee upon the death of the two human trustees. Although the Trust does not have a governing board, the Trustee has convened two advisory boards which review and provide input on strategy and grantmaking.

- Many hospitals set up a foundation to raise funds from individuals and organizations. These **hospital foundations** channel charitable giving to projects aligned with the donors' interests and the hospital's strategic priorities, which might include an expansion of a facility, new equipment, patient support services or subsidies for medical care.

- **Health conversion foundations** (also called "health legacy foundations") are formed when a nonprofit hospital, health care system or health plan is either acquired by a for-profit firm or converted to for-profit status. The proceeds from these transactions are transferred into the endowment of a foundation that maintains the general mission of the entity which was sold (i.e., improving or advancing the health of the population served by the entity). These conversion foundations began emerging in the 1980s as for-profit corporations extended their market reach by acquiring non-profit hospitals, many of them affiliated with religious denominations. A second spate of foundations was formed in the 1990s, including large ones in California and other states through the conversion of Blue Cross Blue Shield plans from nonprofit to for-profit status. Another large cohort has come into existence over the past 5 years as the health care market has adjusted to the Affordable Care Act. The most recent census identified 306 conversion foundations that submitted their annual Form 990 to the IRS in 2010. Together they held a total of $26.2 billion in assets (Niggel & Brandon, 2014). A more recent census is not available, but it is safe to say that at least another 100 have been established since 2010.

The assets of conversion foundations range from less than $10 million (for foundations formed when small hospitals are acquired or closed), to more than $3 billion (for foundations such as the California Endowment and the Colorado Health Foundation, formed when large systems or health plans are sold or converted). The largest conversion foundations typically have a statewide focus, but the majority serve a particular community or sub-state region. Many of these locally oriented foundations award at least $5 million per year in grants.

The most obvious philanthropic partners for Stakeholder Health systems will be the foundations that are affiliated with their collaborating hospital(s). But health conversion foundations may actually be more crucial to the work because, generally, they have more staff and a higher leadership profile in the community. And even non-health foundations, especially community foundations, can add value because they often fund work that addresses various social and economic issues that influence health.

The financial assets that foundations can bring to Stakeholder Health work are obviously valuable, especially because foundations often have a great deal of discretion in deciding how and where to invest their grant dollars. Yet, it is crucial to recognize that foundations are more than funders. They can bring many other resources and can take a variety of actions that enhance the effectiveness and impact of a Stakeholder Health initiative. To better recognize this strategic value, it is useful to take a deeper look at the business of philanthropy.

The Business of Philanthropy

Most foundations disburse their charitable dollars through some sort of grantmaking process. The many different versions of grantmaking depend on a foundation's mission, strategy, size of staff, role of the board, philosophy and culture. The foundation might issue an open request for proposals or it might invite proposals from a small group of pre-screened organizations. It might specify particular types of work that are open for funding or alternatively leave it up to applicants to propose their preferred projects. Grants might support a specific project, the core operating expenses of the grantee organization, or the building of organizational capacity. Some foundations fund the same organizations year after year, while others limit the duration of funding. Some want to invest in innovative project ideas while others are more conservative and focus on evidence-based programs. More generally, each foundation has its own interests, goals and philosophy about what constitutes a "good grant." As such, some foundations will have an affinity for the work of Stakeholder Health while others will regard this as someone else's work.

While grantmaking is the defining element of philanthropy, it is not necessarily the most powerful thing that foundations do. A growing number of foundations view their core business as **catalyzing change**, specifically, change that leads to the impacts referenced in the foundation's mission (e.g., improving health, reducing poverty, creating more vibrant communities, eradicating injustice or racism). They use a variety of strategies that extend well beyond grantmaking to stimulate change at the individual, organizational, community and societal levels. These include: increasing the capacity of nonprofit organizations and government agencies, encouraging these organizations to adopt more effective programs and strategies, establishing new organizations, building the leadership skills of established and emerging leaders, activating local residents and officials to take more initiative and to think more creatively, encouraging changes in public policy (either directly through advocacy or indirectly through policy research and awareness-raising), and leading communities through a process of soul-searching and transformation. Below we present examples of each of these "beyond-grantmaking" strategies.

BUILDING ORGANIZATIONAL CAPACITY

Foundations rely on nonprofit organizations, government agencies and individual people to carry out the day-to-day work that is required to advance their mission, whether it is promoting health, improving educational outcomes, moving people out of poverty, strengthening families, building vibrant communities, creating a more just society, or something else equally as ambitious. This means that a foundation's ability to achieve its goals depends in large part on the capacity of the organizations who serve as its grantees.

National foundations typically have access to a pool of well-established, highly functioning nonprofit organizations interested in carrying out work in line with the foundation's interests. In contrast, foundations operating in a particular community or region may find it much more challenging to find strong nonprofits that are ready to do the type of work that the foundation is interested in supporting. As such, many foundations have gone into the business of building the capacity of nonprofit organizations. This work provides the foundation with more effective partners, while at the same time strengthening the nonprofit sector in communities and regions where the foundation has decided it has an interest.

In a recent survey of foundations (restricted to those that have at least one paid staff position), Grantmakers for Effective Organizations (GEO) found that 77 percent are investing at least some resources in building organizational capacity among their grantees (GEO, 2015). These investments include grants with funding dedicated to training or hiring an organizational development consultant. Alternatively, foundations sometimes hire consulting firms directly and make their services available to a cohort of nonprofits within a community or region. In either case, the intent is to strengthen nonprofit organizations on factors such as program development, strategy, fundraising, communications, technology and evaluation.

The Health Foundation for Western and Central New York (HFWCNY), a health conversion foundation based in Buffalo, established a fairly elaborate capacity building program, GetSET (Success in Extraordinary Times) for health and human service organizations in western New York (HFWCNY, 2015). The impetus for the program was the rapidly changing fiscal environment that is confronting service providers that depend on Medicaid and other government sources for revenue. GetSET uses a team-based approach to assist these organizations in strengthening their strategy, operations and structures. A self-assessment at the outset of the program provides the participating organizations with information on how they are doing with regard to various core competencies. Each organization in the cohort formulates a capacity-building plan and then works on those issues through a process of training, consulting and peer learning. The foundation supports the training and consulting and also provides participating organizations with grants to help implement their organizational changes.

Some foundations have emphasized specific aspects of organizational capacity that they believe are lacking among their grantees and partner organizations. The REACH Health Foundation, a conversion foundation located in Merriman, Kansas, introduced a Cultural Competency Initiative in 2009 which provided health and human service organizations in the Kansas City region with individualized technical assistance to improve their services to uninsured and underserved populations. This assistance included organizational assessment, coaching, policy development and change management. Over time this program has evolved to emphasize peer learning and networking. More than 60 organizations now participate in the Cultural Competency Learning Community. Three other health funders in the region have partnered with REACH to provide additional financial support and in order to spread the program to more organizations and more communities (REACH, 2015).

ESTABLISHING NEW ORGANIZATIONS

As a foundation scans the nonprofit landscape looking for potential grantees and partners, it may find that there are gaps not only in capacity but also in mission. It may have a clear and informed strategy for achieving a particular improvement in health or quality of life, but this approach runs the risk of encouraging the organization to diverge from its mission and goals. One option is to draw a local organization into new work that supports the strategy, but this approach runs the risk of encouraging mission creep, a divergence from original mission goals. Even if the foundation can entice an organization into new territory with a grant, this is arguably an irresponsible use of the foundation's power and resources.

An alternative approach for the foundation is to create a new organization that directly addresses the identified gap. The Rapides Foundation in Alexandria, Louisiana, has exercised this option on a number of occasions because it could not find organizations in its largely rural target area that were suited to carrying out work that the foundation regarded as crucial. In 2001 the foundation established the Cenla Medication Access Program (CMAP) to improve people's access to medication by offering free or reduced-cost prescriptions to eligible clients. Patient Assistance Program specialists employed by the foundation assist rural clinics and primary care practices with accessing these medications. CMAP has grown beyond the foundation's funding region and is now offered statewide (Rapides, 2015).

Edgecombe County, one of the Kate B. Reynolds Charitable Trust's Healthy Places NC communities

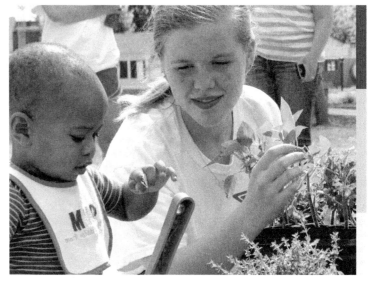

Foundations establish programs to build capacity not only at the organizational level, but also the individual level. The vast majority of these individually oriented programs emphasize leadership skills of one sort or another. The Robert Wood Johnson Foundation and the W.K. Kellogg Foundation each have a long history of leadership development programming to support leaders in fields such as health policy, public health, nursing, academic medicine, health equity and social change. These programs recruit participants nationally or regionally, typically through a competitive process. Some programs are geared towards leaders with established track records and positions of influence, while others are oriented toward emerging leaders or early career professionals who show particular promise. In most cases, the program brings together a cohort of participants in one or more leadership-development training sessions, typically delivered by a highly regarded training group such as the Center for Creative Leadership (CCL) or the Kennedy School of Government at Harvard. Many of these programs also support a process of peer mentoring and learning and some provide each participant with a coach.

While these programs generally provide participants with rich experiences (even life-changing ones), they have been criticized for their focus on individualized development and remote training. Participants come together for intense sessions that leave them with a variety of new skills and tools, but then return to an environment where those skills, tools and new way of looking at the world are foreign and possibly threatening. This makes it difficult for the newly trained leader to apply the competencies that he or she has built. The Kate B. Reynolds Charitable Trust in Winston-Salem, North Carolina, addressed this issue by organizing leadership development sessions within the counties where it seeks to build capacity through its Healthy Places NC (HPNC) initiative. The Trust contracted with the Center for Creative Leadership, which is headquartered in nearby Greensboro, to design and deliver a leadership program appropriate to organizational leaders in rural communities who can play a role in improving population health. It brings together participants with a shared interest (e.g., behavioral health, childhood obesity) in an intensive experiential program to develop "boundary-spanning leadership," which CCL defines as "the capability to establish direction, alignment, and commitment across boundaries in service of a higher vision or goal" (Yip, Ernst & Campbell, 2016). CCL also provides individual coaching and consulting support to help the cohort develop a collective project or strategy

Foundations around the country have established such regionally or locally oriented leadership development programs. Many focus on civic leadership rather than organizational leadership. For example, the Blandin Foundation in northern Minnesota has trained more 7,000 residents from 600 rural communities in creating shared meaning, building social networks, and mobilizing people, resources and power (Blandin, 2015). Other rural funders, such as the Ford Family Foundation in Roseburg, Oregon have developed similar programs, taking advantage of what their peers have learned over the years.

Conversion foundations in particular have come to recognize that leadership development is one of the critical strategies for improving the health of communities. The Kansas Health Foundation is arguably the greatest proponent of this pathway to health. It established the Kansas Community Leadership Institute in 1992, attracting a range of leaders, including hospital administrators, public health officials, nonprofit leaders and county extension agents. That program proved insufficient to meet the demand for leadership development across the state, so in 2005, the foundation invested $30 million to establish the Kansas Leadership Center. The Center has developed its own model of civic leadership (built on the concept of "adaptive leadership"), and a multi-layered curriculum to train leaders from multiple sectors and with different levels of experience as leaders (Chrislip & O'Malley, 2013).

Community change occurs through the actions of many people who display varying levels of leadership. Some will feel comfortable participating in leadership development training, but others view themselves as just doing the necessary work. In at least a few communities, foundations have played a key role in activating residents and mobilizing neighborhoods to take action to improve their health and well-being.

One example is the Greater Rochester Health Foundation in upstate New York which uses a community organizing strategy to improve the physical, social and economic environments of neighborhoods (Zappia, Puntenney & Snyder, 2013). This grassroots orientation grew out of the foundation's experience in working with local residents to carry out a program to remove lead-based paint from homes throughout the city. With its Neighborhood Health Status Improvement initiative, the foundation funded a community organizer position in 10 neighborhoods and rural communities throughout the region. The organizers are trained in the Asset-Based Community Development (ABCD) paradigm of Kretzman and McKnight (1993), reviewed in Chapter 6 of this volume, which focuses on resident-led efforts to improve the quality of life by drawing on the community's own assets.

The ABCD approach has attracted the attention of a number of foundations across the country, especially community foundations. Beginning in the 1980s, community foundations in Denver, Colorado and in Winston-Salem and Greensboro, North Carolina began training residents and nonprofit leaders on the ABCD model and funding the asset-mapping work that is central to it.

FACILITATING PLANNING AND PROBLEM SOLVING

Foundations promote improvements in health beyond individual and neighborhood levels. Health conversion foundations especially have developed initiatives that bring local stakeholders together to identify critical health issues that need resolving on a community-wide level. These initiatives require multiple organizations to sign on for a long-term process of collaboration, planning, and carrying out coordinated work. During the planning phase, the group typically assesses the community's health issues, prioritizes a limited number of focus areas, identifies underlying factors that offer opportunities for improving health, and selects a set of programmatic and policy strategies that operate on those leverage points. At the end of the planning process, the group generates a plan that lays out what each of the participating organizations will do to advance the overall strategy. This typically is submitted to the funder with a proposal for grant funding to support specific elements of the plan. The funder then reviews the products of the planning process and decides which programs, activities and organizations to support through an "implementation grant." These grants typically cover expenses over at least two years, and sometimes up to five.

These planning-based health initiatives began to take root in the early 1990s with The California Wellness Foundation's Health Improvement Initiative (Cheadle, Beery, Greenwald, Nelson, Pearson & Senter, 2003); The Colorado Trust's Colorado Healthy Communities Initiative (Conner & Easterling, 2009); Sierra Health Foundation's Community Partnerships for Healthy Children Initiative (Meehan, Hebbeler, Cherner & Peterson, 2009); Robert Wood Johnson Foundation's Urban Health Initiative (Silver & Weitzman, 2009); and the Community Care Network demonstration program developed by the Health Research and Education Trust in partnership with the American Hospital Association, VHA Inc., and the Catholic Hospital Association (Hasnain-Wynia, 2003). More recently, foundations such as the Kansas Health Foundation, the Health Foundation of South Florida, the New York State Health Foundation and The Duke Endowment have launched additional initiatives that call for a variety of local organizations to come together to create a shared strategy for improving the health of their community. This recent spate of activity has been driven at least in part by the introduction of "collective impact" as a strategy for achieving large-scale change (Kania & Kramer, 2011).

Foundation-sponsored community health initiatives often fall into the category of disruptive innovations. By bringing a more comprehensive, intentional and data-driven approach to strategy design, they disrupt the community's prevailing way of advancing health. And they are innovative in the sense that local actors engage in a form of thinking, problem-solving and planning that departs from normal practice. Though the planning model might not be innovative in an absolute sense, it is novel to the particular community where it is introduced.

Foundations are well-positioned to identify innovations and introduce them into community decision making, problem-solving and strategizing. Their staff often have at least some content expertise in health care, public health and social change, and more specifically, are usually familiar with current research literature on evidence-based and emerging practices. More than most nonprofits, foundations are able to set aside dollars for staff development and attending national meetings. The philanthropic sector is rich with affinity groups that organize annual conferences, facilitate peer learning and disseminate research findings (e.g., Grantmakers in Health, Grantmakers for Effective Organizations, Council of Foundations, Neighborhood Funders Group). This provides foundation staff with multitudes of ideas to enhance the work of grantee organizations and communities, including practices that highlight the benefits and evidence associated with innovation and incentivizes grantees to adopt it.

Innovations that foundations have brought to local organizations, institutions and collaborative bodies include: evidence-based programs to improve child development, practice guidelines for clinicians, tools for assessing clients' needs and goals, quality improvement processes, model legislation to reduce tobacco use and financing reform that encourages cross-agency collaboration.

New frameworks for thinking and problem-solving are a powerful but often overlooked form of innovation. Achieving meaningful progress on entrenched problems invariably requires more than finding and implementing an effective program or two. The critical work happens upstream when actors are analyzing the situation and formulating strategy. Whether those actors find breakthrough strategies depends more on their mindset than the specific programs they come up with. A systems-level framework can provide them with a wide-angle lens that illuminates the local landscape and shows how people, organizations and issues inter-connect with one another (Easterling, Arnold, Smart & Jones, 2013).

One of the most innovative and powerful of these conceptual frameworks comes from County Health Rankings & Roadmaps (CHR&R), a program of the University of Wisconsin Population Health Institute in collaboration with the Robert Wood Johnson Foundation. Building on the pioneering work of Michael McGinnis and William Foege (1993), the CHR&R framework recognizes that the health of a population is determined in large part by factors that fall outside the realm of clinical care, including health behaviors, the physical environment, and social and economic factors. Each year, the CHR&R program uses an algorithm that reflects what they view to be the actual determinants of health to compute a Health Outcomes score and a Health Factors score for every U.S. county. Counties are then ranked from most to least healthy within each state. These CHR&R data generate a great deal of local and national media attention, and also serve as the basis for health planning in communities throughout the country. According to the CHR&R website, "the Roadmaps are helping communities bring people together from all walks of life to look at the many factors that influence health, focus on strategies that we know work, learn from each other, and make changes that will have a lasting impact on health" (UWPHI, 2015). While the groups typically begin with an emphasis on their county's ranking, the exploration process is guided by the expanded conceptualization of health articulated in the CHR&R framework.

The Kate B. Reynolds Charitable Trust has incorporated CHR&R into its Healthy Places NC (HPNC) initiative. Shortly after the launch of HPNC in each county, a representative from the CHR&R project comes to present the conceptual model, along with detailed health data for that specific county (typically in three separate forums targeted to different audiences). The CHR&R data and conceptual framework spur new thinking, conversation, innovation and cross-sector networking, and this materially changes how local actors are tackling the health issues facing their communities. In particular, it fosters more comprehensive, systems-level strategizing. The Clinton Foundation has adopted a similar approach, incorporating the CHR&R framework into its Clinton Health Matters Initiative, which supports community-based assessment and planning across the U.S.

RAISING PUBLIC AWARENESS OF KEY ISSUES

The CHR&R example illustrates another strategy available to foundations: raising public awareness and consciousness on critical issues. Foundations across the country (especially national and state health foundations) have built sophisticated communications departments that devise and deliver campaigns aimed to reach specific target audiences with key messages about particular health issues. These campaigns have helped to elevate onto the public agenda issues such as homelessness, childhood obesity, suicide, opioid abuse, teen pregnancy and bullying. Such awareness-raising has paid off with wide-ranging investments and programming on the part of government agencies, nonprofits, businesses and coalitions.

Foundations have been particularly active in raising public awareness about access to health care. For more than two decades, the Commonwealth Fund and the Kaiser Family Foundation, working with nonprofits such as Families USA, have visibly publicized the proportion of Americans without health insurance. A number of state-level health foundations have stepped into this arena too and commissioned studies that provide a more fine-grained picture of who does and doesn't have insurance coverage within their own state. For example, The Colorado Trust in 2008 funded the Colorado Department of Health Care Policy and Financing to develop and implement the Colorado Household Survey (COHS), which asks multiple questions about insurance status (Colorado Trust, 2009). This survey was able to demonstrate how insurance status varied by region and demographic group—in a much more precise manner than had been previously known. Moreover, these data helped set the stage for a more informed and objective debate around the value of proposals such as the Affordable Care Act.

ADVOCATING FOR POLICY CHANGE

As foundations get into the business of raising issues on the public agenda, they naturally (and sometimes intentionally) find themselves in the midst of policy advocacy. Depending on their tax status (either private foundation, public charity or 501(c)(4) organization) and the risk tolerance of their boards, foundations can be either upfront or behind-the-scenes when advocating for a particular policy.

Some health foundations have been particularly active in advocating for their state legislatures and governors to expand Medicaid as permitted under the Affordable Care Act. For example, the Colorado Trust joined with the Colorado Health Foundation to support advocacy and organizing efforts throughout the state. This included messaging and analysis provided to lawmakers, as well as a more broad-based campaign to build "public will" for Medicaid Expansion. The foundations provided funding and technical assistance to advocacy organizations around the state to build their capacity. Elsewhere, foundations have sponsored studies that provide evidence of the various benefits that will accrue to states if they expand Medicaid (e.g., increased proportion of residents have access to health care, more federal dollars coming into the state, more jobs for health professionals, better balance sheet for rural hospitals).

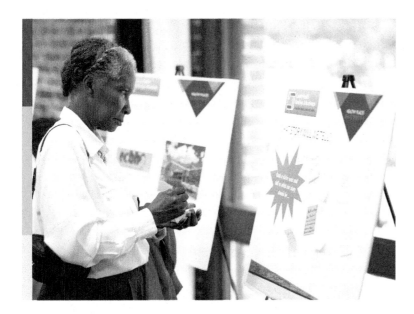

Using the Community Health Rankings & Roadmaps model to support community health planning

Foundations have also taken the lead in advocating for policy change that goes well beyond Medicaid and the Affordable Care Act. One example is The Con Alma Health Foundation, a statewide health conversion foundation based in Santa Fe, New Mexico, which has publicized the detrimental public and environmental effects of a proposal to downgrade New Mexico's water quality standards. The change would potentially affect wildlife, ranchers, and a number of indigenous communities that depend on the Pecos and Rio Grande Rivers for drinking water. In addition to its own role in raising public awareness, the foundation funds Amigos Bravos, a conservation organization guided by social justice principles, to organize political participation within the affected communities (Con Alma, 2015). As a public charity, Con Alma cannot lobby for or against particular pieces of legislation (or fund other organizations to do so on its behalf), but it can carry out and support a broad range of advocacy initiatives that raise public awareness around the underlying issues.

LEADING STRUCTURAL CHANGE

The strategies described so far correspond to various leverage points for improving community health and quality of life—strengthening the capacity of people and organizations, expanding and improving the mix of programs and services that are available to local residents, promoting more deliberate and informed planning, bringing more residents into the life of the community, and changing policy so that it better supports the health of local residents. A handful of foundations have gone even further and taken the lead in changing the fundamental character of the communities they serve.

Leading such community change is illustrated by the Incourage Community Foundation in Wisconsin Rapids, Wisconsin (Easterling & Millesen, 2015). The economy of the region, devastated by a downturn in the papermaking industry and a crash in the price of cranberries in the early 2000s, hemorrhaged not only jobs but also the business executives who had served as civic leaders. The community foundation, working together with the local economic development agency, promoted the idea that the region would not recover by trying to recruit new firms, but instead needed to encourage entrepreneurship and collaborative problem-solving among local residents. More radically, they argued that this recovery would require a shift in the local culture. The traditional economy and political structure had fostered a paternalistic culture that had created a sense of dependency among residents. It designed a new leadership development program—Advanced Leadership Institute—that challenged established leaders to think more inclusively and emerging leaders to step forward with their own ideas and initiative. This was one aspect of a 4-year Community Progress Initiative, which also included community planning processes, the creation of local charitable funds, training programs for fledgling entrepreneurs, venture capital funds, mentoring for business owners, the creation of industry clusters, and study tours to other communities suffering economic upheaval. This work has since led to the emergence of new leaders, increased collaboration across institutions, reduced divisiveness, and nationally recognized initiatives to retool the local workforce and promote new industry. Changes occurred not only among individual participants, but also at a structural level, with the culture beginning to shift from one defined by dependency and paternalism to one where all residents feel personal responsibility and take initiative.

RELEVANCE TO STAKEHOLDER HEALTH INITIATIVES

These examples illustrate a variety of ways in which foundations can support a community-wide or society-wide effort to improve health. Many of these strategies can be directly applied to the work of Stakeholder Health. Some examples of how a foundation could add significant value to a local Stakeholder Health initiative include:

• Providing **targeted funding for key projects** or programs included within the health-improvement strategy. Foundation funding is particularly valuable when setting up a new program or service.

BEHIND THE SCENES CONVENING

Comprehensive solutions require full and serious participation from all organizations that have influence over the issues at hand. In practice most community-based planning efforts will have at least a few holdouts and disengaged participants. Foundations can use their position as community leaders to draw these organizations into the process and to encourage them to participate more enthusiastically and collaboratively. This role is particularly valuable in communities that have competing healthcare systems.

The Mid-Iowa Health Foundation in Des Moines played this neutral convener/arm-twister role in a collaborative effort that brought together the local health department, an affordable housing organization, and all three of the community's hospitals to address the issue of asthma in low-income children. Their effort began when the foundation staff attended a meeting organized by local school nurses to hear about the health issues facing Burmese refugees. According to the CEO, Suzanne Mineck,

> "We were discussing helping the Burmese refugee population identify a medical home and there was a Burmese mom that was sitting in on the conversation with the head of all of the school nurses. We were almost done with the meeting and then this lovely Burmese mom who spoke very little English turned to me and, she knew we were funding the project, and she said first how grateful she was for our support and how much she and the Burmese community appreciated it, but that I needed to know that her son would never be healthy. She could take her son to the doctor every day but if she brought him home to a home that has cockroaches and no heat he would never be healthy. That was profound moment for me. It's one thing to hear yourself talk about social determinants. It's another to really feel them and what that means.

> That was well over 3 years ago. I started having conversations with the Polk County Housing Trust Fund and the public health department. 'What do we do here?' This led to developing a successful proposal to the 'BUILD Health Challenge' program. All three of our hospital institutions came together to participate in the initiative. Our health department, the housing world, our schools have come together and we're doing a project to reduce the cases of chronic pediatric asthma in a poor zip code area in our community. We are working with the hospitals and school nurses to identify kids with chronic pediatric asthma. We go into their homes and do an environmental scan and also a social needs scan.

> The hospitals each put in dollars and in-kind support. More importantly, Build Health was interested in data, which required that hospital leaders be at the table throughout the implementation of the program."

When asked how she was able to get all three hospitals to join together on a common project, Suzanne replied that it was all about relationships. "The public health director had a good relationship with one CEO. I had good relationship with another CEO. And at some point it came down to positioning. We made an invitation to become part of something that was noticeable if they were not involved."

- Supporting the **development of organizational capacity** among any or all of the organizations involved in carrying out the strategy. Capacity building is particularly important for organizations that have new programs to deliver or that need to expand their operations and staff to meet the new expectations assigned to them. This could come in the form of grants that fund new positions, technology, training and coaching. Alternatively the foundation might create a capacity-building program that serves the interests of multiple organizations from across the community.

- Supporting the **development of needed leadership skills** among actors who are key to implementing the strategy. As with organizational capacity, the foundation can either provide funding for leadership training to the organizations where these actors are based, or alternatively, sponsor a leadership program that trains an entire cohort of key actors.

- Sponsoring **community assessments and other research** that allows for a smarter strategy. These studies can take a number of forms, including a drill-down on how specific health issues manifest themselves in the community, a root cause analysis of thorny problems, a mapping of community assets, and an analysis of how various information systems and operational procedures need to adapt in order to support shifts in institutional strategy. Foundations can also pay the costs associated with co-learning, both within and between communities.

- Supporting **awareness raising, agenda setting and policy advocacy** that, taken together, creates an "enabling context" for the new way of thinking and working that Stakeholder Health seeks to cultivate. Such educational and advocacy work can be carried out either by the foundation directly or by nonprofits that the foundation supports. Alternatively the foundation can support a community organizing process that brings residents throughout the community into advocacy roles.

One of the most crucial functions that foundations can play in a Stakeholder Health initiative is to **facilitate the overall process of collaborative problem-solving and collective action**. Stakeholder Health explicitly acknowledges that hospitals and healthcare organizations do not have influence over most of the factors that influence the health of the community—or even the health of their patients. We need to engage in "transformative partnerships" with a broad range of organizations working in the areas of housing, education, transportation and economic development.

Foundations are, in fact, well positioned to convene cross-sectoral partnerships, especially where there are turf issues, competing interests, power differentials and/or oversized egos. These situations call for institutional leaders who are well known and widely respected throughout the community, who are focused on the community's overall well-being rather than their own parochial interests, and who are willing and able to create an open and inclusive problem-solving space. In most cities of any size, there is at least one foundation that has the standing and credibility to play this role. And, because foundations are connected to a multitude of local organizations, while also being politically and financially independent,they have a number of advantages over hospitals, health departments and other institutions that typically take the lead over community planning efforts.

Foundations can continue to play an active leadership role once the key players have come together to look at what they might do to improve community health. This can include facilitating meetings and keeping the process moving toward informed and strategic solutions. Foundations often talk about their role as a "neutral convener," signifying that they are able to stay above the fray and focus on larger goals and the community's overall interests. While one might argue about whether they are really "neutral," it is fair to say that foundations are uniquely situated to serve as guardians of planning processes, ensuring that all partners are heard and that the group doesn't head toward a solution that disregards legitimate interests and perspectives.

In addition to their out-in-front role facilitating and maintaining the integrity of a process, foundations can also operate behind the scenes to bring key players to the table and keep them there when the

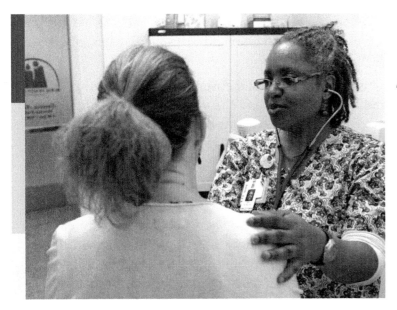

process gets dicey. In this sense, foundations sometimes serve as chaplains, allowing partners to vent their frustrations while bringing them back toward their mission and the opportunities at hand.

OCCASIONAL TENSIONS BETWEEN HOSPITALS AND LOCAL HEALTH FOUNDATIONS

The previous section demonstrated that foundations can contribute to Stakeholder Health efforts, not only with financial resources, but also a broad array of "beyond-grantmaking"strategies. Many communities will have at least one foundation with considerable experience in the business of facilitating collective problem-solving, building organizational capacity, developing community leaders, and cultivating systems change.

If foundations have such a vital role to play in Stakeholder Health, then the logical question is why hospitals have so far neglected to fully engage them? One answer is that hospital executives don't fully recognize what foundations are capable of doing. Foundations are often viewed as organizations that have money to contribute to charitable projects and not much more. This may be true for the hospital's own internal foundation (which typically disburses funds according to the hospital's strategic plan), but other foundations in the community may well operate quite differently. Many of them, as we have noted, are highly strategic entities with ambitious goals and a broad ability to catalyze change.

There is a second important reason that hospitals often might not reach out to include foundations as co-designers or co-leaders of an initiative: hospitals tend to operate autonomously. Because of their extensive financial resources and their status as an economic engine for the community, hospitals have grown accustomed to deciding for themselves what they want to accomplish and how they will go about getting there. Partnering with a foundation on a large-scale initiative requires reaching out in unfamiliar ways and letting go of some of the control they are accustomed to exercising.

What would happen if hospitals were able to acknowledge the value that foundations can bring to their Stakeholder Health work? Would foundations take them up on the invitation? This certainly occurs in some communities. For example, Interact for Health, a health conversion foundation in Cincinnati, developed a partnership with Cincinnati Children's Hospital to increase the number of school-based health centers operating within public schools in the region. The foundation has long been active in establishing and funding school-based health centers. The children's hospital has a special interest in preventing and managing childhood asthma, and saw the value of school-based health centers as a means to advancing this interest. As a result of their collaborative efforts, the hospital took over the management of a center in a school that serves low-income students. The foundation provides funding to support the center (Interact, 2015).

While examples like this demonstrate the benefits of foundations and hospitals working together around a common agenda, we have also witnessed skepticism, suspicion and chagrin on the part of foundations when it comes to the idea of partnering with hospitals. Especially among health foundations that make grants in one particular community, the staff and board sometimes believe that hospitals too often ask for outsized grants for projects that are entirely within the hospitals' own self-interest.

Consider a typical health conversion foundation that has a pool of $10 million to grant each year to improve health in its service area (often a county or multi-county region). Is it surprising that the staff and board will hesitate to fund the local medical center's multi-million dollar request for capital expansion or an endowed chair? A million dollar grant proposal might look "normal" to a medical center (it submits hundreds of these per year to the National Institutes of Health), but it may stir resentment among the foundation's program officer who reviews a hundred proposals from local nonprofits in the $30,000 to $50,000 range.

Another factor that makes foundations disenchanted with hospitals and academic medical centers is the central role of development offices as intermediaries between hospitals and foundations. Many hospitals treat "foundation relations" as completely under the purview of the development office, which acts as the gatekeeper for any and all requests or inquiries that originate within the hospital. Development staff may or may not have a solid understanding of the projects that are being proposed for funding, especially research studies.

CREATING A NEW EQUILIBRIUM

The tension between hospitals and foundations that occurs in many communities is unfortunate in many respects. Hospitals and foundations are, in fact, natural allies when it comes to any large-scale effort to improve community health. Equally important, there is reciprocal value when they work together: foundations can help hospitals achieve their goals, and hospitals can help foundations achieve theirs.

Hospitals can benefit in a number of ways from the expertise, experience and relationships that local foundations have built in carrying out their work. Especially with the emphasis on value-based care under World 2.0 (see chapter 10), hospitals need to expand and adapt their strategies for patient care and transitional care. They also need to establish networks of community-based supports to promote the health of patients before and after their hospital stays. The partnerships that foundations already have with service agencies, faith-based organizations, coalitions and grassroots groups are precisely what hospitals need as they create accountable care organizations and enter into contracts that require them to effectively manage population health. Hospitals can also benefit from foundations in terms of learning about the social determinants of health and how to influence those determinants, given that foundations operate within and across multiple systems, providing them with a rich understanding of how health is created and which roles that various local agencies play in that process.

Foundations likewise have much to gain from partnering more closely with hospitals. While foundations are in the enviable position of having large sums of discretionary funds to invest each year, they are inherently constrained in their ability to achieve their strategic goals. Their staff make grants, lead community-change efforts and connect people and organizations to capacity-building opportunities, but they do not directly carry out the on-the-ground work that brings services to residents or changes conditions within the home or the neighborhood. Foundations rely on their grantees and partner organizations to act as agents in implementing their strategies and to sustain programs that the foundation has helped create. Because of their size, resources and reach, hospitals are thus potentially one of the most important organizations that foundations can work with to achieve their goals.

Given that hospitals and foundations have mutually reinforcing interests, how can we encourage productive partnering? We offer three modest proposals.

First, **we advise hospitals and foundations to take a second look at one another, and a deeper look at one another's assets and interests**. It is crucial for hospitals to recognize that foundations are more than funders. While their financial resources often attract the most attention, foundations can have an even greater impact on community health through their convening, advocacy, capacity building and influence. We recognize that foundations are in the business of making grants and that this is what makes them important and appealing to organizations throughout the community. Conversely, foundations would be well-served in recognizing the role that hospitals can play when they move beyond their own walls. Especially with the advent of accountable care organizations and other innovations in the insurance marketplace, we are beginning to observe hospitals and healthcare systems focusing on community health and social determinants of health in previously unimaginable ways. Foundations may discover that at least some hospitals are coming around to a perspective that aligns with their own.

Second, **we encourage the leaders of hospitals and foundations to reach out to one another on a periodic basis to explore their respective and shared interests**. Hospitals and foundations each have a tendency to act autonomously when developing large-scale initiatives. These two institutions can strengthen their strategies by listening to one another and incorporating each other's perspectives and expertise. The more that local organizations understand one another's interests, strategies and plans, the more that they can find shared opportunities, leverage one another's work and create synergy. This applies not only to hospitals and foundations, but to all organizations that are developing large-scale strategies to improve community health and well-being.

Third, **we recommend using the Stakeholder Health's perspective as a guide for developing shared strategy**. One reason that hospitals and foundations have historically taken different paths to improve community health is that they have been following different road maps. Hospitals are guided by the idea of delivering services to patients one at a time. This is the paradigm of clinical medicine and until recently it provided the framework for invoicing and receiving payment. Foundations in contrast have sought to maintain and improve health at a population level, which has led them to the paradigm of public health which emphasizes prevention, health education, policy approaches to behavior change, community-based organizations and social determinants of health.

Stakeholder Health brings the public health paradigm squarely into healthcare organizations, while still finding an important place for their medical care and the substantial financial, human and physical resources. Just as importantly, Stakeholder Health frames the business of health improvement as a partnership among multiple organizations that complement one another. It also serves as a blueprint for a theater where hospitals, foundations and many other organizations have their own distinct role to play. While some of these players may try to outmaneuver one another to be the lead actor, the real test of a well-functioning ensemble is its ability to draw out the best from one another.

REFERENCES

Blandin Foundation. (2015). *Blandin Community Leadership Program*. Retrieved from http://leadership.blandinfoundation.org/programs/bclp

Cheadle, A., Beery, W. L., Greenwald, H. P., Nelson, G. D., Pearson, D., & Senter, S. (2003). Evaluating the California Wellness Foundation's health improvement initiative: a logic model approach. *Health Promotion Practice,4* (2), 146-156.

Chrislip, D.D. & O'Malley, E. (2013). *For the common good: Redefining civic leadership*. Wichita, KS: KLC Press.

The Colorado Trust. (2009). *Colorado Household Survey Issue Brief*. Retrieved from http://www.coloradotrust.org/sites/default/files/COHS_Overview_Final.pdf

Con Alma Health Foundation (2014). Healthy People, Health Places Grantees: Amigos Bravos. Retrieved from http://conalma.org/hphp-grantees/

Conner, R., & Easterling, D. (2009). The Colorado Trust's Healthy Communities Initiative: Results and lessons for comprehensive community initiatives. Foundation Review, 1(1), 24-42.

Easterling, D., Arnold, E. M., Jones, J. A., & Smart, A. J. (2013). Achieving synergy with collaborative problem solving: The value of system analysis. *The Foundation Review*, 5(1), 105.

Foundation Center. (2015). *Foundation Stats*. [Data file]. Retrieved from http://foundationcenter.org/gainknowledge/research/nationaltrends.html

Easterling, D., & Millesen, J. L. (2015). Achieving Communitywide Impact by Changing the Local Culture: Opportunities and Considerations for Foundations. *The Foundation Review, 7*(3), 5.

Grantmakers for Effective Organizations. (2015). *Strengthening Nonprofit Capacity*. Retrieved from http://www.geofunders.org/resource-library/all/record/a066000000IbGXCAA3

Hacker, K., & Walker, D. K. (2013). Achieving population health in accountable care organizations. *American Journal of Public Health, 103*(7), 1163-116.

Hasnain-Wynia, R. (2003). Overview of the community care network demonstration program and its evaluation. *Medical Care Research and Review, 60*(4 suppl), 5S-16S.

Health Foundation for Western and Central New York (2015). *GetSET*. Retrieved from http://www.hfwcny.org/Tools/Broadcaster/frontend/itemcontent.asp?reset=1&ItemID=395

Health Systems Learning Group (HSLG). (2013). *Health Systems Learning Group Monograph*. Retrieved from http://stakeholderhealth.org/pdf/

Interact for Health. (2015). *School-based health centers in Greater Cincinnati: Improving student health to promote community well-being*. Cincinnati: Interact for Health. Retrieved from: https://www.interactforhealth.org/upl/SBHC_report_with_map_101615.pdf

Kania, J., & Kramer, M. (2011). Collective impact. *Stanford Social Innovation Review, 9(1),* 36-41.

Kretzman, J. P., & McKnight, J. L. (1993). *Building communities from the inside out*. Evanston, IL: Northwestern University.

MacFarquhar, L. (2016, January 4). What money can buy. *The New Yorker*. Retrieved from http://www.newyorker.com/magazine/2016/01/04/what-money-can-buy-profiles-larissa-macfarquhar

McGinnis, J. M., & Foege, W. H. (1993). Actual causes of death in the United States. *JAMA*, 270(18), 2207-2212.

Meehan, D., Hebbeler, K., Cherner, S., & Peterson, D. (2009). Community building for children's health: Lessons from Partnerships for Healthy Children. *Foundation Review, 1(1),* 43-54.

Niggel, S. J., & Brandon, W. P. (2014). Health legacy foundations: a new census. *Health Affairs,* 33.1, 172-177. doi: 10.1377/hlthaff.2013.0868

Rapides Foundation. (2015). *Cenla Medication Access Program*. Retrieved from http://www.rapidesfoundation.org/Newsroom/News/TabId/121/ArtMID/474/ArticleID/108/Cenla-Medication-Access-Program.aspx

REACH Healthcare Foundation. (2015). *Cultural Competency Initiative*. Retrieved from https://reachhealth.org/goals/cultural-competency-initiative/

University of Wisconsin Population Health Institute. (2015). [Model of population health]. County Health Rankings. Retrieved from http://www.countyhealthrankings.org/our-approach

Silver, D., & Weitzman, B. C. (2009). The pros and cons of comprehensive community initiatives at the city level: The case of the Urban Health Initiative. *Foundation Review, 1(1),* 85-95.

Tipirneni, R., Vickery, K. D., & Ehlinger, E. P. (2015). Accountable communities for health: moving from providing accountable care to creating health. *The Annals of Family Medicine, 13*(4), 367-369.

Yip, J., Ernst, C., & Campbell, M. (2016). *Boundary spanning leadership: Mission critical perspectives from the executive suite*. Greensboro NC: Center for Creative Leadership. Downloaded at: http://insights.ccl.org/wp-content/uploads/2015/04/BoundarySpanningLeadership.pdf

Zappia, B., Puntenney, D. & Snyder, L. (2013). Neighborhood Health Status Initiative – Information Sessions. [PowerPoint slides]. Retrieved from http://www.thegrhf.org/funding/neighborhood-health/reports/

FULL AUTHORSHIP LISTING

Doug Easterling, PhD, Professor, Wake Forest School of Medicine, Div. of Public Health Sciences, Dept. of Social Sciences and Public Policy, Winston Salem, NC

Allen Smart, MPH, Interim President, Kate B. Reynolds Charitable Trust, Winston Salem, NC

Laura McDuffee, MPA, Research Associate, Wake Forest School of Medicine, Div. of Public Health Sciences, Dept. of Social Sciences and Public Policy, Winston Salem, NC

For more information about this chapter, contact **Doug Easterling** at e-mail, dveaster@wakehealth.edu or phone, (336) 716-9213.

CHAPTER 10

Global Dynamics At Home

James R. Cochrane and Gary Gunderson, with Jerry Winslow and Heather Wood Ion

Overview

Stakeholder Health began when a White House delegation came to Memphis to see how an African model of "religious health assets mapping" might be adapted in the US context. As in Africa, the Memphis assessment unveiled about six times as many generative partners as the prevailing official maps showed. In Memphis that meant a huge number of "faith forming things" (congregations), while elsewhere such as in North Carolina the surprise is the number of faith-based community organizations one finds.

"If you do not set high, high ambitions, people won't change the way they work."

(World Bank Group President Jim Yong Kim on what he learned from the 3x5 HIV goals set by the WHO. Task Force for Global Health, 2015)

The ability to perceive the full range of health assets, and how to align, animate and release them, especially in troubled neighborhoods, underpins everything else Stakeholder Health tries to learn. Because this is precisely what is needed anywhere in the world for transforming health care, it makes Stakeholder Health part of a global learning community. The mother lode for this kind of learning is post-colonial Africa, where the health of its people rests heavily on their own energy, intelligence and liberation. That is also true for South Memphis, San Bernardino, or the left-behind urban areas of Detroit and West Baltimore. Stakeholder Health learns the most in, from and with those working in tough places—a very global kind of work.

In this chapter, we open our imagination to think about the increasingly rich, dynamic interactions that are occurring between locally acquired knowledge and global health systems and experiences. Although as Stakeholder Health leaders we are responsible for institutions in the USA, we are also well aware of the challenges of global health. We apply international standards in dealing with certain diseases or epidemics and commonly engage in professional exchanges with other countries and international partner health systems. Increasingly we are learning how to extend our horizons beyond national borders—boundaries that are now obviously imaginary.

Neither the movement of human beings across territories and continents nor the interaction between them across astonishing distances is new. Today, however, this movement and interaction are unprecedented in scope and scale and they are escalating to obscure formal borders. The local and the global are ineluctably and increasingly intertwined. People, ideas, practices, technologies and goods flow from one place to another in progressively complex networks of actions and interactions.

This has major implications for health. Radiologists in Bangalore read X-rays in the middle of the night for hospitals in Akron. Infectious diseases like Ebola show how the effects of particular events can cascade across traditional institutional, geographical and policy boundaries. The relationship between the local and global, is in fact, to use a metaphor from quantum physics, increasingly "entangled."

This "entanglement" goes well beyond links between discrete areas of thought and operation. The dramatic and increasing compression of time and space that marks the globalization of every sphere of human activity virtually guarantees growing entanglement. It forces us to think not just of global health but also of local health in terms of "complex living human systems" that have cascading network effects.

These effects, from the local to the global and vice-versa, include vital network pathways between them that configure the way people access and use health services.

Healthcare must cope with this increasing complexity. And local delivery systems will and do find themselves coping with global challenges in ways that are not only unexpected, but confront mission-driven priorities.

What Do We Mean by Global Health?

What is now described as "global health" used to be called "international health," which was largely focused on controlling the spread of epidemics (Beaglehole & Bonita, 2010). More than a terminological shift, "global health" signals:

- A better grasp of the interconnectedness of health and its contributory factors across national and other boundaries

- Recognition that extra-local, global movements and flows influence local health factors

- Awareness that solutions to population health at local level in one place are not disconnected from those in another place.

"Global health" also signals another crucial shift—from mere disease-control to a conception of health as a human right (Gruskin, Mills & Tarantola, 2007). This is captured in the WHO's post-World War II vision of "health for all." It is echoed now in questions on the availability, affordability, and acceptability of health provision (who.int/mediacentre/factsheets/fs323/en), and underlined in what we know of the social determinants of health (who.int/social_determinants/thecommission/finalreport/en/). In 1984, Bill Foege founded the Task Force on Global Health (first called the Task Force on Child Survival)—which now reaches people in 135 countries (http://www.taskforce.org/)—with the global human rights goal of ending preventable and treatable diseases that assault people living in extreme poverty.

In this context, questions of human dignity and equity are prominent. They are equally relevant to any conception of mission by local healthcare systems that embraces a vision of "health for all" those who live in the areas they reach. They also push us beyond "service delivery"— where, in principle, the deliverer is always the agent and the recipient a patient—to consider how everyone is an agent in her or his own right, capable jointly of achieving the outcomes desired by all. Equity not only signifies the redressing of disadvantage and the promotion of inclusion, a formal feature of justice, but as a critical dimension of any healthy community, "it also helps to create confidence, and a sense of participation and belonging" (Kalula, 2013, p.16). Commitments to preserve human dignity and establish equitable social institutions are constitutive virtues of any society deserving to be called good.

Why Does Global Health Matter?

Health care, then, beyond the provision and application of brilliant technological and managerial capacities to combat disease and illness, is a crucial support for the "living human system." To define it as a *human* system and not simply a delivery or health system (or the like) calls forth a commitment to dignity and equity in partnership with all stakeholders. Fundamentally, then, it is not *just* about individuals, but also about establishing the healthy communities within which those individuals live and must find and sustain their own health with others.

Here we face the "constituency problem." Who are the relevant people or partners to whom one owes such a commitment? Does the constituency encompass one's own clients, a service area, a regional authority, a nation-state, or all of humanity? If geographical and even cultural boundaries increasingly turn out to be irrelevant (as in the Ebola cascade noted above; or in the sharing of human organs for transplantation, for example), where are the limits on what we consider the relevant constituency? As the movement of people grows, who has access to care and who does not?

> "Global health, in this sense, is not about something somewhere else but about one's own location in a much larger, complex reality that has to do with one's own long-term impact and sustainability."

Such questions, cutting across all traditional boundaries, are central to global health—but they are equally applicable locally. The issue becomes clearer when we think of mobility, risk management and strategies of planning, all of which transcend local realities. In short, not only every government or public health system but also every private healthcare system in the world:

- … *struggles* with how to prioritize healthcare spending—especially in the tension between the dramatic needs of the poorest for basic primary care and the massive costs of managing the growing array of chronic conditions;

- … *confronts*, at some level, market pressures governing access to quality high-tech healthcare and expensive drugs and treatments (often restricted to the upper middle classes);

- … *must find* legislative and/or other means to address the social demand for health and well-being;

- … *faces* the tension—directly impacting upon the provision and acceptance of healthcare—between the powerful medical, technical, and operational instruments it wields (which tend to view a patient as a composite of materials and processes to be managed or repaired), and the complex, socially formed, relationally embedded, and self-directed persons that human beings actually are (see HSLG, 2013, Ch.5).

Notwithstanding different political frameworks and regulatory milieus, we have much to learn in all these respects from what others are doing elsewhere in the world and we hope that they may indeed have something to learn from us.

Movement and dynamic interaction across existing borders and boundaries—geographical, disciplinary, institutional and social—are not exceptions but, now more so than ever, definitive. Global health, in this sense, is not about something somewhere else but about one's own location in a much larger, complex reality that has to do with one's own long-term impact and sustainability. Most fundamentally, it has to do with the "just and equitable distribution of the risk of suffering and of tools to lessen and prevent it" (Farmer, Kleinman, Kim, & Basilico, 2013, Preface). This basic vision of health binds the global to the local and the local to the global, and it incorporates both nation-states and non-state institutions such as non-governmental organizations (NGOs) or non-profits, private philanthropists, and community-based organizations.

Pathologies of Global Health

Just as no one escapes the effects of global ill-health in the end (Kim, Millen, Irwin, & Gershman, 2000), so no one escapes the global marketing and pricing realities that are rapidly emerging in healthcare. The human capacity to invent new and costly healthcare interventions greatly outstrips the human capacity to pay for these interventions.

> Consider just one recent example: the production and selling of a molecule called sofosbuvir, marketed as Sovaldi by an Israeli company called Gilead (see http://chisite.org/research/the-value-of-sovaldi). This drug is phenomenally successful in treating Hepatitis C. Gilead sells the drug in the U.S. for $1000 per pill. This means that the treatment of one patient will cost about $80K or more. With about eight million Americans infected with the disease, it is easy to see that this one new drug will add billions to our healthcare costs. And this is just one example of which there are many.

Such considerations drive us to think about the language of life (see further below on Leading Causes of Life) rather than just the language of fighting disease or death. Adopting a more global perspective on such matters, it is readily evident that our current efforts in and dialogues about addressing questions of justice or fairness when it comes to the distribution of great benefits and great burdens are deeply inadequate. We need vital ideas and new frameworks to address these issues, as well as ways of rethinking old models that have not been fully realized.

Think, for example, of the core principles that supported the rise of primary health care (PHC). Its origins lie precisely in an earlier conundrum about the high cost of tertiary (especially) and secondary care in contexts where, for one reason or another, despite the availability of world-class medicine and professional staff, many still had no adequate access to it. PHC was not just a management solution but also a different vision of the place and purpose of tertiary and secondary institutions. Originally propagated by the WHO in its 1978 Alma Ata Declaration of "health for all by 2000," its vision was partly inspired by the Christian Medical Commission, which included leading US figures, working under the World Council of Churches in Geneva (McGilvray, 1981). And it already contained a clear view on what we today call the "social determinants" of health. Stripped of such elements and reduced largely to silo-based interventions (Cueto, 2004), the grand dream of PHC has largely fallen short of its promise—not for technical reasons but for watered down goals and naiveté about the fundamental complicities of power and privilege that create institutional inertia.

The history of PHC also reflects a more general reality. The emphasis of the WHO Social Determinants Commission (2008) on population health has enormous sway in health policy (bleeding over in the USA into notions of "population health management"). As important as it is, it still conceptualizes health care less fully than was done forty years ago. It identifies several key actors (global institutions and agencies, government, civil society, research and academic communities, and the private sector [WHO, 2008, p. 44]) and "three principles of action" (see sidebar on the next page), but it largely overlooks the significance of the communities per se within which people find their lives and their health. In over 200 pages, it only very briefly refers to "the importance of including intended beneficiary groups in all aspects of policy and programme development, implementation, and evaluation" (p. 96). It also barely mentions the need to enact "legal changes to recognize and support community empowerment initiatives will ensure the comprehensive inclusion of disadvantaged groups in action at global, national, and local levels concerned with improving health and health equity" (p.162).

Just as limited as the WHO's discussion of social determinants in this respect is the CDC perspective. It has identified six critical areas for "health systems strengthening" (HSS, another new catch phrase in global health), namely: Epidemiologic information, institutions and infrastructure, laboratory networks, capable workforce, programs, and research (Bloland, Simone, Burkholder, Slutsker, & Cock, 2012). None come close to incorporating in any meaningful way ALL those for whom it is meant. It remains a technical, managerial approach that limits our ability to figure out how to work across systems in their fullness—including with the communities served in "population health."

Assessing the state of global health research and practice at the beginning of the Twenty-First Century, Panter-Brick et al. (2014) thus forcefully argue that:

- Global health falls prey to deadly sins—coveting silo gains, lusting for technological solutions, leaving broad promises largely unfulfilled, and boasting of narrow successes.

- Global health needs to transform its current landscape to keep faith with its core mandate of promoting health equity.

- Principled action is grounded in ethical values that put front and center the quality of our relationships with the communities served.

- Articulating a coherent global health agenda will come from virtuous courage and prudence in decision-making, fostering people-centered systems of care, and addressing health needs over the entire lifespan.

Stakeholder Health wants to understand how to approach health care provision and access for complex people in complex communities. The idea that anyone, or any one entity can simply "manage" a population to achieve health is inadequate for leaders trying help their institutions and communities adapt. Worse, it could draw leaders into further complicity regarding the ills that are ascribed to global health but that affect us all locally too. Hospital leaders must acknowledge that they are in relationship with their nearby communities. And, as noted in earlier chapters, most hospital relationships with their communities have been marked, when examined honestly, by historical events that merit lament about the past and demand rigor in present day dealings.

Perhaps the time has come to fulfill what was imagined a half century ago. One key shift—still a new thought even for Stakeholder Health—is that a global vision doesn't apply just to "Third World" or "developing countries" (as the CDC position and others describe it), but to the whole global community.

Grasping the Promise: The Future Present

We should speak not only of the "sins" of global health but also of ways of re-orienting action. Right now, perhaps more than ever before, there are particularly good reasons to do so:

- With applied will and intelligence the possibility now exists within global health of a "Grand Convergence"—a realistic chance of reducing infections and child and maternal mortality to low rates universally, and of tackling non-communicable diseases and the impoverishing effects of health expenditures within a generation (Lancet Commission, 2013; Dybul, 2013; Kim, 2013).

- The raised emphasis on the social determinants of health coincides with a global commitment to new "sustainable development goals" (Open Working Group on Sustainable Development Goals, 2014) that include numerous and ambitious measurable aims relevant to health and health equity.

- A specific concern to address diseases that affect the poor is manifest in The Global Fund to Fight HIV, TB and Malaria. As a major 21st Century initiative, it actively promotes and supports an idea of partnership in health that rests on continual growth, driven by mutual respect, shared responsibility and a strong commitment by all (www.theglobalfund.org/en/overview/).

- A rapidly growing interest in health systems research—astonishingly, largely absent before the first meeting of the First Global Symposium on Health Systems Research in Montreux in 2010 (two held since in Beijing and Cape Town, a fourth soon in Vancouver)—signals a deep concern for the interlinked aspects of health care, with working groups on finance, medicine, quality, evidence, ethics, community care and more (www.healthsystemsglobal.org/twg/).

- Widespread and increasingly central chronic conditions that extend over increasingly long periods of peoples' lives call forth a global rethink of costs and the nature of health services. Critically, this pandemic of chronic conditions also highlights the crucial role of appropriate local signaling mechanisms—ways in which families, friends, attentive local leaders or community groups are alert to what is happening to someone around them—and of the accompaniment of people who live with these conditions that hospitals and clinics cannot achieve on their own.

- Our earlier publication (Health Systems Learning Group, 2013) and this volume (Ch. 6: Community Asset Mapping), directs us to think of how one accesses and supports the already existing assets and agency in the communities served, including those inspired and sustained by faith commitments and networks (Olivier et al., 2015; ARHAP, 2006). As such, herein lies the greatest challenge in how we understand individual health in relation to community health on the one hand, and community health to formal institutions of health provision on the other.

GLOBAL HEALTH ACTION

Current literature has highlighted at least six ways to re-orient global health action. Specific future steps are to:

- Strengthen institutional leadership

- Follow a people-centered and life-course agenda

- Theorize global health in a manner which robustly integrates structural and behavioral change in systems of care

- Espouse a coherent strategic frame for financial incentives and effective leadership

- Deliver with more consistency on medical and public health promises

- Listen more carefully to what locally matters in everyday life.

(Panter-Brick, Eggerman, & Tomlinson, 2014, p. 23411)

Seeing the Local Relevance

Many of the issues and concerns that shape transformations in global health are not simply global; they arise from and return to local contexts. The global and the local are not really opposed, then, but "different sides of the same coin" in which general insights and knowledge become available even as "all ideas and practices have to adapt to [particular] contexts and niches" (Robertson & White, 2007, p.62-3). Learning between contexts happens by diffusion and adaptation. There are thus several ways in which the insights from global health have relevance for Stakeholder Health members (and vice-versa).

The first is the changed environment in the USA. The Affordable Care Act has introduced concepts and operational demands that force a reconsideration of health care provision and its accountability structures as a whole, whether public or private. The ideas suggested as crucial for global health action (see sidebar on "Global Health Action") are directly translatable into local contexts, and the ACA pushes in this direction. Second, worldwide, this has given new impetus to the role of community health workers (see HSLG, 2013, p.59-62; this volume, Chapter 5), but also extended it beyond the provision of a service to the idea of 'transformative partnerships' (HSLG, 2013, Ch.6).

Still fully to be grasped is the complexity this involves (as noted in Chapter 1), taking us beyond the walls of our formal health care facilities, in operational and governance terms. Here we add a deeper awareness that many of us already have surprising partnerships beyond the local that can contribute to our mutual learning.

Partnerships Again

Many questions have been raised about partnerships in the context of global health, particularly some of their critical shortcomings. Power dynamics favor the financially and politically strong partner's ability to dictate the terms of partnership, creating an unproductive and ultimately unsustainable one-sidedness in the relationship. "Forming partnerships" is not enough even when those involved genuinely have good intentions and want to move towards equitable relations through these partnerships. Whereas medical education is now moving toward collaboration rather than competition, few great examples exist to define what authentic collaboration means between health systems and communities they serve. Collaboration in health care raises issues of shared responsibility and mutual accountability that have not been addressed in most discussions of the changing nature of delivery systems.

In fact, the relevant learning partnerships are often found by following the threads of existing relationships. These can be surprising; instead of just following them home to a nearby neighborhood, we might well follow them home to a neighborhood a few thousand miles over the horizon. The Somalis out the window in Minneapolis are already a live bridge to northeastern Africa. Look out the other window and the Hmong neighbors are a bridge to Southeastern Asia. Those bridges tend to be marked by "mission" and care for the needy, but they are also clues to where to find resilience and adaptive practices relevant to many challenges in Minneapolis—or Atlanta, Winston, San Bernardino, Miami or Houston.

Key Reference Points

The globe is round and if we go far enough one way we will actually come back home—all of the lively domains of global health learning and policy elsewhere are alive and contentious in every county in the United States. Some are particularly relevant to the learning process upon which Stakeholder Health has embarked. We introduce them here, adding our own thoughts about potentially fruitful directions of thought and learning.

A. NEITHER UPSTREAM NOR DOWNSTREAM: PRIORITIZING MEDICINE IN THE 21ST CENTURY

How do we prioritize services in the face of growing and aging populations, shifting patters of life-long chronic illnesses, rising costs, changing professional goals, and increasing specializations (Cochrane, 2015)? Neither "vertical prioritization" (a hierarchy of choice within a special field or group of patients) nor "horizontal prioritization" (a hierarchy of choice between special fields or types of illness or disease) is best.

Arriving at a fitting answer is confounded by the conceptual split between "upstream" (distal) and "downstream" (proximal) interventions, which imposes a linear logic on the way we do things. This prevents a clear grasp of the interacting causal pathways that operate at multiple levels (body, person, family, community, society, polity, economy and environment), sequentially or simultaneously, to shape health and ill-health. We tend to emphasize one against the other and allocate our resources and energies accordingly. So we fail to account for or adequately respond to the full ecology of human health (Krieger, 2008; Manchanda, 2013).

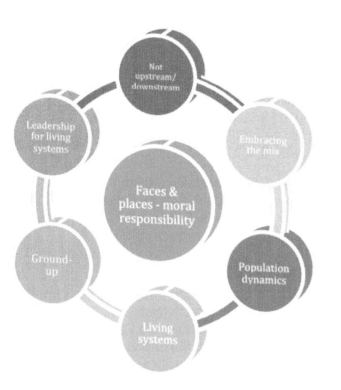

We could think in terms of turbulent circles of interacting energies, of a vortex rather than a linear stream, of whirls with continually shifting centers moving in constantly interacting ways. That would mean paying attention to the dynamic whole within which any particular level can have a direct impact on any other even when they are not "proximate" in space and time. Reimaging health care along such lines would force us to reorganize the way health care delivery is understood, over the lifespan of individuals and of populations, as an ecological whole. Within this ecological whole, we would need to identify both pathological patterns, but also generative ones, beyond the limited set of levels and limited range of responses that hospitals can address on their own.

B. EMBRACING THE MIX: TRANSCULTURAL "HEALTHWORLDS"

Part of that turbulent vortex includes increasingly diverse people or groups who hold visions of health and well-being that are often not compatible with what a hospital or its professional staff think they are about, yet which can and do have considerable impact on if, how and when someone accesses any formal health care services and what else they do "out of sight" of the formal protocols. Health system providers have looked for ways of providing culturally competent or culturally sensitive healthcare delivery but this only goes part of the way. We expand this to include the idea of "healthworlds": the ways people construct their understandings of health and illness in local contexts through coherent, organized patterns of interpretation that guide their health-seeking behavior, as shaped by culture, sociopolitical context and environment (Germond & Cochrane, 2010). These healthworlds reflect a transcultural reality with which health care providers have to come to terms, paying attention to them critically but also insightfully and appreciatively. This also reflects a growing movement in healthcare delivery to focus on dyadic partnerships between activated, informed patients (who are increasingly accountable to outcomes) and providers (Epping-Jordan, et al., 2004).

C. POPULATION DYNAMICS: TRANSNATIONAL MOVEMENT

The migrant has been called the "political figure of our time" (Nail, 2015). Migration has always been with us across the globe, but qualitative shifts are affecting the way this plays itself out. These shifts impact upon local realities as more people move more frequently, while greater diversity (with all its challenges) in local populations increasingly becomes a norm. Migration is no longer the exception but increasingly the rule in matters of polity and citizenship, with direct impact on health systems and nation-state understandings. Sociologists speak of "transnational" flows that, despite controls, do not obey the constraints imposed by existing nation-state boundaries (Vertovec & Cohen, 1999). Moreover, thanks to contemporary modes of travel and communication, people who migrate now move less from one place to another and more in an oscillating pattern between places, exchanging material and immaterial goods across space and time in unprecedented ways.

Health care provision is also affected by this oscillating system of ties, interactions, fluid exchanges and high levels of mobility that are often intensive, function in real time and impact upon the numerous spaces that people on the move now occupy. We do not yet know how important this is and to what extent it affects population health (either negatively or positively). The USA is a country built up-on migrant populations but with policies and programs largely still framed within the traditional, more static view of what migration means. Global health research suggests that the phenomenon may become more important, especially as diseases and illnesses migrate more easily for the same reasons, in complex ways and in multiple directions. What is true of disease and illness would be true of both tangible and intangible assets for supporting and enhancing health as well.

D. LIVING SYSTEMS: PATTERNS, NODES AND PATHWAYS

We need a more mature science of complexity around health systems, including a more complex view of what we mean by a health system. Our earlier document began to consider some dimensions of what this might mean (HSLG, 2013, Ch.3: "Leading Health Structures", & Ch.6: "Integrating Community & Health Systems") and Chapter 2 in this volume alluded to the foundational frameworks needed as we begin this task.

Sir Muir Gray (2011) thinks that "If the 20th century was dominated by bureaucracies and markets, the 21st century will be dominated by collaboratives, cooperatives, networks or complex adaptive systems." He thus advocates a "systems approach'" to health care, defined as a set of activities with a common set of objectives, focused on particular illnesses or diseases but cutting across the traditional division between primary, secondary and tertiary healthcare. It is thus still limited to the delivery of health services by professional providers through what he calls "care pathways" that navigate patients between the levels of care.

Besides really still representing a focus on "illness care" rather than "health care," there is only limited discussion of how, if at all, others outside of the formal healthcare facilities might be part of this. Currently, some of this focus already exists in many community health centers in the USA, whose Boards consist of local citizens.

Unfortunately, our understanding of a health system still revolves primarily around an inside-out approach (from provider to client). As long as this functions as our primary intellectual model, we cannot adequately take account of the complexity of health challenges and opportunities, nor of our relationship to communities we serve. Whether we are speaking of medicine or of care and health more generally, our interventions are in living systems. Without understanding more about such systems, we will not be able to achieve the goal of health for all that meets our mission.

Here sciences of complexity such as neurology provide us with useful (and applicable) metaphors for rethinking the way we organize ourselves. In particular, complex systems are networks of nodes and pathways, varying in density or impact. The hospital, clinic or dispensary are only some of the nodes that matter, and the pathways to health they provide are not only relatively limited but often even not the most important ones except at critical moments.

A further implication follows: complex living systems also generate qualities that are an expression of the system as a whole and not of particular nodes or pathways. This thought has important implications for how one might understand population health, including how one might measure its status. In these metaphors, three ideas are worth exploring: patterned complexity, generative nodes, and effective pathways (see Sidebar).

- **PATTERNED COMPLEXITY** - Complex systems are dynamic, emergent and partly unpredictable, but they also exhibit regular and repeated patterns at multiple levels (they are 'fractal') that can be grasped and worked with to advance health. The 'leading causes of life' framework captures on such a set of patterns that are applicable from the biological to the global level.

- **GENERATIVE NODES** - By generative nodes we mean those organizations where differing streams of thought, innovations, and relationships come together to form a hub capable of generating fresh approaches to community health development. Networked living systems survive and flourish because of the presence of generative nodes (one may also speak of 'keystone species' in some contexts). It would be valuable and possible to identify these nodes and nurture them towards 'life.'

- **EFFECTIVE PATHWAYS** – Network pathways that connect nodes in differing ways represent crucial communication and action channels. Again, it should be possible to track the most effective pathways between generative nodes within the system while identifying those that are degenerative, ineffective or redundant. This could be key to adaptive and more durable health care practices and interventions.

Living human systems are dynamic, ever-evolving, self-organizing networks that have a "logic" of their own. They include a degree of unpredictability and their processes are out of our immediate or direct control. Yet the more we grasp and adaptively work with them, the more we may be able to look forward to a time, even if still a distance away, when quality is normal and care is rationally aligned. We need better ways of understanding the impact of interdependent variables, context-dependent network relationships, time-dependent variation and forms of local control. Yet it is common to discuss them, particularly within hospitals, as designed institutions: predictable and serving efficiencies.

In a hospital institution dedicated to preserving itself, predictability and related resource allocation will seem dependent on a precise knowledge of averages and aggregations. In the complex system, averages and aggregations may be relatively meaningless because of the interactions and relationships of the parts. This has enormous implications for health system operations, accounting and research. We should be able to understand human living systems with a rigor to match that applied in understanding pathologies. We should also be able to rethink accordingly the meaning of the "data-information-communication-understanding" continuum of learning. All of this also has critical implications for the way we lead our institutions, with a view that encompasses a far more expansive approach than traditional accounting and modes of operational functioning allow.

As discussed in Chapter Three on "Leading Health Structures", we advocate that health system leadership recognize what has already been stressed repeatedly in this volume: markets, persons served or populations, migrant streams, infectious disease and chronic disease patterns, data and payer panels and more, exist in living systems that are in constant chaos or flux, and cannot be controlled or managed. These factors must be dealt with adaptively and proactively rather than reactively. This is possible not only because of our own institutional capabilities but also because complex adaptive, living systems possess the capacity to change and learn from experience. This calls for what we have in Chapter Three described as an inside out approach to leadership, in which the intelligence of the community outside the health systems guide our work as it expands beyond the hospital walls.

At the same time and in reality, healthcare systems are themselves complex adaptive human living systems. As such, they are also messy, unpredictable, and fraught with multiple and diverse relationships and meanings. The adaptive nature of these systems, both within and outside hospitals, means that as externalities change, so too do the relationships among the elements change.

In this respect, a "living systems" approach also confronts the harmful assumption that positional power is the only form of power that matters in an organization. Yet there are many forms of power. Leaders with a "living systems" view will seek to identify these kinds of power and those who use them as an important step in building cohesion and stability. They will humbly seek out those who understand and wield these differing kinds of power and reinforce the continuous learning necessary to support, encourage and realign practices. This will often require that we intentionally and without guile flip the power dynamics and turn them upside-down, that we as providers and the hospital as institutions cede power to those typically marginalized both within the hospital and outside in community, valuing and honoring the intelligence of those persons and communities.

F. FACES & PLACES: MORAL RESPONSIBILITY

At the heart of the vision of medical science and of those whose passion is to work for the health of individuals and the health of all is the question of means and ends. For Stakeholder Health, the overarching end is health for all, which is of course very different from merely "health care for all". Though no single institution or even network of institutions can assure this end, it serves as the universal lodestar for understanding our particular contribution and must take into account all those who have a stake in their own health and well being.

Here the question of accountability and its mechanisms becomes central for any particular leader or institution. We deal with this in two ways below: a consideration of what we might understand by working with the complexity of human life ("World Three" and a "language of life"), and in some implications for how we might understand accountability as going beyond the institutions or organizations for which we are responsible.

FROM WORLD ONE TO WORLD THREE: COMPLEX LIVING SYSTEMS

- The promise of **World One** is arriving at the point where all the component tools and practices for improving health are dependably competent, efficient and fairly available to those who need them. We cannot treat lightly the successes of process improvements that have been achieved in this regard, though it remains only a first basic step.

- **World Two** is marked by thoughtful gains and synergies achieved by integrating and aligning the many tools, procedures and techniques for detection, prevention, treatment and management of disease conditions. This is within the range of most schemes of population health management and their common focus on illness and disease.

- The essence of **World Three** is that its primary organizing logic rests on the causes of life rather than the causes of death—a fitting language for the complex, fluid social life of human populations. Here the many parts of our institutions, guilds, networks and relationships, including the huge array of now-relevant community partners and social assets, find alignment in contributing to the life of people and the life of the social whole.

World Three: Working with the Complexity of Human Life

Global health emphasizes health as a human right and aims at "health for all." In both respects the last two centuries has seen major advances, yet much remains a hope rather than an achievement. A lesser, seemingly more reachable, golden goal of global health is disease eradication. Here current developments in science, technology and funding are promising but not enough. As a recent high-level international assessment confirms, "Even when the biological, technical and operational criteria are by and large favourable" the eradication of a disease will also depend upon non-biological "critical enabling factors" (Cochi & Dowdle, 2011, p. 99), like social complexity, political will and moral judgments—in short, vital qualities of a human living system. A good example is the ongoing campaign to eradicate polio, always affected by local human realities and large system rigidity or brittleness in changing methods.

The future in global health/local health, then, may well in part depend upon conceiving not just of morbidity and mortality (or pathologies and "death") as key points of engagement and investment, especially because now chronic disease and mental health issues are so dominant. Equally rigorous attention needs to be given to leading causes of life: generative processes—biological, personal, relational and social—that sustain and enhance health and well-being in the first place. We think of this as moving from World One to World Three (Gunderson, Cutts & Cochrane, 2015).

A Language of Life

With such a vision, we begin to see people and their groups in terms of how they find their life by identifying and tracking a select but operationally meaningful set of factors that "cause" life. This opens up a significantly different way of organizing the strengths, structures and assets of the health sector with people for whom they might be relevant.

A "language of life" conceptualizes a living human being, beyond mechanics and disease, as a complex, adaptive, choice-making, meaning-rich, generative, future-seeking creature that is alive. Not able to be controlled rigidly, not merely following instructions or prescriptions, perhaps as likely to be non-compliant as not, a human person is alive, filled with the potential of creative freedom ("spirit") and capable of more life. That energy, expressed at social scale of community and populations, allows us to think of healthy human populations and not just of managing the care of a group of mammals.

The Supporters of Health Initiative has identified trusted connectors to the people in census tracts that represent the high cost outliers with chronic and costly Emergency Department and hospital use. These Supporters are long-term employees of the hospital who, as identified by their former supervisor M. Smallwood, are trustworthy listeners, energetic advocates, and brilliant field workers.

They are the "embedded reporters" who can not only identify the priority of necessary supports for individual clients, but also can coordinate (and discover) community services which can deliver components of support. They are constantly evaluating what is offered, what is delivered, and with what impact, for the survival of the most vulnerable populations in Winston-Salem served by Wake Forest Baptist Medical Center.

The pioneering Supporters apply the approach of Leading Causes of Life (LCL) by:

- Establishing connections on behalf of their patients, and among community entities serving the vulnerable

- Creating coherence for those whose illness or vulnerability have challenged their sense of meaning by accompanying them on their life journeys

- Advocating self-reliance as awareness of agency both for their patients and for service providers who may not be aware that they are part of a network of care

- Reinforcing hope by their daily presence, and by the intimate actions they take on behalf of a future of health and engagement

- Identifying and exemplifying intergenerativity by seeking out the lessons to be learned from those serving and being served by community efforts and by expanding the impact of each of those efforts.

(Wood Ion, 2015)

Harnessing, nurturing, encouraging and creating space for this life, and then aligning it with all that we have gained from Worlds One and Two, is the task of World Three health systems (Gunderson, Cutts & Cochrane, 2015).

Here we are also talking about a conversation to share and explore an entirely new healthcare vocabulary—new words that guide decisions and interventions to improve well-being and vitality. Among the words in this new vocabulary of a language of life are connection, coherence, agency, intergenerativity and hope (Gunderson & Pray, 2006; Gunderson & Cochrane, 2015, p.59-79).

In healthcare and medicine we often use the word system in the sense of "an assemblage of parts" that describes discrete units of understanding to form a unitary whole. The task of the Supporters of Health (see sidebar above) is different: it is both to discover and to strengthen the unitary whole, and to do it by finding connections, etc. among the discrete units or issues of care and community. These staff work with a "living system."

Implications for Stakeholder Health?

The implications we draw here from our whole discussion of global health are easier to write down than act upon. Even conceptualizing these ideas may be difficult for leaders who must contend with a failed model of fee-for-service healthcare and who are trying to operate demanding and busy hospitals and clinics in the face of what often appear as impossible complexities and competing or conflicting agendas. Moreover, in any institution dedicated to its own preservation, careful attention will be given to the sources of funding for paying the bills. Funding arrangements do more to structure healthcare systems (or the lack of a system) than most other factors. We are beginning to see this point in action, as the major governmental sources of funding begin to shift their reimbursement schemes.

So perhaps our experience might be described as having one foot firmly planted on the dock of World One, and the other on a bobbing boat headed slowly toward World Two with World Three barely in view as yet, if at all. Yet sooner or later World Three will be the future. How then does one jump into the future without drowning?

Perhaps this work we are doing in Stakeholder Health can help. Thinking about how global dynamics "come home" in local healthcare systems is more than an exercise in comparing local and global realities or distinguishing between different levels of decision-making and action. It means thinking of a "fractal reality" in which patterns at one level (e.g. global) reappear at every other level (e.g. regional, local, or even in the guise of a single individual human being). As long as we are taking seriously the complex entanglement that shapes the health of individual human beings, of groups of human beings and of populations as a whole, what is learned at one level is intrinsically relevant to another. The lessons learned from cardiac care and recovery, for example, have been essential foundations of the wellness movement. Another example is the mass immunization campaigns have taught even small hospitals the importance of checklists, supply chain integrity, and so on.

On that basis, we identify at least six key implications for thought and practice around health and health care at both global and local level.

1ST IMPLICATION: PRIORITIZE LIVING SYSTEMS

To evaluate effectiveness a hospital system may seek measures of financial impact or indices of increased health literacy, and these measures will serve short-term goals; but real evaluation will only be valid in a perspective of long-term emergent change and the learning that has resulted. This takes patience and courage, as well as a profound and humble willingness to abandon what is comfortable and challenge what is denied. Then, we can discover what is at this point invisible to us, yet critical to health, and we can learn from ambiguity within the realization that we must remain uncertain out of our respect for the life in the living system.

2ND IMPLICATION: EXPAND THE UNDERSTANDING OF ACCOUNTABILITY

To whom am I or are we accountable for what? This can be answered narrowly but we pose the question broadly, framing it in terms of the differences between 'internal accountability', 'bureaucratic accountability,' and 'external accountability.'

- **Internal accountability** – being answerable for one's skills or expertise (as a scientist, a technician, an administrator, a health care professional, etc.)

- **Bureaucratic accountability** – answerability between different levels of the formal health system

- **External accountability** – answerability between health provider and community.

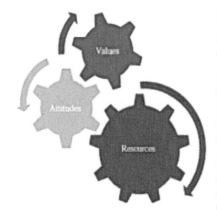

How do the **values**, beliefs, and culture of system actors interface with the accountability mechanism? How does the system and accountability mechanism interface with the values and beliefs of citizens and patients?

How do the **attitudes** and perceptions of providers, managers, bureaucrats and policymakers interface with the accountability mechanism? How does the system and accountability mechanism interface with the attitudes and perceptions of citizens and patients?

How do **resources** and capacities in the system interface with the accountability mechanism? How does the system and accountability mechanism fit with the resources and capacities of citizens and patients?

Figure 2 Factors influencing the functioning of accountability mechanisms. *(Cleary, Molyneux & Gilson, 2013)*

Internal accountability is obviously what one wants at the highest possible level and we take that for granted. Of greater relevance to us here is the tension between bureaucratic and external accountability. Cleary, Molyneux and Gilson (2013), who are on the cutting edge of new health systems research work, note that how one regulates this tension using which 'governance' tools is deeply affected by a combination of values, attitudes and resources (figure 2 above).

In this view, a key consideration is the link between organizational culture, relationships and accountability processes. Here Cleary, Molyneux and Gilson speak of the importance of the "decision space" that one enables. Commonly, to create some accountability between the health provider and the community it serves, the decision space is constructed by seeking community representation on clinic committees, by presenting reports, and by instituting complaint mechanisms. This is too limited an understanding of accountability, however. In practice it readily leads the patient/individual to false expectations and flawed optimism even as it leaves the formal health system wholly "in charge." And the notion of credible and fruitful partnerships is almost entirely absent.

The size and scope of private and public formal health care systems, and the influence and money they wield, gives them significant power and money to affect people's lives and well-being. As noted before, this power differential acts as a barrier between citizens and providers and limits, sometimes severely, any adequate functioning of external accountability mechanisms (Brinkerhoff, 2004). To balance this with stronger citizen engagement, involvement or participation is a challenge as we aim at "deep accountability" (Gunderson & Cochrane, 2012, Ch.9) for the health of the population we serve. Here "system learning" could become a key aspect of enhancing accountability in both directions, and as a way of handling the tensions and conflicts between them that are inevitable.

3RD IMPLICATION: DEVELOP THE NECESSARY SCIENCE OF COMPLEXITY

In working with living systems, we need evidence that matches their emergent, adaptive, dynamic and entangled yet always partially indeterminate complexity (think of a detective weighing clues) rather than data derived from tools designed for nonliving systems. Sorting evidence rather than data is important especially when we recognize that interconnectedness means that there will be increasing variation in any living system. Evidence includes narrative, reflections and deep searching for tacit knowledge beyond instrumental measures and a stronger valuing of these qualitative metrics. Evidence-based medicine tells us what to do, not how to do it.

4TH IMPLICATION: ADVOCATE "NURTURE" ABOVE "CONTROL"

The great virtue of scientific medicine is that it helps us identify particular health problems with increasing precision and explanatory capacity, while giving us measurable outcomes. This tends to drive from sight, however, the communicative and relational nature of human life. Equally virtuous then is a focus instead on the practical, on "what works" to establish, sustain and enhance health for individuals or communities, how they can and do draw on their own creativity and resources for health in the living system they inhabit. Here we face the tension between the skills that experts and organizations need to function well with financial accountability, and the creative capacities and living assets that communities can leverage as co-creators of their health and well-being.

Surely, though, we are able to imagine and invent ways of turning this either/or into a both/and? To do that we would need simultaneously to cultivate the skills of instrumental reason in both our scientific activity (medicine) and our organizational operations (administration) even as we act to nurture the creative capacities that reside in the human beings both inside organizations and in the communities to which they relate. These life capacities are not limited to intellectually or scientifically trained experts or confined to particular institutions or guilds. They are present everywhere, and they are the stuff that allows for invention and innovation.

To nurture the whole as a living system is to honor not just what the scientist and the administrator brings but also lay competence in communities (even among one's own employees as shown by the experience of the Supporters of Health at Wake Forest Baptist Health; see sidebar, "The language of life in action," above). This redefines the relationship between providers and recipients of health care as one of mutual learning and mutually acknowledged responsibility for the health of the whole.

5TH IMPLICATION: GO BEYOND SIMPLE PARTNERSHIPS AND EXCHANGES

Stakeholder Health, as in its first learning document (HSLG, 2013), continues to explore the meaning of partnerships and further thoughts on what they are or could be and mean. So we re-emphasize how important it is to include uncommon and unanticipated partners, including those with their own set of assets and community benefits levers, such as banks.

Given the complications of power and money in every context, it is in and through partnerships that we necessarily face the issue of health equity, so crucial to contemporary concerns in global health but no less relevant in almost every local context (Daniels, 2007). We need more conceptual and practical work on health equity, and we need more imagination around what it means for our systems. Partnership, as Paul Farmer has said, is "not just forming a task force or a multi-sectoral approach, it's a lot more than that. It's understanding when we get stuck …. [the need] to imagine a world in which we don't need to be socialized for scarcity. That's the biggest problem, that we have this profound failure of imagination …." (Task Force for Global Health, 2015).

6TH IMPLICATION: ACT LOCALLY, COMMUNICATE GLOBALLY

Local learning as we have said is not simply local, and Stakeholder Health is a prime example of that. It is not surprising that Stakeholder Health's earlier HSLG document has garnered interest from others in other parts of the world. Despite different regulatory, political or economic environments, many of the same concerns are present well beyond the particular peculiarities of the USA or North America. What we learn is not only of potential significance to those with whom our own institutions are linked across the globe, but to many others as well in the context of global health.

One of the great positive lessons of the Primary Health Care movement is the fact that it rested on a non-hierarchical and open-ended global sharing of local learning out of which arose its vision of the possibility of health for all. In the more recent global fight against HIV and AIDS, notes Matshidiso Moeti (World Health Organization Regional Director for Africa), "What we started to learn was that … there are certain things that need attention ethically – justice, inclusiveness, dealing with everybody – and paying particular attention to these, not hoping that by accident in enlarging and scaling up services that … things would trickle down …." (Task Force, 2015).

One of the great strengths of Stakeholder Health is that we mirror both a similar commitment to learning within the USA, and across our member institutions, and a similar awareness of the relationship between the moral demand shaped by our mission and professional demand to honor high quality science and deeply accountable management for health care. Through the living dynamic of the learning process we have put in place for ourselves and the global awareness of many of us and our partners, we represent and model an ethos and commitment that is open, in the spirit of collaborative learning, to others elsewhere in the world who share a similar vision. In a world where borders and boundaries are less and less relevant to health care, this can only benefit and even inspire all the many stakeholders found in our "living systems," not least we ourselves.

REFERENCES

African Religious Health Assets Programme. (2006). *Appreciating assets: the contribution of religion to Universal Access in Africa*. Report for the World Health Organization, retrieved from http://www.irhap.uct.ac.za/pub_WHO2006.php.

Beaglehole, R., & Bonita, R. (2010). What is global health? *Global Health Action, 3*. Retrieved from DOI: 10.3402/gha.v3403i3400.5142.

Bloland, P., Simone, P., Burkholder, B., Slutsker, L., & Cock, K. M. D. (2012). The role of public health institutions in global health system strengthening efforts: the US CDC's perspective. *PLoS Medicine, 9*(4), e1001199.

Brinkerhoff, D. W. (2004). Accountability and health systems: toward conceptual clarity and policy relevance. *Health Policy and Planning, 19*(6), 371–379.

Cleary, S. M., Molyneux, S., & Gilson, L. (2013). Resources, attitudes and culture: an understanding of the factors that influence the functioning of accountability mechanisms in primary health care settings. *BMC Health Services Research, 13(320)*. Retrieved from http://researchonline.lshtm.ac.uk/1300563/

Cochi, S. L., & Dowdle, W. R. (Eds.). (2011). *Disease eradication in the 21st Century: implications for global health*. Cambridge, MA & London: MIT Press.

Cochrane, J. R. (2015). Fundamental evaluation criteria in the medicine of the 21st Century. In E. Nagel & M. Lauerer (Eds.), *Prioritization in medicine: an international dialogue* (11-37). New York: Springer.

Cueto, M. (2004). The origins of primary health care and selective primary health care. *American Journal of Public Health, 94*(11), 1864-1874.

Daniels, N. (2007). *Just health: meeting health needs fairly*. New York: Cambridge University Press.

Dybul, M. (2013). A grand convergence and a historic opportunity. *The Lancet, 382*(9908). Retrieved from e38-e39. DOI: 0.1016/S0140-6736(13)62344-2.

Epping-Jordan, J. E., Pruitt, S. D., Bengoa, R., & Wagner, E. H. (2004). Improving the quality of health care for chronic conditions. *Quality and Safety in Health Care, 13*, 299–305.

Farmer, P., Kleinman, A., Kim, J. Y., & Basilico, M. (2013). *Reimagining global health: an introduction*. Berkeley: University of California Press.

Germond, P., & Cochrane, J. R. (2010). Healthworlds: conceptualizing landscapes of health and healing. *Sociology, 44*(2), 307-324.

Gruskin, S., Mills, E. J., & Tarantola, D. (2007). History, principles, and practice of health and human rights. *The Lancet, 370*(August 4), 449–455. Retrieved from www.thelancet.com.

Gunderson, G., Cutts, T., & Cochrane, J. R. (2015). *The health of complex human populations*. Institute of Medicine, Washington D.C.

Gunderson, G. R., & Cochrane, J. R. (2012). *Religion and the health of the public: shifting the paradigm*. New York: Palgrave MacMillan.

Gunderson, G. R., & Pray, L. (2006). *Leading causes of life*. Memphis, TN: The Center of Excellence in Faith and Health, Methodist Le Bonheur Healthcare.

Health Systems Learning Group (HSLG). (2013). *Strategic investment in shared outcomes: transformative partnerships between health systems and communities*. Retrieved from http://stakeholderhealth.org/wp-content/uploads/2013/09/HSLG-V11.pdf.

Kalula, E. (2013). *The Will to Live and Serve*. Farewell lecture, Faculty of Law, University of Cape Town.

Kim, J. Y. (2013). Time for even greater ambition in global health. *The Lancet, 382*(9908), Retrieved from e33-e34. DOI:10.1016/S0140-6736(13)62374-0.

Kim, J. Y., Millen, J. V., Irwin, A., & Gershman, J. (Eds.). (2000). *Dying for growth: global inequality and the health of the poor*. Monroe, ME: Common Courage Press.

Krieger, N. (2008). Proximal, distal, and the politics of causation: what's level got to do with it? *American Journal of Public Health, 98*, 221-230.

Lancet Commission, T. (2013). Global health 2035: a world converging within a generation. *The Lancet*. Retrieved from http://dx.doi.org/10.1016/S0140-6736(13)62105-4.

Manchanda, R. (2013). *The upstream doctors: medical innovators track sickness to its source*. Amazon Digital Services: TED Books.

McGilvray, J. C. (1981). *The quest for health and wholeness*. Tübingen: German Institute for Medical Mission.

Muir Gray, J. A. (2011). *How to build healthcare systems*. Oxford: Offox Press.

Nail, T. (2015). *The figure of the migrant*. Palo Alto, CA: Stanford University Press.

Olivier, J., Tsimpo, C., Gemignani, R., Shojo, M., Coulombe, H., Dimmock, F., Nguyen, M.C., Hines, H., Mills, E. J., Dieleman, J. L., Haakenstad, A., Wodon, Q. (2015). Understanding the roles of faith-based health-care providers in Africa: review of the evidence with a focus on magnitude, reach, cost, and satisfaction. *The Lancet, 386*(10005), 1765–1775. Retrieved from http://dx.doi.org/10.1016/S0140-6736(15)60251-3.

Open Working Group on Sustainable Development Goals. (2014). *Final compilation of amendments to goals and targets*. Retrieved from https://sustainabledevelopment.un.org/content/documents/4438mgscompilationowg13.pdf

Panter-Brick, C., Eggerman, M., & Tomlinson, M. (2014). How might global health master deadly sins and strive for greater virtues? *Global Health Action, 7*(23411), 1-5.

Robertson, R., & White, K. E. (2007). What is globalization? In G. Ritzer (Ed.), *The Blackwell companion to globalization* (pp. 54-66). Malden, MA; Oxford, UK: Blackwell Publishing.

Task Force for Global Health. (2015). Panel Discussion: A Celebration of Three Decades of Contributions to Global Health, October 12. Retrieved from https://www.youtube.com/watch?v=24YkghgecNo.

Vertovec, S., & Cohen, R. (Eds.). (1999). *Migration, diasporas and transnationalism* (Vol. 9). Cheltenham, U.K.: Edward Elgar Publishing.

Wood Ion, H. (2015). *The lens of Leading Causes of Life: working in living systems*. Wake Forest Baptist Health, FaithHealth Division. Winston-Salem, NC.

World Health Organization (WHO). (2008). *Closing the gap in a generation: health equity through action on the social determinants of health*. Commission on Social Determinants of Health. Retrieved from http://www.who.int/social_determinants/final_report/csdh_finalreport_2008.pdf.

FULL AUTHORSHIP LISTING

James R. Cochrane, PhD, Professor, Dept. of Family Medicine and Public Health, University of Capetown, South Africa

Gary R. Gunderson, MDiv, DMin, DTh [Hon], Vice President of FaithHealth, Wake Forest Baptist Medical Center and Wake Forest School of Medicine, Public Health Science, Winston Salem, NC

Gerald Winslow, PhD, Vice President of Mission and Culture, Loma Linda University Health, Loma Linda, CA

Heather Wood Ion, PhD, Executive Director, Epidemic of Health, Badger, CAs

For more information about this chapter, contact **Jim Cochrane** at e-mail, jrcochrane@gmail.com.

CHAPTER 11

Mission and the Heart of Healthy Communities

Gerald Winslow with Fred Smith, Don Stiger, Dora Barilla and Cynthia Carter Perrilliat

Introduction

In our previous monograph, we gave brief expression to the core convictions that have empowered the mission of faith-based and charitable health systems in their work for community health development. We reflected on the essential values and beliefs that have led health systems to work for the health of whole communities, and to create what we called "the beloved community of health." We wrote that "we accept our responsibility to lead organizations that will pioneer new ways of achieving truly healthy communities. We know we have a significant role in helping to create and sustain communities that invite the engagement of all members—communities that sense both their shared heritage and their shared future" (Health Systems Learning Group, 2013, p. 82).

The exploration of our founding principles, and the sense of calling they represent, renewed our appreciation of what gives heart to our work in communities of great need. This, we believe, is what furnishes durability to efforts that are often gritty and difficult. It is also what makes this work joyous, even when it is hard. In the present chapter, we give further attention to the mission, purpose, and power of the organizations that have chosen to be generative nodes in the growing network of Stakeholder Health.

By generative nodes we mean those organizations where differing streams of thought, innovations, and relationships come together to form a hub capable of generating fresh approaches to community health development. Such nodes create new connections and facilitate the exchange of creative ideas and new energy. Thus they add life to the growing Faith and Health Movement. The goal of this network is to learn from each other not only how to do the work of building more whole communities, but also to learn more about why this work is essential to our mission.

In the time since writing the earlier monograph, the importance of creating a network of health systems that share a commitment to the development of healthy communities has become even more evident. The energy generated in recent years by healthcare reform or, perhaps more accurately, the reform of healthcare reimbursement, has led to increased attention on the part of healthcare systems to "population health."

Often this expression refers to little more than hospitals' attempts to improve traditional case management. But the transformational work of creating a culture of health for whole communities will require far more fundamental changes—particularly, more effective and efficient coordination of care. Collaborative networks of organizations, including communities of faith, can help us move toward the goal in demonstrably effective ways. While we celebrate the fact that millions of fellow citizens have received health insurance coverage for the first time, we know that more health care does not always lead to healthier communities. For this, we need the collaboration of all segments and supporting systems of the community. Communities of faith and charitable health care will continue to play a critical role in this transformational and fundamental change, if we are to create a beloved community of health.

During this same time period, some formidable challenges and risks for charitable health care have also become more apparent. The rapid strides toward mergers and acquisitions, leading to ever larger, bureaucratized and more commoditized systems, threaten to undermine the identity of health care institutions with long traditions of faith-inspired, benevolent missions (Panicola & Hamel, 2015). It is thus important to reconsider the basic commitments to human wholeness, compassion and social justice that fuel our willingness to become integrally united with the communities we serve, for the sake of strengthening health, hope, and healing.

Heritage of Faith and Health

From its beginnings in our culture, health care has had strong, organic links to religious faith. Early examples include Egyptian and Greek temples where people sought cures for their diseases. Notable among these were the temples dedicated to Asclepius, the god of healing in Greek mythology (Rosen, 1999; Edelstein & Edelstein, 1998). To this day, the snake-entwined rod of Asclepius remains one of medicine's most recognized symbols. And the time-honored Oath of Hippocrates, still adapted for use in some medical schools (Orr, Pang, Pellegrion, & Siegler, 1997), begins by swearing allegiance to Asclepius and his daughters, Hygeia and Panacea. Some of the initial steps to systematize the healing arts also arose in the context of Greek temples of healing, where attempted remedies, including the therapeutic energies of music, were carefully observed and documented (Risse, 1990).

Throughout Jewish history, as evidenced in sacred writings, health and healing have been understood as direct manifestations of what it means to be created "in the image of God" (Hebrew *b'tzelem Elo-him*). In the tradition of inclusive Abrahamic hospitality, health care is not a privilege for a few, but should be equitably available to all. Judaism continues to hold wholeness and completeness (*shalom bayit*) at the center of its teaching and practice. Shalom is realized through faithful, loving-kindness (*chesed*). Important dimensions of contemporary Jewish life include the concepts of repairing what is broken in the world (*tikkun olam*) and whole-person care for the sick (*bikkur holim*), remaining mindful of the abiding promise: "For I am the LORD who heals you" (Exodus 15:26, *New Revised Standard Version*).

With the rise of Christianity, the story of organized health care often involved members of the faith community creating institutions in which ministry to the sick could be provided. By the fourth century, hospitals were being established in the larger cities where there was also a cathedral. The most prominent of these came to be known as "Basilicas" founded by St. Basil in Cappadocia in 369 (Walsh, 1910). This institution was eventually organized as a small city with homes for physicians and nurses, and a variety of buildings for persons with differing needs, including those with leprosy. The name given to such institutions came from the Latin root *hospes* that referred both to guests and to hosts, and appears in other words today such as hostel and hospitality.

Established in mercy to care for those who were in need, early hospitals provided shelter not only for the sick but also traveling pilgrims, the homeless, and the destitute. The religious impulse to provide hospitality to those in need continued with the development of monastic orders throughout the Middle Ages. Monasteries and convents often included facilities that were designed to give both physical and spiritual care to the needy. For example, the Alexian Brothers risked their own lives in order to provide care for victims of the Black Plague in Europe (Alexian Brothers, 2016). Another of these religious orders, San Spirito (the Order of the Holy Ghost) founded hospitals first in Rome and then in many other European cities (Moeller, 1910). These facilities provided food, clothing, and shelter for the poor and typically gave some medical and nursing care.

Within Islamic history, there has also been a very close relationship between religion and medicine. In the Qur'an and other teachings, Muhammad includes instructions for sick persons to take medicine, as he did himself through expert physicians. Muslims have traditionally placed strong emphasis on charitable care, as well as the disciplined practice of preventative measures in healthcare. Islam has particularly been known for a refreshing openness to accept, use, and improve upon non-Muslim, as well as pre-Islamic, health and healing practices.

The religious impulses of Western health care have been prominent in the development of health care in America, which was predominantly built on the commitments of religious faith to offer charitable care. The tradition of religious almshouses, or "poor houses," which had begun in Europe, was continued in the U.S. Eventually, these institutions began adding wards in which the sick could receive care. In the Nineteenth Century, both Catholics and Protestants established hospitals intended primarily to care for the poor. During this time period, wealthy people who became ill were typically treated in their own homes by physicians and nurses who were paid to engage in home care, including surgery (Wall, n.d.) Today, many of the health care systems in the U.S. bear the names of their founding Roman Catholic religious orders, such as the Congregation of the Sisters of Bon Secours, or Sisters of Providence, or their parent Protestant denominations such as Lutheran, Methodist, Presbyterian, Baptist, or Adventist. Several of the organizations affiliated with Stakeholder Health have their roots in this tradition of faith-based and charitable health care. care (see Appendix 3 for full vision and mission statements from select faith traditions).

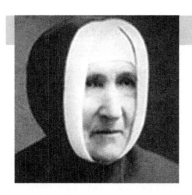

MOTHER JOSEPH OF THE SACRED HEART

Mother Joseph arrived at Fort Vancouver in the Washington Territory on December 8, 1856. Following her profound belief in Divine Providence and faith in the Sacred Heart of Jesus Christ, she began her work to serve those suffering the misfortunes of life. When she first arrived she discovered a land with no hospitals, and insignificant schools and charitable organizations for those suffering hardships on the frontier. With an attic as home for herself and her fellow sisters, she immediately embarked upon her purpose. Their mandate and their desire was to care for the poor and the sick, to educate the children, and to bring the light of Christ into the lives of all they met.

Born and raised in Quebec Canada, Mother Joseph only spoke French upon her arrival in Vancouver; this issue was only the smallest of stumbling blocks as she traversed the territory and petitioned for funding. Until she learned the language, two bilingual sisters facilitated communication and taught her English. Her first project, after hearing the desires of the people of Vancouver, was to found and construct a boarding school, most recently known as Providence Academy. The citizens were now also clamoring for a hospital; with the assurance the women of Vancouver would pay for poor patients to receive treatment, Mother Joseph converted a building into the first permanent hospital in the Northwest, St. Joseph Hospital. The corporation Mother Joseph established in 1859 is acknowledged as a "Pioneer Corporation in Washington State," and is one of the oldest in the Northwest.

As the more people moved into the territory, Mother Joseph was tireless in her efforts, traveling by horse to communities across what is now Washington, Oregon, Idaho, Montana, and British Columbia.

As a child, she was instructed in design and the industrial arts by her father, an expert coach builder. These skills and knowledge would serve her repeatedly in her mission of service. She was an exacting supervisor and took personal interest in all of the projects she oversaw; people would recount seeing her climbing and inspecting construction quality, or working long into the night herself to repair poor build quality. The design and quality of her buildings led the American Institute of Architects to declare Mother Joseph "The First Architect of the Pacific Northwest".

She worked tirelessly for over 45 years and is responsible for opening over 30 hospitals, schools, and homes for orphans. Even as her strength failed and she was treated for breast cancer she considered it only "inconveniences" and continued her work traveling to support the work of the Sisters of Providence. She was known for her political acumen, intelligence, and compassion; these traits paled in comparison to her faith and devotion to the Sacred Heart of Jesus. With her final breath she spoke these words, "My dear sisters, allow me to recommend to you the care of the poor in our houses, as well as those without. Take good care of them; have no fear of them; assist them and receive them. Then, you will have no regrets. Do not say: ah! This does not concern me, let others see to them. My sisters, whatever concerns the poor is always our affair."

The Language of Mission

Among the gifts bequeathed by the heritage of faith-inspired and charitable health care is language that shapes our moral imagination. The words we use to express the meaning of health care are not mere linguistic decorations. The words have a powerful capacity to support or to undermine commitments to provide charitable care. The philosopher, Jeffrey Stout, observes this about the moral power of the language we choose: "The idea that there are distinct moral languages, disparate conceptualities within which to understand and appraise conduct, character, and community, has become a commonplace in recent humanistic scholarship" (Stout, 1988, p. x). This means that faith-based and charitable healthcare organizations would do well to attend to the dominant language used to describe their work (Winslow, 1996). Some healthcare systems, such as that of Providence Health & Services, whose founder, Mother Joseph, in described in the sidebar above, have been careful to retain that language of service and caring.

As we have seen, one of the oldest ways to frame health care in Western culture (and perhaps in most human societies) is as sacred service. Consider, for example, the prayer attributed to the legendary medieval Jewish physician, Maimonides, which ends with these words: "Thou, All-Bountiful One, has chosen me to watch over the life and death of Thy creatures. I prepare myself now for my calling. Stand Thou by me in this great task, so that it may prosper" (Lyons & Petrucelli, 1978, p. 315). Similarly, in Christianity the connection between faith and the ministry of healing has remained strong. In the Christian testament, for example, one word (Greek *sozo*) means both "to heal" and "to save." Jesus commissioned his followers to teach the news about salvation and to heal the sick (Luke 9:1-2).

The evidence of health care's roots in religious faith remains, even if sometimes muted, in the languages of today's Western cultures. In Germany, for instance, nurses are still referred to as *Krankenschwestern*, or "sisters for the sick." In England, nurse managers are still called "ward sisters." Hospitals named for saints, or called Good Samaritan, Deaconess, or Sacred Heart are still common. Air ambulances in some areas fly through the sky with the name "Mercy" emblazoned on them. Multitudes of healthcare professionals in our society still understand their work as a vocational calling that is first and foremost a sacred ministry to those in need (Chapman, 2006). A prime example of this was the founder of NYU Brooklyn Lutheran Hospital, Sister Betty, a Lutheran visionary (see sidebar below).

I WAS A STRANGER AND YOU WELCOMED ME. (MATTHEW 25)

As waves of new immigrants struggled to survive in America's largest cities during the latter half of the 19th century, several faith groups were among the charitable organizations that stepped forward to create much-needed safety nets of health and human services. The depth and breadth of social ministries sponsored by the Catholic Church soon became an inspiring model for many other denominations. Norwegian American Lutherans alone sponsored 28 hospitals, 20 hospices, 20 "homes for the aged," 14 children's homes, and a home-placement service for orphaned children.

A predominant number of these health and social ministry services were founded and operated through the Protestant Deaconess movement, with scores of women trained in "motherhouses" to serve as nurses and healthcare providers. The Norwegian churches in America established 3 such motherhouses in Brooklyn (1883), Minneapolis (1889) and Chicago (1897). These faith-grounded communities, centered in nurturing vocation and practical training, served as "nodes" for a widespread array of healthcare ministries, reaching inestimable numbers of unserved and underserved persons. For them, mission, meaning, and motivation were all grounded in faith, core values, and a deeply felt commitment to religious vocation.

A Norwegian Deaconess Nurse, Sister Elisabeth Fedde, stands prominently among those who literally immersed themselves—body, mind, and spirit—in providing medical care not only to their own particular ethnic group, but who also actively addressed the underlying "social determinants" of health/well-being encountered throughout the multi-cultural communities they served. In Fedde's case, The Norwegian Relief Society—the fledgling mission she founded with local congregations in 1883 in a 3-room boardinghouse—soon became known not only for providing medical care to Scandinavian seafarers, but also as a wider mission marked by whole person care throughout south Brooklyn— particularly benefitting the disenfranchised and impoverished. That included spiritual care, work in homes, prisons and congregations, financial relief, and placement services for orphans and the unemployed. The mission quickly evolved into a 50-bed hospital with both an ambulance service and nursing school. Now incorporated as "NYU Lutheran," its mission to the underserved immigrants of south Brooklyn *has virtually not changed*. Today it comprises one to the busiest Level I Trauma Centers in New York City, serving all 5 boroughs through one of the oldest and largest Federally Qualified Health Centers in the United States.

There are, of course, alternative ways to describe the work of health care. During the second half of the 19th Century, for example, a novel way of talking about health care arose—it became *war* against disease. One author suggests that this language coincided with the arrival of germ theory, the bacterial enemies viewed as threatening invaders capable of overwhelming the body's defenses (Sontag, 1978). It is also the case that much of what medicine came to know about trauma surgery, triage, and the control of infections during this time was being learned on the battlefields of Europe. In the military manner of speaking, health care's mission was to combat diseases with batteries of tests and arsenals of drugs, sometime referred to as the physicians' armamentarium. Doctors write "orders," and younger staff physicians are still called house "officers." It is also telltale that patients who leave hospitals are discharged. Nurses, who work at stations, take orders when they are on duty. Sometimes they refer to the injections they give as "shots." Today the military language is so pervasive that what was once novel has become common.

The widespread adoption of military language in the provision of health care has had powerful effects in creating a shared understanding of the work's meaning. Its use helps to ensure the expectation of loyal obedience to authority along with courageous, self-sacrificial service against a common enemy. Such language supports a willingness to take risks, work long hours, and create a tightly knit team in the noble battle against illness.

Today, the languages of the ministry and of the military have largely yielded center stage to the language of the market. The 1980s witnessed the appearance of the "health care industry." One of the first persons to notice such language and complain about it in print was Rashi Fein who wrote: "A new language is infecting the culture of American medicine. It is the language of the marketplace ... and the cost accountant" (Fein, 1982, p. 863). At the heart of his complaint was the belief that such language "depersonalizes both patients and physicians" (Fein, 1982, p. 863). Now, more than 30 years later, the idioms of business tend to dominate much of our talk about health care. In this business-like way of speaking, health care professionals became providers and patients became customers or, especially in the language of some nurses, clients. Discussions among health care executives are filled with references to market share, productivity measures, and product lines. Such language is borrowed substantially from economics and marketing. Those who cannot or choose not to speak this way are likely to be written off as lacking necessary, hard-edged economic realism. In sum, today's health care increasingly runs the danger of losing its charitable soul, devolving into yet another commoditized industry.

The distance from the ministry of healing to the health care industry is great. It is not measured in years or miles but in the way people understand the essence and meaning of what they are doing when they care for the health of another person, and *why* such care is offered. Each of the three ways of characterizing health care's purpose as described above discloses some important truths about caring for the health of whole communities and for their members who become ill. No one can deny, for example, that medicine today is big business, and growing bigger all the time. The financial resources required to keep such efforts going are enormous. No one who cares about the viability of today's health care can ignore the pervasive financial realities. And whether it is a battle against an outbreak of the Ebola virus or a fight against cancer, there are certainly analogies to marshalling the troops to win the war. Physicians will still give orders, and patients will still hope to be discharged, as opposed to "checking out."

What about health care as the response of faith, hope, and charity to people's often inconvenient pleas for mercy? One of the critically important roles for Stakeholder Health is strengthening the self-understanding of faith-inspired and charitable health systems as they develop more effective ways to care for the health of whole communities. This requires more than the preservation of nostalgic language or storied past. Together, the participants in this learning collaborative can find new language that powerfully expresses our commitments to charitable service in the 21st Century with all its cultural and religious diversity. Finding fresh ways to explain the core value of health care understood as spiritually meaningful service is a welcome opportunity. There is good reason to hope that creative communities of spirit will find those fresh ways to grow their centuries-old legacy of health care as the service of mercy, such as that emerging in Alameda County, California (see Alameda County Care Alliance Advanced Illness Care Program™ sidebar).

THE ALAMEDA COUNTY CARE ALLIANCE ADVANCED ILLNESS CARE PROGRAM™: A FAITH LED COMMUNITY-FAITH-HEALTH SYSTEM PARTNERSHIP

The Alameda County Care Alliance (ACCA) is a coalition of five churches representing over 35,000 people in Alameda County. Together, the Pastors and congregation members with experience in healthcare and healthcare administration have designed The Advanced Illness Care Program™. This program provides persons needing advanced illness care and their caregivers with navigation assistance to local resources and information to manage spiritual, social, health, and planning for advanced care needs. With support from Kaiser Permanente, the Advanced Illness Care Program™ has been developed as a partnership of the ACCA with local clinical, academic, and public health institutions.

ACCA utilizes a three-pronged approach to improving care management for persons with advanced illness and their caregivers by training 1) church-based community care navigators, 2) pastors and faith leaders, and 3) family caregivers. Through a series of 10 in-person and telephone interactions, ACCA care navigators and faith leaders link persons needing advanced illness care and family caregivers to needed resources, including transportation and meal preparation, support for advanced care planning, and to address identified physical, psychological, and spiritual needs. The Advanced Illness Care Program™ will enroll 500 persons needing care and caregivers, tracking program feasibility, process implementation measures, and satisfaction, quality of life, and experiences of care for persons with advanced illness, their caregivers, pastors and faith leaders, and navigators. ACCA will serve as a national resource and knowledge base for a faith led community-faith-health system partnership to improve advanced illness care management.

Building off the community health worker model of community health clinics, the ACCA has developed the community care navigator role from a faith-based perspective within all Hub churches. Community care navigators are not medical professionals, but are trusted, well-respected individuals in their ACCA church. Having undergone extensive training with a curriculum developed by the ACCA and the Allen Temple Leadership Institute, community care navigators work closely with their churches, ministries, and community organizations to align advanced illness care resources and associated information to the needs of persons needing care and caregivers. The ACCA has also developed a Care Ministry of dedicated volunteer congregants who work with the ACCA and care navigators to support programmatic needs. Seven care navigators have been trained and are working with over 300 persons needing care and caregivers through the 5 ACCA Hub Churches in Alameda County. Additionally, 61 volunteers are assisting with the program. Over 98 individuals participated in a 2-day care ministry volunteer training at the end of July 2015 on advanced illness care, interviewing skills, and roles and responsibilities of volunteers in the ACCA AIC Program™.

The ACCA program has comprehensive outreach efforts in place for recruitment of participants, communications with local media and partner organizations, and is building partnerships with health systems and hospitals, hospices, and community organizations. On August 30, 2015, the ACCA and its partners hosted a Caregiver Recognition Celebration and Health Expo bringing together 1100 people across Alameda County to honor the dedication and support that caregivers provide to loved ones. Over 25 local, regional, and national organizations attended this event.

The ACCA is part of a national movement to transform care for those with advanced illness, and is a member of the Coalition to Transform Advanced Care (C-TAC), a national, non-partisan, non-profit coalition of 120+ organizations. ACCA shares the C-TAC vision that all Americans with advanced illness, especially the sickest and most vulnerable, should receive comprehensive, high-quality, person-centered and family-centered care that is consistent with their personal goals and values and honors their dignity. ACCA looks to expand the program within the Hub churches and beyond, partnering with community organizations and health systems to support advanced care planning. For more information on the ACCA Advanced Illness Care Program™, Hub churches and Partners, sponsorship opportunities, and the Caregiver Recognition Celebration and Health Expo, please visit www.accarealliance.org or contact Rev. Cynthia Carter Perrilliat, Executive Director, 510-427-4624.

Moral Vision

The moral vision of Stakeholder Health continues to be best expressed in the expectation of creating the beloved community of life, health, and hope. Both the heritage and language of faith-based and charitable healthcare institutions grow out of the compelling moral vision of grace, sacrifice, compassion, and abundant life. This is a vision of life over death—a vision of health continually coming to life within communities of spirit. The vision of the beloved community of health is the yearning expression of faithful people to create better health outcomes for all.

We believe the current period of America's story represents what may be called a *Kairos* moment— the right time for renewing the moral vision of faith-shaped and charitable healthcare. Alternatives to the complete commodification of healthcare are needed now more than ever. Health care envisioned as the business of waging war against death, in the most cost-efficient manner, will not provide the transformative power that will lead to the beloved community of health. What is needed, instead, is an abiding commitment to social justice and a firm unwillingness to accept health disparities as inevitable. This is the vision that has enlivened the participants in Stakeholder Health at their best.

Such vision is exemplified beyond the normal boundaries of healthcare in the growing movement called "Black Lives Matter" which challenges the notion that the lives of African American are in any way less valuable than other lives in our society (Day, 2015). The movement seeks to address the issues of violence and discrimination in the administration of criminal "justice." The need for such a movement is a reminder of the depth of social injustice that is still pervasive in our social institutions, including health care. As Dr. Martin Luther King, Jr. (1966) once said, "Of all the forms of inequality, injustice in healthcare is the most shocking and inhumane." Inexplicable and inexcusable unfairness in healthcare is now so much a part of the fabric of our society that it may cease to shock our collective conscience.

Part of the prophetic core mission of Stakeholder Health is to remind society that the social determinants contributing to poor health are the products of intentional behaviors and policies. These policies are often rooted in soil that includes white supremacy, male dominance, and pervasive xenophobia. This is the soil of death and destruction. The moral vision of Stakeholder Health emboldens us to stand against such injustice and take the side of life.

Choosing Life

In this chapter, we have set forth some of the central values that can guide the work of creating and sustaining the beloved community of health. We have also attended to the ways in which our language is shaped by a moral vision of mercy and justice and, in turn, how our choice of language may extend or diminish the moral vision. We conclude this chapter with a renewed expression of commitment to this vision. As leaders of organizations that participate in Stakeholder Health, we are devoted to investing our creative energy to *build a future in which whole communities choose life over death*.

As we wrote in our previous monograph, "We have the audacity to believe in a future in which a healthy, beloved community is an achievable reality" (Health Systems Learning Group, 2013, p. 82). We will continually refresh our covenant to learn from each other how we can best accomplish this goal.

REFERENCES

Alexian Brothers (2016). History of the Alexian Brothers. Retrieved from Alexian Brothers website: http://alexianbrothers.ie/our-history

Chapman, E. (2006). *Sacred Work.* Nashville: Baptist Healing Trust.

Day, E. (2015, July 19). Black Lives Matter: The Birth of a New Civil Rights Movement. *The Observer.* Retrieved from website: http://www.theguardian.com/world/2015/jul/19/blacklivesmatter-birth-civil-rights-movement

Fein, R. (1982). What's Wrong with the Language of Medicine? *The New England Journal of Medicine, 306,* 863-864.

Health Systems Learning Group (2013). *Monograph.* Retrieved from Stakeholder Health website: http://stakeholderhealth.org/wp-content/uploads/2013/09/HSLG-V11.pdf

King, M. L. (1966). Informal speech. Retrieved from Health Justice CT website: https://www.healthjusticect.org/of-all-the-forms-of-inequality-injustice-in-healthcare-is-the-most-shocking-and-inhumane-mlk/

Lyons, A. S. & Petrucelli, R. J. (1978). *Medicine: An Illustrated History.* New York: Abradale Press.

Moeller, C. (1910) Orders of the Holy Ghost. *The Catholic Encyclopedia.* Vol. 7. New York: Robert Appleton Company. Retrieved from website: http://www.newadvent.org/cathen/07415a.htm

Orr, R., Pang, N., Pellegrino, E. & Siegler, M. (1997). Use of the Hippocratic Oath: A Review of Twentieth Century Practice. *Journal of Clinical Ethics,* 8, 377.

Panicola, M. & Hamel, R. (2015). Catholic Identity and the Reshaping of Health Care. *Health Progress,* September-October, 46-56.

Risse, G. B. (1990). *Mending Bodies, Saving Souls: A History of Hospitals.* Oxford: Oxford University Press.

Sontag, S. (1978). *Illness as Metaphor.* New York: Farrar, Straus and Giroux.

Rosen, G. (1999). *A history of public health.* Baltimore, MD: Johns Hopkins University Press.

Stout, J. (1988). *Ethics after Babel.* Boston: Beacon Press.

Wall, B. M. (n.d.). History of Hospitals. Unpublished manuscript retrieved from University of Pennsylvania website: http://www.nursing.upenn.edu/nhhc/Welcome%20Page%20Content/History%20of%20Hospitals.pdf

Walsh, J.J. (1910). Hospitals. *The Catholic Encyclopedia.* New York: Robert Appleton Company. Retrieved from New Advent website: http://www.newadvent.org/cathen/07480a.htm

Winslow, G. R. (1996). Minding Our Language: Metaphors and Biomedical Ethics. In E. E. Shelp (Ed.). *Secular Bioethics in Theological Perspective.* pp. 19-30. Boston: Kluwer Academic Press.

FULL AUTHORSHIP LISTING

Gerald Winslow, PhD, Vice President of Mission and Culture, Loma Linda University Health, Loma Linda, CA

Fred Smith, PhD, Co-Chair Health Equity, Insitute for Healthcare Improvement, 100 Million Lives, Oakland, CA

Don Stiger, MDiv, BCC, Senior Vice President, Mission and Spiritual Care, NYU Lutheran, Brooklyn, NY

Dora Barilla, DrPH, President, HC2 Strategies, Inc. and Executive Leader, Community Investments, Providence Health and Services, Tacoma, WA

Cynthia Carter Perrilliat, MPA, Executive Director, Alameda County Care Alliance, Oakland, CA

For more information about this chapter, contact **Gerald Winslow** at e-mail, gwinslow@llu.edu.

APPENDICES

Stakeholder Health: Our Story

Gary Gunderson, Teresa Cutts, Heidi Christensen and Tom Peterson

Stakeholder Health (SH) is a learning group of hospitals (with the benefits of other private and public partners along the way) distinguished by what we are trying to learn and who is doing the learning. The focus is simple and profound: can faith-based and mission oriented institutions deliver what we were created to do? Most of our institutions were founded several generations ago by people of faith or with deep community vision who thought a hospital would advance the general health and well-being of some place they loved, whether in Detroit, Winston-Salem or the wilds of West Baltimore or Tacoma.

Fast forward to the 21st century, and the technology of these hospitals would be almost unrecognizable to those founders. The public health field has come almost full circle in the era of the Affordable Care Act and as a result of advances in health science for prevention, early detection and long-term management of so many conditions that were once death sentences. But what about the mission? How does that go forward? Maybe now we can do what we were created to do a century ago: learn the things that make not just for good *hospitals* but for the full *health* of all.

The Stakeholder Health learning collaborative is also distinctive in who is asking and answering that profound question. Many of us work at fairly high levels in the hospitals, often for most of our careers. We know health systems from investing our time, energy and mind in them at all hours on the clock, year after year. We hope for them as we hope for the communities they—we—serve. So we know the traps, complicities, perversities and inertia involved as these massive institutions—usually the largest in their communities—refocus, remember their purpose, and try to align themselves with the noble work of health at large scale. We, the learners writing here, are far removed from naiveté—but not from hope. At any gathering and in every collaborative chapter in the path of SH you'll see intellectual generosity and courage born of that hope that can only be nurtured and made real by working with others who themselves are moved by it.

This appendix gathers the remarkable bundle of threads of the learning journey of SH to date. We are early on that journey in many ways, so the previous chapters look down the road and around the world for clues to where we must go next. Here we sum up what we have come to learn so far.

The learning group that became SH emerged when a White House delegation came to Memphis to see how an African model of "religious health assets mapping" was being adapted into the US context. As was true in Africa, the Memphis assessment unveiled about six times as many generative partners as the prevailing official maps showed. In the case of Memphis, that meant hundreds of faith-forming things (congregations), while elsewhere, such as in North Carolina, the surprise is the number of faith-based community organizations at work (details of the African mapping model and others are in Chapter 6 in this work). How to see, align, animate and release these assets, especially in troubled neighborhoods, lies beneath everything Stakeholder Health tries to learn. Given that these key resources are needed worldwide, this makes Stakeholder Health part of a global learning community. The motherland for this kind of learning is post-colonial Africa, which knows that the health of its people rests on their own energy, intelligence and, yes, liberation. That's true for South Memphis, San Bernardino, the left-behind urban areas of Detroit and West Baltimore, too. Stakeholder Health learns the most in, from and with those working in tough places—a very global kind of thing to do.

It wasn't just the huge connectional network of Memphis that caught the attention of HHS, but creative data gathering that showed powerful effect where you wouldn't expect it. The community partnerships were moving hospital data. That's the other consistent Stakeholder Health focus—a constant search for real-time evaluation so that all of the stakeholders in and around the healing enterprises called hospitals could test their best intentions against actual results as quickly as possible. We know that health is mostly the result of long trajectory "determinants" (which we consider variables), so we know our efforts will take decades. This puts additional intellectual pressure on us to find the earliest reliable indicators to steer our partnerships so they might, as Martin Luther King would want, "bend the arc of history toward justice." That's what we want to learn. We want our lives as professionals and that of our institutions, professing mercy and justice, to learn the things that will bend the long arc of what we care the most about. The learning this book outlines was done on the way with little patience for our own pace. We know we will need to know more and learn faster as we go further toward accomplishing our original goals. The rest of this document, far from complacent then, is even less patient.

Brief History

The site visit to Memphis from Feb. 6-8, 2011 that led to Stakeholder Health was an exploratory consultation led by the White House Office and HHS Center for Faith-based and Neighborhood Partnerships. They brought leaders from other governmental agencies too: Administration on Aging, Agency for Healthcare Research and Quality, Health Resources Services Administration, Office of Minority Health, Regional Health Administrator, Office of the Assistant Secretary for Health Substance Abuse and Mental Health Services Administration. These leaders arrived in Memphis just as the first data from the Congregational Health Network became available and this shifted the energy to exploring practices of innovative health systems interested in partnering more intentionally with vulnerable populations.

To tap into that innovative partnership energy the February meeting was followed by a national gathering in Sept. 2011 at the White House co-hosted by its Office of Faith Based and Neighborhood Partnerships and the HHS Partnership Center, attended by senior representatives of 22 different health systems. Besides the Memphis Model's Congregational Health Network, the Camden Coalition's hotspotting and South Central Foundation (NUKA) integrated health systems approaches were highlighted. Since then, the HHS Partnership Center has coordinated and walked alongside this voluntary, peer-led learning collaborative of hospital health professionals motivated by the ACA to accelerate their institution's progress in transforming the health of their communities. Initially called the Health Systems Learning Group (HSLG), it shifted its name to Stakeholder Health in 2013.

Stakeholder Health Partners

To date Stakeholder Health has enjoyed the participation of over 90 organizations across diverse sectors (53 are hospital health systems), including governmental and community partners, denominational partners, other initiatives or coalitions (e.g. , 100 Million Lives), as well as policy, research institute and think tank partners (e.g. IOM Roundtable on Population Health, ReThink Health, and RWJF). With past or current contributing partners bolded, they include:

- **Adventist Health Central Valley Network, CA**
- **Adventist HealthCare, MD/NJ**
- **Adventist Health System, Orlando, FL**
- **Advocate HealthCare, Chicago, IL**
- Allen Temple Baptist Church, Oakland, CA
- American Muslim Health Professionals (AMHP)
- **Ascension Health, St. Louis, MO**
- Aurora Health System, Milwaukee, WI
- Baptist Health (Northeast Florida & Southeast Georgia)
- Baptist State Convention of North Carolina
- **Baylor, Scott & White Health System, Central Dallas, TX**
- **Bon Secours Health System, Inc.**
- Bon Secours Baltimore Health System, Baltimore, MD
- Bon Secours Richmond Health System, VA
- Bread for the World
- California Endowment (The)
- Camden Coalition of Health Care Providers
- Catholic Charities, USA
- Catholic Health Association
- **Catholic Health Initiatives, Franciscan Health & MultiCare Health System (joined SH together), Tacoma, WA**
- Carter Center (The)
- Centers for Disease Control and Prevention
- Centers for Medicaid and Medicare, DC
- Central Dallas Ministries
- Centura, Englewood, CO
- ChangeLab Solutions, Oakland, CA
- CHE/Trinity Health System, Livonia, MI
- CHRISTUS Health, Irving, TX
- CitySquare, Dallas, TX
- Clark University, MA
- Community Catalyst
- Dept. of Health and Human Services
- Democracy Collaborative, (The)
- **Dignity Health, San Francisco, CA**
- Duke University Hospital, Raleigh, NC
- EMORY Interfaith Health Program
- Fairview Health Services, Minneapolis, MN
- George Washington Department of Health Policy, School of Public Health and Health Services, DC
- Gordon-Conwell Seminary, Charlotte, NC
- **Henry Ford Health System, Detroit, MI**
- Hood Theological Seminary, Salisbury, NC
- Hope *worldwide*
- Howard University and University Hospital, Washington, DC
- **Indiana University Health, Indianapolis**
- Inova Health System, Fairfax, VA
- Institute for Healthcare Improvement, 100 Million Lives, Boston, MA
- Institute of Medicine, DC
- Islamic Society of North America;
- Jewish Community Center Association of North America (JCCA), NY
- Johns Hopkins University School of Medicine
- Intermountain Healthcare, Salt Lake City, Utah
- Kaiser Permanente, Oakland, CA
- **Kettering Health Network, Dayton, OH**
- Kresge Foundation
- Leadership Foundation, Knoxville, TN
- **Loma Linda University Health, CA**
- Lutheran Healthcare, Brooklyn, NY
- Lutheran Services of America, DC
- Lutheran Services of Florida
- **Lutheran Social Services, Illinois**
- Medical Network Devoted to Service (MiNDS)
- MedStar Health, MD, DC
- Memorial Hospital of South Bend, IN
- **Methodist Le Bonheur Healthcare, Memphis, TN**
- NAD Seventh-day Adventists, Adventist Health Ministries
- National Association of Hispanic Nurses
- National Baptist Convention
- **Nemours, DEL, Fl**
- OhioHealth, Columbus, OH
- Penrose-St. Francis Health Services, Colorado Springs, CO
- People Improving Community by Organizing Network (PICO)
- Pinnacle Health Systems, Harrisburg, PA
- **ProMedica Health, Toledo, OH**
- Providence Hospital, Washington, DC
- **Providence Health & Services, Tacoma, WA**
- Prevention Institute, Oakland, CA
- Public Health Institute, Oakland, CA
- ReThink Health, The Fannie E. Rippel Foundation
- **Robert Wood Johnson Foundation**
- Serve West Dallas, TX

- Shawnee Mission Medical Center, Kansas
- Sibley Hospital, Washington DC
- St. Joseph Health System, Sonoma County, CA
- Southcentral Foundation, Alaska
- **Summa Health System, Akron, OH**
- **Texas Health Resources, Dallas/Ft Worth**
- The Bridgespan Group
- The California Endowment
- Trinity Health System, Livonia, MI
- Trust for America's Health, Washington, DC
- Union Theological Seminary, Dayton, OH
- United Methodist Committee on Relief (UMCOR)
- United Way Worldwide
- United Way Santa Cruz
- **University Health, Cleveland, OH**
- UMASS Memorial Health System, Worcester
- University of Illinois Health and Hospital System, Chicago, IL
- Urban Strategies, DC
- **Wake Forest Baptist Health, Winston-Salem, NC**
- Wesley Theological Seminary, Washington DC
- YMCA of the USA

Stakeholder Health Structure and Function

SH was initially funded by a few contributing hospital systems per their CEOs' discretion: Methodist Le Bonheur Healthcare, Texas Health Resources, Henry Ford Health System, Advocate Healthcare, Indiana University, Loma Linda University Health, Adventist Florida, Dignity Health and Summa Health System. Funding from CEOs started in December 2011 and continues currently with these partners: Methodist Le Bonheur Healthcare, Wake Forest Baptist Medical Center, Henry Ford Health System, Advocate Healthcare, Bon Secours System, Baltimore and Richmond, Adventist West, Adventist Maryland, Adventist West, Loma Linda University Health, Adventist Florida, Dignity Health, Ascension Health, University Health in Cleveland, ProMedica, Nemours and Providence Health & Services. Recently Catholic Health Initiative (CHI) Franciscan Health & MultiCare Health System from Tacoma (WA) joined SH together in an unprecedented model of two competing health systems joining as one.

Stakeholder Health is now administered by a Secretariat housed at Wake Forest Baptist Medical Center in partnership with the HHS Partnership Center, with Gary Gunderson serving as the Secretary of the group and Teresa Cutts as staff liaison, along with Tom Peterson (Communications Director), Fred Smith (Faith Community Liaison) and Heidi Christensen (HHS Partnership Center Liaison). Jerry Winslow serves as Chair of the Stakeholder Health Advisory Council (SHAC).

Formed in 2014, the SHAC serves as an informal council without by-laws or regulations, though members serve as the decision-making body of SH. The contributing health systems (bolded in the participant grid above) have representatives on the SHAC. SH prides itself on keeping a lean and nimble infrastructure and not being grant or philanthropy dependent. Funds beyond grant monies are used to subsidize regional meetings and travel, as well as to support communication efforts.

Stakeholder Health Mission and Focus

Stakeholder Health is a voluntary movement of people working within hospital health systems who see in the current policy environment the opportunity to address the underlying causes of poor health in their communities by strategically shifting existing resources and partnering with diverse stakeholders.

Stakeholder Health participants are committed to **open source learning** and **a shared mission** articulated initially in a co-created 80-page monograph that was presented to their senior leadership at HHS in April 2013. In it, they outlined a framework for the health outcomes of the broader population, including its most vulnerable citizens. Stakeholder Health members are promoting three foundational strategies that will achieve greater health, particularly in the most vulnerable neighborhoods:

- **Address the social complexity of the most challenging patients** by engaging them at **the "neighborhood" level,**
- Work with **large-scale community partnerships**, and
- Proactively use **existing resources such** as charity care or community health assets.

(See 2016 updates from select case studies presented in the HSLG Monograph in Appendix 3.)

HHS Partnership Center and Stakeholder Health Convenings and Site Visits

SH and the HHS Partnership Center have coordinated national and regional convenings and site visits to health systems demonstrating exemplary practices advancing population health efforts since 2011. To date, these convenings and site visits have included:

NATIONAL:

- **Improving Health Outcomes through Faith-Based and Community Partnerships,** White House, September 20, 2011 **(65 participants)**

- **Improving Health Outcomes through Faith-Based and Community: Best Practices from the Field,** Dept. of Health and Human Services (HHS), DC, February 16-17, 2012 **(61 participants)**

- **Strategic Investment in Shared Outcomes: Transformative Partnerships between Health Systems and Communities, HHS**, April 4, 2013 **(40 participants)**

- **Mission, Purpose and Power, Loma Linda University Health,** Feb. 17-18, 2014 **(29 participants)**

- **Chawumba (informal gathering of the SH "tribe"),** July 2015, Winston Salem, NC **(38 participants)**

- **Stakeholder Health Advisory Council Retreat,** Institute of Medicine, October 21, 22, 2014 **(12 participants)**

- **Health IT— Accounting for Social and Behavioral Factors,** Dept. of Health and Human Services, September 18, 2014 **(57 participants)**

- **Listening sessions with CDC and CMMI,** HHS, September 18, 2014 **(25 participants)**

- **Partners in Health: Aligning Clinical Systems and Community Health Assets,** White House, April 15, 16, 2015 **(70 participants)**

(See 2016 updates from select case studies presented in the HSLG Monograph in Appendix 3.)

REGIONAL:

- **Memphis System of Health: Mapping and Aligning the Health Assets,** Feb. 6-8, 2011, Methodist Le Bonheur Healthcare, Memphis, TN **(30 participants)**

- **Health Systems Learning Group Regional Meeting,** Henry Ford Health System, Detroit, MI. October 9-11, 2012 **(65 participants)**

- **Expanded Models of Community Partnership: Securing a Return on Investment,** Loma Linda University Medical Center, San Bernardino, CA. June 28, 29, 2013 **(36 participants)**

- **Leadership through Partnership**, Advocate Healthcare, Chicago, IL, Sept. 24-25, 2015 **(43 participants)**

For all convenings held before 2013, the agendas and PowerPoint presentations can be found at the Center of Excellence in Faith and Health website, Methodist Le Bonheur Healthcare
http://www.methodisthealth.org/about-us/faith-and-health/research/learning-collaborative/

Group field site visits encourage deeper "cross-pollination" or learning and sharing best practices from site to site, as well as expansion of SH membership. These visits are usually initiated by Secretariat staff or our SH members. Visits to date, attended by one or more of the Secretariat, include:

Adventist Health, Orlando Florida (December 2013)

Bon Secours Richmond, VA (November 2013)

Bon Secours Baltimore, MD (March 2014)

UMass Memorial Health, Worcester, MA (September 2014)

Henry Ford Health System, Detroit (April 2015)

Loma Linda University Medical Center, San Bernardino (December 2014)

MultiCare Health & Catholic Health Initiatives, Franciscan, Tacoma, WA (May 2015)

Mt. Sinai, Icahn School of Medicine (November 2015)

NYU Brooklyn Lutheran (November 2015)

Providence Health & Services, Tacoma, WA (January 2016)

Stakeholder Health Forum Series

Led and managed by The HHS Partnership Center, SH produced and co-hosted a monthly web-based Stakeholder Health Forum from Fall 2013 through 2014. Presentations by participants focused on sharing concrete, granular intelligence on their efforts to reform systems from within their institutions. An impressive 800 persons in total participated, ranging from 30 to a high of 90 per Forum. The Forum formally ended in December 2014. Its topics included:

- **IT Working Group report-out/ Propeller Health** (Loma Linda, Wake Forest, Dignity, 9/25/2013). Presenters: Dora Barilla and Eileen Barsi

- **Institutionalizing Strategies for Population Health: How ProMedica Achieved Consensus for a Hunger-Free Community** (ProMedica, 10/2/2013). Presenters: Barb Petee and Randy Oostra

- **Exploring Stakeholder Health website** (12/4/2103). Presenter: Tom Peterson

- **"It's about Geography": Place and Person-centered Community Health Development** (Loma Linda, Adventist Health System, 1/8/2014). Presenters: Dora Barilla and Maureen Kersmarki, Tim McKinney

- **Community Health Asset Mapping: Moving from CHNA to Sustainable Networks of Community Health Assets** (Wake Forest, Advocate Health Care, 2/5/2014). Presenters: Teresa Cutts and Kirsten Peachey

- **Prioritizing Equity and Wellness: Reducing Infant Mortality by Meeting Women's Needs** (Henry Ford Health System, 3/5/2014). Presenters: Kimberlydawn Wisdom and Jaye Clement

- **Connecting Performance Incentives to Community Health Outcomes** (Nemours, 4/2/2014). Presenters: Debbie Chang and David Bailey

- **Proactive Mercy: Community Investment Grants that Promote Population Health and Expand Access To Care** (Dignity, 5/7/2014). Presenters: Eileen Barsi and Pablo Bravo

- **Financing Population Health Improvement** (Public Health Institute, Wake Forest, Loma Linda,6/04/2014). Presenters: Kevin Barnett, Gary Gunderson, and Jerry Winslow

- **Community Rx: Connecting People to Community Health Resources** (Univ. of Chicago Medicine, 9/3/2014). Presenter: Stacy Lindau
- **Trauma's Toll on Health: A Community-wide Response** (Memorial Hospital South Bend, 10/1/2014). Presenter: Margo DeMont
- **Designing "Outside-In" Health IT Measurement Frameworks** (Dignity Health , Loma Linda, 11/5/2014). Presenters: Dora Barilla and Eileen Barsi
- **CDC Community Health Improvement (CHI) Technical Package** (Centers for Disease Control and Prevention, 12/3/2014). Presenter: Denise Koo

All Forum presentations are available on the SH website. In addition to acting as a convener and coordinator, The HHS Partnership Center took a key role in SH. It supported existing network of participants and recruited new health system members and other relevant stakeholders. Additionally, the HHS Partnership Center contributes to the ongoing content for the website, Stakeholderhealth.org, which acts as a disseminating platform for exemplary practices and models.

Several exemplars were featured on RWJF's New Public Health daily blog that records and showcases innovative and noteworthy practice in the population health movement. These include:

- Health Systems Learning Group: New Public Health Q&A with Gary Gunderson (Sept. 16, 2013)
- Stakeholder Health: Q&A with Kimberlydawn Wisdom (Nov. 6, 2013)
- How Do You Transform a Community After a Century of Neglect? (Nov. 20, 2013)
- A Hospital Helps Revitalize the Community Outside Its Walls: Q & A with George Kleb and Christine Madigan (March 25, 2014)
- A Trauma Informed Community, Margo De Mont (Oct. 1, 2014)

Website, E-Zine and Communication Strategy

As a learning collective, Stakeholder Health is a forum for sharing and questioning together. Our website (www.stakeholderhealth.org) is where the face-to-face meetings are captured and reflections posted. For most convenings, agendas and presentations are posted along with notes. In November 2013, SH launched a website to host an online conversation. Through stories, blog posts, and Q&A's with thought leaders, the site shares struggles of the community with a focus on what's working, challenges and questions. The site also serves as the main avenue to alert the learning community about upcoming webinars, workshops, trainings and other kinds of meetings. Since it was set up, the site has had around 20,000 user sessions, more than 160 posts and filled 110 pages. In addition, a monthly online newsletter goes to subscribers. As this has evolved, it has taken on particular themes such as navigation networks, aligning community assets, overcoming the transportation barrier, and community health workers.

FULL AUTHORSHIP LISTING

Gary R. Gunderson, MDiv, DMin, DTh (Hon), VP of FaithHealth, Wake Forest Baptist Medical Center and Professor, Faith and Health of the Public, Wake Divinity School and Wake Forest School of Medicine, Winston Salem, NC

Teresa Cutts, PhD, Asst. Research Professor, Wake Forest School of Medicine, Div. of Public Health Science, Dept. of Social Sciences and Health Policy, Winston Salem, NC

Heidi Christensen, MTS, Associate Director for Community Engagement, U.S. Dept. of Health and Human Services, Office of Faith-based and Neighborhood Partnerships, Washington, DC

Tom Peterson, MDiv, Adjunct Instructor, Clinton School of Public Service; Principal, Thunderhead Works, Little Rock, AR

For more information about this chapter, contact **Teresa Cutts** at e-mail, cutts02@gmail.com or phone, (901) 643-8104.

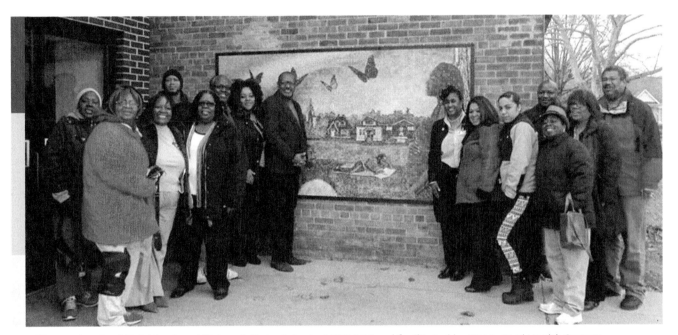

Women-Inspired Neighborhood Network-Detroit Project SNAP Mural facilitated by Henry Ford Health System

Population Health Screening Tools

Adverse Childhood Experience (ACE) Questionnaire Finding your ACE Score

While you were growing up, during your first 18 years of life:

1. Did a parent or other adult in the household often ...
   Swear at you, insult you, put you down, or humiliate you?
   or
   Act in a way that made you afraid that you might be physically hurt?
   Yes No If yes enter 1 _____

2. Did a parent or other adult in the household often ...
   Push, grab, slap, or throw something at you?
   or
   Ever hit you so hard that you had marks or were injured?
   Yes No If yes enter 1 _____

3. Did an adult or person at least 5 years older than you ever...
   Touch or fondle you or have you touch their body in a sexual way?
   or
   Try to or actually have oral, anal, or vaginal sex with you?
   Yes No If yes enter 1 _____

4. Did you often feel that ...
   No one in your family loved you or thought you were important or special?
   or
   Your family didn't look out for each other, feel close to each other, or support each other?
   Yes No If yes enter 1 _____

5. Did you often feel that ...
   You didn't have enough to eat, had to wear dirty clothes, and had no one to protect you?
   or
   Your parents were too drunk or high to take care of you or take you to the doctor if you needed it?
   Yes No If yes enter 1 _____

6. Were your parents ever separated or divorced?
   Yes No If yes enter 1 _____

7. Was your mother or stepmother:
   Often pushed, grabbed, slapped, or had something thrown at her?
   or
   Sometimes or often kicked, bitten, hit with a fist, or hit with something hard?
   or
   Ever repeatedly hit over at least a few minutes or threatened with a gun or knife?
   Yes No If yes enter 1 _____

8. Did you live with anyone who was a problem drinker or alcoholic or who used street drugs?
   Yes No If yes enter 1 _____

9. Was a household member depressed or mentally ill or did a household member attempt suicide?
   Yes No If yes enter 1 _____

10. Did a household member go to prison?
    Yes No If yes enter 1 _____

Now add up your "Yes" answers: _____ This is your ACE Score

SBIRT Screening Tools

PREFACE:

Would you mind if I ask you some personal questions that I ask all my patients?

These questions help me to provide the best possible care.

You do not have to answer them if you feel uncomfortable.

ALCOHOL: FREQUENCY

1. On average, how many days per week do you drink alcohol? (beer, wine, liquor)

ALCOHOL: QUANTITY

2. On a typical day when you drink, how many drinks do you have?

HEAVY EPISODIC DRINKING (HED)

3. In the last month: What is the maximum number of drinks you had in a 2-hour period?

DRUGS: ANY USE

3. In the past year: How many times have you used an illegal drug, or used a prescription medication for nonmedical reasons?

_____ **Drinking-Days per Week x** _____**Drinks per Day =** _____ **Drinks per Week**

NIAA GUIDELINES FOR LOW-RISK DRINKING

	Risky Drinking	Heavy Episodic Drinking (HED)
Men	> 14 drinks/week	5+ drinks in 2 hours
Women	> 7 drinks/week	4+ drinks in 2 hours
Pregnant	Any	Any

Audit

Box 4

The Alcohol Use Disorders Identification Test: Interview Version

Read questions as written. Record answers carefully. Begin the AUDIT by saying "Now I am going to ask you some questions about your use of alcoholic beverages during this past year." Explain what is meant by "alcoholic beverages" by using local examples of beer, wine, vodka, etc. Code answers in terms of "standard drinks". Place the correct answer number in the box at the right.

1. How often do you have a drink containing alcohol?

   (0) Never [Skip to Qs 9-10]
   (1) Monthly or less
   (2) 2 to 4 times a month
   (3) 2 to 3 times a week
   (4) 4 or more times a week

2. How many drinks containing alcohol do you have on a typical day when you are drinking?

   (0) 1 or 2
   (1) 3 or 4
   (2) 5 or 6
   (3) 7, 8, or 9
   (4) 10 or more

3. How often do you have six or more drinks on one occasion?

   (0) Never
   (1) Less than monthly
   (2) Monthly
   (3) Weekly
   (4) Daily or almost daily
   Skip to Questions 9 and 10 if Total Score for Questions 2 and 3 = 0

4. How often during the last year have you found that you were not able to stop drinking once you had started?

   (0) Never
   (1) Less than monthly
   (2) Monthly
   (3) Weekly
   (4) Daily or almost daily

5. How often during the last year have you failed to do what was normally expected from you because of drinking?

   (0) Never
   (1) Less than monthly
   (2) Monthly
   (3) Weekly
   (4) Daily or almost daily

6. How often during the last year have you needed a first drink in the morning to get yourself going after a heavy drinking session?

   (0) Never
   (1) Less than monthly
   (2) Monthly
   (3) Weekly
   (4) Daily or almost daily

7. How often during the last year have you had a feeling of guilt or remorse after drinking?

   (0) Never
   (1) Less than monthly
   (2) Monthly
   (3) Weekly
   (4) Daily or almost daily

8. How often during the last year have you been unable to remember what happened the night before because you had been drinking?

   (0) Never
   (1) Less than monthly
   (2) Monthly
   (3) Weekly
   (4) Daily or almost daily

9. Have you or someone else been injured as a result of your drinking?

   (0) No
   (2) Yes, but not in the last year
   (4) Yes, during the last year

10. Has a relative or friend or a doctor or another health worker been concerned about your drinking or suggested you cut down?

   (0) No
   (2) Yes, but not in the last year
   (4) Yes, during the last year

Record total of specific items here

If total is greater than recommended cut-off, consult User's Manual.

An AUDIT score ≥ 8 is recommended as an indicator of hazardous or harmful alcohol use, as well as possible alcohol dependence. Since the effects of alcohol vary with average body weight and differences in metabolism, establishing the cut off point for all women and men over age 65 one point lower at a score of 7 will increase sensitivity for these population groups.

Audit-C

Please circle the answer that is correct for you.

1. **How often do you have a drink containing alcohol? SCORE**
   Never (0)
   Monthly or less (1)
   Two to four times a month (2)
   Two to three times per week (3)
   Four or more times a week (4)

   _____

2. **How many drinks containing alcohol do you have on a typical day when you are drinking?**
   1 or 2 (0)
   3 or 4 (1)
   5 or 6 (2)
   7 to 9 (3)
   10 or more (4)

   _____

3. **How often do you have six or more drinks on one occasion?**
   Never (0)
   Less than Monthly (1)
   Monthly (2)
   Two to three times per week (3)
   Four or more times a week (4)

   _____

TOTAL SCORE
Add the number for each question to get your total score. _____

Maximum score is 12. A score of > 4 identifies 86% of men who report drinking above recommended levels or meets criteria for alcohol use disorders. A score of > 2 identifies 84% of women who report hazardous drinking or alcohol use disorders.

Patient Health Questionnaire (PHQ-9)

Over the last 2 weeks, how often have you been bothered by any of the following problems?
(Use "✔" to indicate your answer)

	Not at all	Several days	More than half the days	Nearly every day
1. Little interest or pleasure in doing things	0	1	2	3
2. Feeling down, depressed, or hopeless	0	1	2	3
3. Trouble falling or staying asleep, or sleeping too much	0	1	2	3
4. Feeling tired or having little energy	0	1	2	3
5. Poor appetite or overeating	0	1	2	3
6. Feeling bad about yourself — or that you are a failure or have let yourself or your family down	0	1	2	3
7. Trouble concentrating on things, such as reading the newspaper or watching television	0	1	2	3
8. Moving or speaking so slowly that other people could have noticed? Or the opposite — being so fidgety or restless that you have been moving around a lot more than usual	0	1	2	3
9. Thoughts that you would be better off dead or of hurting yourself in some way	0	1	2	3

FOR OFFICE CODING 0 + _____ + _____ + _____

=Total Score: _____

If you checked off any problems, how difficult have these problems made it for you to do your work, take care of things at home, or get along with other people?

❑ Not difficult at all
❑ Somewhat difficult
❑ Very difficult
❑ Extremely difficult

Developed by Drs. Robert L. Spitzer, Janet B.W. Williams, Kurt Kroenke and colleagues, with an educational grant from Pfizer Inc. No permission required to reproduce, translate, display or distribute.

PHQ-9 Patient Depression Questionnaire

For initial diagnosis:

1. Patient completes PHQ-9 Quick Depression Assessment.

2. If there are at least 4 ✔'s in the shaded section (including Questions #1 and #2), consider a depressive disorder. Add score to determine severity.

Consider Major Depressive Disorder

- if there are at least 5 ✔'s in the shaded section (one of which corresponds to Question #1 or #2)

Consider Other Depressive Disorder

- if there are 2-4 ✔'s in the shaded section (one of which corresponds to Question #1 or #2)

Note: Since the questionnaire relies on patient self-report, all responses should be verified by the clinician, and a definitive diagnosis is made on clinical grounds taking into account how well the patient understood the questionnaire, as well as other relevant information from the patient.

Diagnoses of Major Depressive Disorder or Other Depressive Disorder also require impairment of social, occupational, or other important areas of functioning (Question #10) and ruling out normal bereavement, a history of a Manic Episode (Bipolar Disorder), and a physical disorder, medication, or other drug as the biological cause of the depressive symptoms.

To monitor severity over time for newly diagnosed patients or patients in current treatment for depression:

1. Patients may complete questionnaires at baseline and at regular intervals (eg, every 2 weeks) at home and bring them in at their next appointment for scoring or they may complete the questionnaire during each scheduled appointment.

2. Add up ✔'s by column. For every ✔: Several days = 1 More than half the days = 2 Nearly every day = 3

3. Add together column scores to get a TOTAL score.

4. Refer to the accompanying PHQ-9 Scoring Box to interpret the TOTAL score.

5. Results may be included in patient files to assist you in setting up a treatment goal, determining degree of response, as well as guiding treatment intervention.

Scoring: add up all checked boxes on PHQ-9

For every ✔ Not at all = 0; Several days = 1;
More than half the days = 2; Nearly every day = 3

Interpretation of Total Score

Total Score Depression Severity

1-4 Minimal depression

5-9 Mild depression

10-14 Moderate depression

15-19 Moderately severe depression

20-27 Severe depression

Generalized Anxiety Disorder-7 (GAD-7)

Over the last 2 weeks, how often have you been bothered by any of the following problems?
(Use "✔" to indicate your answer)

	Not at all	Several days	More than half the days	Nearly every day
1. Feeling nervous, anxious or on edge	0	1	2	3
2. Not being able to stop or control worrying	0	1	2	3
3. Worrying too much about different things	0	1	2	3
4. Trouble relaxing	0	1	2	3
5. Being so restless that it is hard to sit still	0	1	2	3
6. Becoming easily annoyed or irritable	0	1	2	3
7. Feeling afraid as if something awful might happen	0	1	2	3

FOR OFFICE CODING 0 + _____ + _____ + _____

=Total Score: _____

Developed by Drs. Robert L. Spitzer, Janet B.W. Williams, Kurt Kroenke and colleagues, with an educational grant from Pfizer Inc. No permission required to reproduce, translate, display or distribute.

Updates from the Field

Approaching Social Determinants at the Population Scale by "Sewing Up the Safety Net"- Collaborating with Competitors to Save Infant Lives

The CEOs of four major health systems serving Detroit (Henry Ford Health System, Detroit Medical Center, Oakwood Healthcare System, and St. John Providence Health System) committed their organizations to find enduring, collaborative solutions to reduce the city's infant mortality—among the highest in the nation. In 2008, they commissioned the Detroit Regional Infant Mortality Reduction Task Force, under the leadership of Henry Ford's Kimberlydawn Wisdom, MD, to develop an action plan.

A true public-private partnership, the Task Force represents a range of expertise and perspectives, from clinical to community, and from programmatic to policy, environment and behavior change. The health systems bring the strength and size of their provider networks, and their ability to reach women and families at multiple points across the clinical spectrum. Public health leaders from state and local health departments provide population-based perspectives and a focus on the social determinants of health—racism and its relentless cascade of socioeconomic factors influencing the life course. Agency members provide further policy expertise and links to organizations conducting synergistic work. An equally important cadre of community partners—neighborhood organizations and stakeholder groups —joined the Task Force in designing an innovative grassroots approach.

The result—the $2.6-million grant-funded Sew Up the Safety Net for Women & Children—demonstrates place-based population health management; innovative, sustainable service delivery models; high-tech/high touch social marketing; provider education on the health equity framework; and institutional alignment—even amongst competing health systems.

Sew Up the Safety Net is funded by the Robert Wood Johnson Foundation, The Kresge Foundation, W. K. Kellogg Foundation, PNC Foundation, University of Michigan School of Public Health, and the four health systems.

Infant mortality is known as a "sentinel" health indicator—the infant mortality rate correlates with the health status of the community. In Detroit, infant mortality hovered around 14.4/1000 for the past three years, or about 200 babies each year who do not survive their first birthday. Higher than some developing countries and over twice the U.S. rate, these statistics are cogently painful when the racial health disparity of 15.9/1000 for black babies is compared to 5.6/1000 for white infants for the same period.

According to a 2009 survey conducted by the Detroit Regional Infant Mortality Reduction Task Force, many local programs and services to support women at risk for infant mortality were significantly underused. It was then that the Task Force conceived Sew Up the Safety Net, to tighten this loose web of disconnected medical, social, and community organizations into an accountable network of care.

The project works in three neighborhoods to connect women at risk for infant mortality with community health workers, known as Community & Neighborhood Navigators ("CNNs"), framed by three key objectives:

- The first objective centers on the CNN-participant relationship. Trained as community health workers by a specialist from the Detroit Department of Health & Wellness Promotion with additional education in maternal-child health, the CNNs mentor participants by helping them learn to navigate an array of socially and economically appropriate healthcare services, tailored neighbor¬hood resources, and phone and Web-based information. Moreover, the CNNs provide the vital validation that says "I believe in you" amidst the oft-discouraging, lonely life journeys that many young women in poverty describe facing. In turn, participants become empowered to link their own social networks to similar resources for long-term success and improved health and well-being of women, families (including men), neighborhoods and communities. Over three years, 1,500 women—375 pregnant and 1,125 nonpregnant women of childbearing age—will participate.

- The second objective is providing education on the health equity framework to 500 physicians and other healthcare professionals. Built on a tested, successful Henry Ford healthcare equity CME course, the interactive, challenging workshops are designed to improve awareness of health equity and racial disparities, result¬ing in increased understanding of how life's difficult circumstances impact health. Resources such as MIBridges and United Way 2-1-1 are shared in a case study approach. A train-the-trainer course also is being offered to expand provider education reach.

- The third objective is to establish technologically relevant products to engage the broader community in promoting good health status prior to and during pregnancy. Social media, a program website and text messaging are being used to connect women to the program, link to related services, and provide a virtual "living room" for sharing and learning. Project planners learned in early focus groups that the name "Sew Up the Safety Net" was not as relatable for the target population as for health professionals. A CNN proposed the new name, Women-Inspired Neighborhood Network Detroit (WIN Network Detroit) to very positive reception from program members, and it is now used.

At a neighborhood health fair, a CNN recruited "Sonya," 27, a single mom pregnant with her second child. The CNN learned that Sonya and her 5-year-old son "Derek" are "couch-homeless"—living with various relatives for short periods. Sonya opened up to the CNN about the hardships and disappointments of moving her life from house to house whenever a family member was "tired of having them." The CNN immediately referred Sonya and Derek to a shelter program that is assisting them with permanent housing. Sonya told her CNN that before her involvement with Sew Up the Safety Net, she felt lost and unsupported. Thanks to her CNN, she said she now "feels hope" and is making plans to become a registered nurse after her second child is born. Meanwhile, the CNN continues to mentor Sonya, connecting her with other needed resources including food, clothing, and a referral to a college counselor. In a sign of her growing sense of optimism and self-efficacy, Sonya has already enrolled in college classes.

While too early for reportable outcomes, as of February 2013, the project had enrolled more than 135 pregnant women and engaged hundreds of women who are pre-pregnancy or between pregnancies. Sew Up the Safety Net is measuring impact around three distinct yet interdependent metrics: 1) no preventable infant deaths among participants—with measures including the effectiveness of community-based referrals, increased social support, and behavior change; 2) knowledge and behavior change on equity-promoting strategies among the 500 healthcare professionals participating in health equity education; and 3) knowledge and behavior change on prenatal care, preconception health, interconception health, and access to community services via the social media campaign.

- Zero preventable infant deaths amongst program participants.

- Average birth weight of infants was 6.79 pounds with only 12% at low birth weight. 89% had full-term gestation.

- To date, 364 pregnant women and 900 non-pregnant women were enrolled in WIN Network programs.

- As of March 2015, 477 professionals participated in our healthcare equity training; 97% plan to incorporate the information learned in to their respective practices.

- Since launching our website in July 2013, we have had over 12,000 visits, and our Facebook page has grown to over 600 likes, reaching thousands of people in Detroit.

- The Detroit Regional Infant Mortality Reduction Task Force has received numerous awards and recognitions including but not limited to being featured in the University of Kentucky's national study on successful partnerships, the Jackson Healthcare Hospital Charitable Services Award, and a variety of journal, newspaper and television features.

Transforming a Forgotten Community

Bithlo is a semi-rural community in Orlando (FL) that resembles parts of Appalachia. Poverty is the norm for most of its 8,200 residents. The issues that segregate families of poverty in Bithlo are many and complex—and generational. Residents struggle each day with basic survival needs: food, clothing and shelter. Jobs are scarce, and the major industry is junk yards. There is no grocery store, barbershop, library gym, swimming pool, or place to earn a GED. At least 80% of the housing is in dilapidated trailers. Until recently, the nearest bus stop was nine miles along a busy highway with no sidewalks.

Bithlo also faces major environmental issues. Residents rely on well water because there is no public water or sewer. The well water is orange (from iron) and contaminated with known carcinogens from an old gas station and an eight-acre, 25-year-old illegal landfill.

In August 2009, a small 501c3 called United Global Outreach conducted a door-knocking campaign that sparked the "Bithlo Transformation Effort" that focuses on Education, Environment, Transportation, Health Care, Housing, Basic Needs, Building Community, Economic Opportunity and the Arts.

After discussion with UGO leaders, Florida Hospital adopted Bithlo as a local mission project in 2011. The hospital supports UGO's mission of "transforming forgotten communities into places in which we'd all want to live." Most importantly, the hospital committed to supporting UGO's efforts—rather than "taking over" or "doing it the hospital way."

Mitch was a homeless man who came drunk to one of UGO's community suppers. He was belligerent but ultimately begged a UGO volunteer to "please help me." UGO arranged for counseling but Mitch was arrested the next day.

When he was released from jail after a few weeks, Mitch was walking home to his tent in the woods. As he maneuvered along the shoulder of the busy highway that runs through Bithlo, Mitch was hit by a car and died.

Help came in time for another homeless man. James, too, lived in the woods; he is just 45 years old but was blind from cataracts and had lost his job and home. An ophthalmologist donated cataract surgery for both eyes. Today, James is back to his construction job and is a contributing resident of his community.

Helping individuals helps communities. After being an isolated, forgotten community for nearly 80 years, many of Bithlo's issues still loom large. But residents and partners are confident that attention to the root causes of poor health—the physical, built, economic and social conditions—are transforming the Bithlo community into "a place in which we'd all want to live."

- The area's first permanent medical clinic (an FQHC) opened.

- Other medical services include dental care, mental health and substance abuse efforts, vision services, and domestic violence counseling —all free to Bithlo residents.

- The Florida Department of Transportation is widening a dangerous bridge (with an 18-inch pedestrian walkway) in 2014 (instead of 2022).

- The road widening will allow county government to bring clean water to Bithlo.

- Bus service has been restored, and County Government committed to seven miles of sidewalks.

- Florida Hospital provided some dollars, and has leveraged relationships with its construction, fire system and other vendors to donate services. Hospital departments provide hundreds of hours of volunteer time.

- The hospital also serves as the fiscal agent for several grants, a much-needed dental grant that has leveraged over $1 million in dental services for the community.

- UGO operates a 40-student private school for Bithlo children who were not succeeding in public school.

The three-acre "Transformation Village" now anchors a sense of place to Bithlo, with a private school, a hydroponic garden, community meeting space, a library and computer lab, GED classes, social services and Medicaid enrollment, and more. The planned "Dignity Village" will be a small-home community for Bithlo's homeless residents.

Over 100,000 uninsured residents of Orange County have access to affordable primary and secondary care through a "Stone Soup" model that builds on existing assets and has spawned crucial new services.

The Primary Care Access Network (PCAN) was formed in 2001 as a cost-effective, family-friendly, integrated system of care for the county's uninsured residents. PCAN has 22 safety net providers: three hospitals, county government, 13 Federally Qualified Health Centers (FGHCs), a specialty care clinic, a chronic care medical home, five (free) volunteer clinics, the health department, respite care, and others.

PCAN started with a small indigent clinic serving 5,000 people at a cost of $10,000 per year. Today, PCAN serves 92,000 uninsured people 13 primary care medical homes, and over 10,000 secondary care patients—for just a few more dollars.

PCAN partner agencies bring their assets to the table—much like the children's book "Stone Soup" in which villagers add their own vegetables to a simmering pot of water and stones; the result is a pot of soup for everyone to share.

Like the villagers, PCAN builds on existing assets:

- PCAN partners provide nearly $70 million in donated care (excluding hospital charity care).

- The backbone of PCAN is a network of 13 FQHC medical homes and a strong case management effort.

- County Government puts $13 million per year into the state's Inter-Governmental Transfer (IGT) program, drawing down Medicaid match dollars for the two DSH hospitals.

- The DSH hospitals donate back the dollars through an interagency agreement:

  - Some dollars allow the FQHCs to see "additional" uninsured patients.

  - Other IGT dollars pay for non-volunteer specialty care and help support the free clinics.

  - All three hospitals write off needed surgeries and diagnostics as charity care.

- Other PCAN agencies rely on their "usual" funding sources as well as collaborative grants with other PCAN partners.

As new medical homes open, the hospitals see a drop in non-urgent, self-pay ER visits. In addition, Patients also benefit: the FQHC medical homes have seen a 68% decrease in blood pressure, an 83% decrease in cholesterol, and a 95% patient report of personal health improvement.

Informal "parking lot meetings" have generated new services and millions of additional grant dollars. Examples include the Congestive Heart Failure, Lung, Depression and Anxiety, and Family Medicine Residency clinics as well as chronic disease programs.

"Mary" has health insurance. A routine mammogram picked up a suspicious mass (so small it could not be felt) in her left breast, and Mary's family doctor referred her to a surgeon.

The surgeon ordered a diagnostic mammogram, followed by an ultrasound-guided biopsy that determined that the small mass was only pre-malignant. But the surgeon said that the lump needed to come out. Before surgery, he referred her for a breast MRI and then, for implantation of a single radioactive seed. Mary then went to pre-admission testing and finally, outpatient surgery where the seed and the mass were removed.

The co-pays for the five radiology procedures, three physician visits, pre-admission testing and surgery came to $3,700 – with insurance. What if Mary had not had insurance?

The PCAN specialty care clinic cares for women like Mary every day. For many of them, the cost of care frequently means delays in care and, sometimes, their conditions are more urgent and outcomes are not as good. PCAN partners know that their "stone soup recipe" nurtures thousands of low-income, uninsured people in Orange County, Florida.

Advocate Health Care provides a quarter of trauma care for Illinois, mostly unreimbursed. At Advocate Christ Medical Center, a Level 1 Trauma Center, physicians and staff began to recognize patients who were being admitted multiple times and partnered with Chicago-based CeaseFire, which has been effective in reducing community violence rates. The partnership offers services to trauma patients, their families, and communities, within an hour of a violent incident. Conversations happen when patients are willing and able to reflect on the import of retaliation and the cycle of violence they are caught up in. In Chicago, violence is a leading causes of death for people between 15-34 years. The majority are male, low income, young and minorities. This deadly violence is concentrated in communities with high unemployment rates, few business opportunities and limited social service resources. Repeat violent injury patterns are common. According to one study, after being victimized once, a person's risk of being violently re-injured is 1.5 to 2.4 times greater than an individual who has never been victimized. In communities where violence is an accepted method of resolving conflict, victims and their families are also highly susceptible to retaliation. In 2005, Advocate Christ Medical Center, a Level 1 Trauma Center, partnered with CeaseFire to develop the region's first hospital-based gun violence prevention project. CeaseFire, which works in five 'hotspot' communities that overlap with Christ Medical Center's service area, employs trained 'violence interrupters' and 'community-based outreach workers.' The violence interrupters—individuals who may previously have been in street gangs—use cognitive-behavioral methods to mediate conflict between gangs, and intervene to stop the cycle of retaliatory violence that threatens after a shooting. Professionally trained and credible, they are able to work effectively with highest-risk individuals to change thinking around violent behavior. The communitybased outreach workers provide counseling and services to high risk individuals in communities with high violence rates. The program builds on the strong role of chaplains already working in the Emergency Department as part of the trauma care team. When a gunshot victim is admitted, an Advocate chaplain alerts the hospital response coordinator, who is available 24/7, to their pending arrival. Hospital responders immediately work one-on-one with the victim, and family and friends, to diffuse tension and reduce the risk of retaliation. Responders are street-savvy individuals (many are ex-offenders) with strong community ties to the high-risk population. They leverage their network of contacts with CeaseFire 'violence interrupters' to mediate conflicts and squash retaliations. Dante, previously in a gang, forged a strong bond with the hospital case manager, whose own 'street history' allowed Dante to confide about serious family and social issues he faces in his transition away from the street activity. In the course of these conversations, the hospital case manager supported Dante, encouraging him to seek clinical care from a licensed therapist. Due to the stigma associated with mental health issues and treatment within his community, it would have been very difficult for another intervener to successfully connect Dante with the services needed. In 2011, the Christ CeaseFire Violence Prevention Project responded to a total of 580 incidents of violent injury and connected 298 patients to community-based violence interrupters. While unable yet to assess actual impact on costs, Advocate Christ Medical Center invested $120,000 in 2013 to support the case manager role. The program's success has led to its replication at two other Chicago trauma centers.

2016 UPDATE:

Interrupters in the Christ CeaseFire Violence Prevention Project responded to a total of 868 incidents of violent injury and made community-based resource referrals for 766 patients in 2015. Even though some patients were not immediately connected to an interrupter in the hospital, many of them end up working with the case manager later through the trauma clinic. While unable yet to assess actual impact on costs, Advocate Christ Medical Center invests $120,000 each year to support the case manager role. The program's success has led to its replication at trauma centers around the country.

Mission and Vision Statements

The Vision for Adventist Healthcare Ministry in North America*

...seek the peace and prosperity of the city to which I have carried you into exile. Pray to the LORD for it, because if it prospers, you too will prosper." Jer 29:7 NIV

I will bring health and healing to the city; I will heal my people and will let them enjoy abundant peace and security. Jer 33:6 NIV

I am come that they might have life, and that they might have it more abundantly. John 10:10 KJV

...the angel showed me the river of the water of life ... flowing from the throne of God and of the Lamb ... on each side ... stood the tree of life ... And the leaves of the tree are for the healing of the nations. Rev 22:1-3 NIV

...I have set before you life and death, blessings and curses. Now choose life, so that you and your children may live 20 and that you may love the Lord your God, listen to his voice, and hold fast to him. For the Lord is your life, and he will give you many years in the land ... Deut 30:19-20 NIV

"He sent them to preach the kingdom of God, and to heal the sick" Luke 9:2

"During His ministry, Jesus devoted more time to healing the sick than to preaching. His miracles testified to the truth of His words, that He came not to destroy, but to save." Ellen White, The Ministry of Healing

Introduction

Since the 19th Century, Seventh-day Adventists have been developing faithful, innovative approaches to health for the whole person. The successes of the past have laid the foundation for renewing a vision of faith-inspired healthcare in which patients experience seamless excellence, integrating the best of spiritually nurturing care. The challenges of providing health care in the 21st Century make the renewal of this vision imperative. The opportunities for leading our society, as it seeks to reform its health system, are unprecedented.

Developing new forms of collaboration between our Church and its health systems will open new channels for service throughout North America. By embracing the mission and core values we share, we will find new ways to bear witness to our Creator's love, and new avenues for vivifying the prophetic message of the Advent movement. The central convictions of this movement have caused us to plant healthcare institutions in the "furrow of the world's needs." Today, more people come into personal contact with Adventist ministry through our healthcare institutions than in any other way. These institutions, in cooperation with faith communities within their regions, can elevate the health outcomes for countless people with complex needs.

In this brief statement of vision, we express some of the theological and ethical convictions we believe are most essential for faithfulness in our Adventist health ministry. We know that clarity regarding these beliefs is necessary if we are to sustain genuinely faithful Adventist healthcare institutions that are strategically aligned with the mission of our Church.

Convictions

At its best, health care is mission-focused love in action. We believe that we have been created by our loving God as whole persons—each one a unity of body, mind, and spirit, capable of experiencing the joy of wholeness within relationships of trust. Healing ministry, as given to us by Jesus Christ, is the work of helping persons to regain their wholeness. This ministry includes careful attention to the physical, emotional, spiritual, and relational dimensions of a person's life. Such work is always more than business exchanges. Many of the persons who most need care are in socially complex circumstances and have little to offer in the exchange of commodities. We believe that all persons in need of healthcare, regardless of their social or economic status, are beloved of God. Each one presents us with a unique opportunity to serve our Lord Jesus personally.

We are committed to providing the highest quality of evidence-based health care in ways that nurture the human spirit and offer transcendent hope. Because of the vastness of medical needs in today's society, we are also committed to offering care that is efficient and cost-worthy. We are eager to advance effective, new approaches to disease prevention and health promotion. We are convinced that the establishment of trust is crucial to our work, so we are dedicated to principles of transparency and integrity in the communities we serve.

As we live by these convictions, we aspire to serve our Lord and our Church by finding creative approaches to healthcare ministry. Such approaches include developing partnerships between healthcare institutions and communities of faith enabling every congregation to be a center for health, healing and wholeness in the community. We can express this vision with a concluding invitation to imagine a world in which the communities we serve are blessed by the healthcare ministry to which our Creator has called us:

Imagine

- – Incarnational ministry ... becoming one with our community, knowing and understanding their needs and together striving to elevate their well-being.
- M – Making a tangible, measurable and meaningful difference in people's lives.
- A - Actions that are culturally competent, data driven, professionally developed and personally delivered.
- G - Geographically touching every community on this continent with the needed and helpful ministry of Healing.
- I – Inculcating integrative, grace-filled partnerships with community resources, thereby re-envisioning, re-energizing, and leveraging resources to meet the community's need.
- N – Network of congregations and healthcare institutions, partnering as the Church to educate, nurture and inspire a culture of wholeness.
- E – Evangelizing as Jesus did: Seeking first to fill the people's needs, He then invited them to follow Him.

American Muslim Health Professionals (AMHP) Mission Statement

MISSION

American Muslim Health Professionals (AMHP) was created with the intent of bridging the tenets of Islam with key public health issues facing our communities. AMHP aspires to be a leader in improving public health through efforts inspired by the Islamic tradition in three unique ways: 1) professional development of Muslims across health professions; 2) health education and community outreach; 3) state and national advocacy on issues of access and awareness. Over the past 11 years, AMHP has provided outlets for American Muslims who work in the healthcare sector to network and collaborate on issues that operationalize their faith by serving the community.

ACCESS TO HEALTH COVERAGE

AMHP believes that faith communities can and should be major partners in the movement to improve healthcare. It is for that reason that AMHP has spearheaded the "Connecting Muslims to Coverage" campaign for the last three Affordable Care Act (ACA) enrollment cycles. The campaign's objective is to help American-Muslims become informed about their health insurance options and obtain health insurance coverage through the open enrollment periods. The concepts of caring for ourselves and promoting the common good is central to our as well as other faith traditions. It is narrated that the Prophet Muhammad (PBUH) said that "your body has a right over you"; in other words, we have been entrusted with a physical body, and we have an obligation to take proper care of it.

American-Muslims are an especially critical group to target with regards to health insurance coverage since they are often composed of self-employed and under-employed individuals. As a result, they do not have the option of employer-sponsored coverage, which is one of the main avenues through which individuals obtain coverage for themselves and their families. To reach the diverse and widespread Muslim communities in the United States, AMHP hired a team of on-the-ground organizers independently working in their respective states to identify local mosques and community-based organizations where they can host enrollment and outreach events. This grassroots approach has been critical to reaching the uninsured American-Muslims.

Mental Health

Survey done with AMHP membership in 2012 indicated mental health literacy as an area of public health concern among Muslims in the U.S. In response, over the past few years, AMHP has conducted a Mental Health First Aid program for Imams and Chaplains, hosted a series of Mental Health Webinars in partnership with the Department of Health and Human Services and will be launching a series of events to help Muslim youth deal with issues of discrimination, trauma and alienation.

ENABLEDMUSLIM PROGRAM

Another avenue through which AMHP translates their faith into public health and social justice work that benefits the community is through the EnabledMuslim program. EnabledMuslim is an online community that offers spiritual and practical support for Muslims with disabilities and their loved ones. EnabledMuslim provides Muslims with access to relevant information about their situation and the ability to connect and sustain long-lasting relationships with others who have similar experiences. We estimate that there are approximately 600,000 Muslims with disabilities in the United States. Almost one-third of all families in the U.S. have at least one family member with a disability. Through our work with Muslims with disabilities and their loved ones, AMHP learned about some of the most common challenges and opportunities to best address them. It is reported that the Prophet Muhammad (PBUH) once said, "The believers, in their mutual mercy, love and compassion, are like a (single) body; if one part of it feels pain, the rest of the body will join it in suffering" (Sahih Bukhari).

CONCLUSION

For this reason, we believe that as American-Muslims, we have a moral obligation to address the health needs of our communities. As a small community in America (Muslims are roughly 2% of the U.S. population), it hurts us all when even a single brother or sister faces hardship.

Caring for Health: Our Shared Endeavor A Covenantal Rededication to Mission

Lutheran HealthCare, Brooklyn, NY

And what does the Lord require of you but to do justice,
love mercy, and walk humbly with your God."
(Micah 6:8)

PREAMBLE

Upon this, the 130th anniversary of Lutheran Medical Center and 10th anniversary of the adoption of the Evangelical Lutheran Church in America's (ELCA) Social Statement, "Caring for Health: Our Shared Endeavor", Lutheran Health Care (LHC) affirms its ongoing moral partnership in healthcare ministry with the church. As a direct expression of this relationship and our shared heritage, we will actively cooperate together in a vital social ministry of health, healing, and healthcare.

GUIDING PRINCIPLES

Consistent with the nature of this relationship, the integrity and autonomy of each partner is recognized, while at one and the same time an environment of shared mission is nurtured in which each partner acts upon the rich potential for cooperation. This posture recognizes that LHC and the ELCA are each fully responsible for their own management, operations, and financial affairs; further, each is ultimately accountable through its own governing bodies to its respective mission statements, constitutions, and by-laws.

In shaping its ongoing missional life, LHC continues to draw heavily on the ethical and theological framework found in the ELCA's Social Statement, "Caring for Health" (CFH). We reaffirm our shared mission and relationship with the church as being grounded in the following major tenets of that statement:

- Healthcare and healing are concrete manifestations of God's ongoing care for all of creation. (CFH, p.2)

- At the center of the Judaeo-Christian tradition and Jesus' ministry is love … in response to God's love, we work to promote the health and healing of all people. (CFH, pp. 2,18)

- Our commitment is shaped by the witness of Scripture, together with the church's historical and contemporary ministry in healing and health. (CFH, p. 2)

- Health is always a matter of both love and justice … caring for the health of others expresses both love for our neighbor and responsibility for a just society. (CFH, p. 1, p. 18)

- God creates human beings as whole persons—each one a dynamic unity of body, mind, and spirit … concern for health should attend to the physical, mental, spiritual, and communal dimensions of a person's well-being. (CFH, p. 3)

- Healing is restoration of wholeness … it is more than physical cure alone …. we can always care, even when we cannot cure. (CFH, p. 4, p. 15)

- We are committed to equitable access for all people to basic healthcare services. (CFH, p. 3)

- Patients and caregivers are more than consumers or providers; they are whole persons working together in healing relationships that depend on and preserve community … healthcare cannot be reduced to a commodity. (CFH, p. 6)

- Together, we commit to working for and supporting healthcare for all people as a shared endeavor. (CFH, p. 2)

- Caring for health affirms the diversity of our community and the values of its many religious and spiritual traditions. (CFH, p. 5, p. 14)

HALLMARKS OF PUBLIC HEALTHCARE MINISTRY

Just as a craftsperson identifies a work by a hallmark embedded in his/her product, so the work of Lutheran-affiliated healthcare has some essential, identifiable markers embedded in its public ministry of care and hospitality. While we believe that every act of genuine human care is an expression of mission, at LHC we will continue to commit to maintaining the following activities as both intrinsic and vital to our unique heritage, identity, and ongoing mission:

- Promoting an Institutional Climate of Compassionate, Whole-Person Care—one that informs and permeates all that we do and why we do it, including the vital interconnections of health and spirituality.

- Mission Awareness and Integration—intentional and purposeful ways of interpreting and actualizing mission, vision and core values.

- Ethics and Ethics Consultation Services—grounded in the shared core values of LHC and "Caring for Health", nurturing shared moral deliberation with/among all who serve and are served.

- Pastoral/Spiritual Care and Clinical Pastoral Education—including provision of chapel space and regular worship opportunities for persons of all faith expressions.

- Community Congregational Faith/Health Ministries—growing congregationally-based health ministry partnerships with local faith groups.

- Advocacy—active involvement in issues of healthcare justice, equitable access, governmental policy and reform.

- Heritage and Identity—preservation and interpretation of our story and archives as they continue to shape institutional identity and mission-driven service.

- Communication—regular contact with the church and all ministry partners for purposes of sharing vital information and nurturing relationships and cooperation.

National Baptist Congress of Christian Education, Health and Wellness Initiative

The National Baptist Congress of Christian Education Health and Wellness Initiative is a collaborative effort of National Baptist churches, medical professionals, and health related organizations committed to health outreach and prevention education (H.O.P.E.).

VISION

We see a day when all National Baptist churches will have vibrant health and wellness ministries resulting in members being good stewards of their health and wellness.

MISSION

We will achieve this vision by reaching across the depth and breadth of our denomination to inspire and enable our fellow National Baptists to commit to healthier lifestyles through

- health and wellness education;
- resource materials and services;
- support networks of trained resource persons and facilitators; and
- evidenced based outcomes assessment.

CHALLENGE

We want to make the NBCUSA the healthiest major denomination in America over the next ten years as measured by the ABCS (aspirin use for those needing it, blood pressure, cholesterol, and smoking cessation).

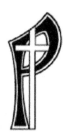

Hopes and Aspirations for Providence Ministries
From the Sisters of Providence, Mother Joseph Province

In establishing Providence Ministries as a public juridic person of the Roman Catholic Church, the Sisters of Providence take another step in our continuing journey with lay persons to provide leadership for the ministry. This is a significant step for our Sisters and our lay colleagues. We have no fixed blueprint for how to express the role and responsibilities of Providence Ministries other than by reading the signs of the time, trusting in Providence, and embracing our Baptismal call to follow Christ. Except for the requirements of canon law, there are but minimal requirements to provide the frame of hope and faith for the Sisters of Providence. We hope this document will capture some of that spirit and offer to future leaders our hopes and aspirations for the ministries we have been entrusted by the Church and blessed to lead for 153 years.

With confidence that our Providential God will continue to bless, guide and pray for you, we ask that you:

Remain Faithful to the Mission

Although expressed in different words in different times, we believe that our Mission as Sisters of Providence is to be the living expression and continuation of the Mission of Jesus. We have taken inspiration from the phrase, "Caritas Christi Urget Nos," which for us means that the love of Christ moves us, even compels us, to follow his example in providing healing, education and service to all we encounter, with a special concern for those who are most poor and vulnerable. Through compassionate service, we believe we continue the Mission of Jesus, bringing forth "the reign of God," helping to make our world a more just, peaceful and loving place for all. We understand this to be the Mission of Jesus so it remains our Mission, and we ask that it be held in trust as the continuing Mission of Providence Ministries.

We ask that you reflect often and deeply on this Mission so it may become a source of inspiration and strength for you and for all who participate in the work of Providence. Be mindful of the values Jesus expressed in the Gospels, and let those values guide all your actions. We hope you will develop regular practices of education and formation so that all who work in Providence Ministries understand the Mission and these values and find in them a source of personal inspiration. At the same time, we expect that you will continue our practice of inviting into this work people of good will who share our commitment to compassionate service and to our values, whether their individual religious and spiritual traditions are the same as or different from our own.

We expect Providence Ministries to be a voice for and a servant to those who are poor and vulnerable among us. This special concern for the poor is at the core of the Mission we share. Like Our Mother of Sorrows, we want to be a sign of compassion and hope to them. Drawing upon the example of St. Vincent DePaul, whose model of service we follow, we first called ourselves, "Daughters of Charity, Servants of the Poor." When Emilie Gamelin was dying, she called us to the virtues of Humility, Simplicity, and Charity as in the legacy of St. Vincent DePaul. In her final words, Mother Joseph also reminded her companion Sisters, "Whatever concerns the poor is always our affair ...". We offer the same words to the future leaders of Providence.

We hope you will also pay special attention to care for those who carry out the work of Providence. Our workplaces should always strive to model the values we profess and be places where each person is treated with dignity, respect, and justice. As you attend to the physical, mental, social, and spiritual needs of those we serve, pay equal attention to the same needs of those who serve in Providence. We must model in our own ministries the values we profess.

We ask you to pay particular attention to the spiritual needs of people. It is often those spiritual needs that make us most vulnerable and that are ignored by our society. Our tradition offers many resources that can help people. May Providence Ministries always be known as a ministry that attends, in a special way, to the spiritual dimension in our lives as well as the lives of those we are called to serve.

We ask that you be good stewards of all we have been given for this ministry—our people, our resources, and our earth. We have been blessed, particularly in Alaska, Washington, Montana, Idaho, Oregon, California, and El Salvador with an abundance of natural resources that have allowed our ministries to flourish. Yet our society has not always been wise in its use of our land, water, and air. We hope Providence will be a model of good stewardship that we may demonstrate faithfulness to our values and that others may learn sound stewardship practices from us.

We have always partnered with people of many faiths and expect the diversity within our ministries to grow in the future. Bringing together people of many backgrounds into a common ministry of service creates an important opportunity to build understanding and community. At the same time we must honor our own heritage and identity. As ministries of the Catholic Church, Providence Ministries is part of a larger community to which it must be faithful and with which it must be in regular dialog.

We expect Providence Ministries to ensure that Providence Health & Services engages in regular practices to help sustain its identity and to celebrate its heritage so the Mission and values come alive in all it does. Today we see evidence of this commitment in programs of formation of leaders, education for employees, rituals and celebrations, decision-making processes, and in many other ways. We hope these efforts will develop even more in the future. As Sisters we have understood that we cannot take for granted our heritage, Mission, or values. Only by responding to the call to education, and to the initial and continuing formation of the members, have we been able to continue our work over generations. We expect Providence Ministries to cherish the Mission and values and develop ways to assess the effectiveness of the people and practices required to sustain them.

To help keep our heritage alive, we expect Providence Ministries will see that our practice of maintaining the Chronicles is continued, preserving for future generations a written history of the good works of Providence Health & Services.

We hope you will also continue to embrace and tell the stories of those who have gone before us, women like Blessed Emilie Gamelin, Mother Joseph, Mother Bernarda, Venerable Mary Potter, and those other religious women, as well as lay men and women who have inspired us and on whose shoulders we stand. These are our ancestors. Honor them and let others know them so they too can draw inspiration from their lives. In your own time celebrate the living legacy of Providence as lived among your colleagues. In this way, Providence lives faithfully.

The Sisters of Providence have always responded to changing times, reaching out to those who are poor and vulnerable. It was this spirit of service that responded to the call of the Bishops to send the first Sisters of Providence to the Oregon Territory in 1852 and 1856. In the same way, Mother Joseph did not remain in the initial foundation in Vancouver but she and her small bands of Sisters continued to respond to serve needs of education, health care, and social services in Walla Walla and Montana that would otherwise have been unmet. Reaching out to new forms of service was done with complete trust in God's Providence as the Sisters moved forward making decisions that were never foolish, but did involve risk. They did all they could for success, but also trusted in Divine Providence. This tradition has continued as we established ministries for vulnerable people who are in need of housing, shelter from violence, education, and pastoral service in El Salvador.

This outreach or "missionary" spirit is fundamental to the Sisters of Providence and to our tradition in the Church. We expect that Providence Ministries will continue outreach to the poor as a central element of the work of Providence Health & Services, responding to emerging needs of the poor and using its resources to address them with wise stewardship, but also with a willingness to take risks. We expect them to reach beyond the borders of our own country as global citizens exemplified through the witness of Providence International Missions. Such efforts provide transformation, not only for the recipients of the services but also for Providence people who provide services.

In the future, collaboration with other Catholic ministries and organizations that share our values will continue to be strengthened. As transportation and communication bring us closer together, we hope Providence Ministries will embrace a spirit of collaboration, not competition, in service of the Mission. Stewardship of the resources of Providence, our communities, and our society require that we work with others to find new ways to advocate more effectively for the poor and to meet their needs and avoid wasteful duplication. We expect Providence Ministries to search for new ways to carry out the Mission, honoring Providence tradition, but not letting past practice constrict the vision of what is best for the future. Changing needs, social structures and institutions will require new and different responses. We expect that you will be open to the call of those who suffer by addressing emerging needs with wise and discerning responses so the poor and vulnerable may be served in new and more effective ways.

As Sponsor of Providence Health & Services, Providence Ministries will address the hopes and aspirations we have outlined through its collaborative work with the governing boards and management. We expect that all in Providence leadership will work to see that these relationships are healthy, creative, and collaborative. We know there will be disagreements on important matters, just as there always have been, but we know too that these will be resolved most effectively when all parties listen carefully to each other in a spirit of discernment and focus on what best serves the Mission.

Providence Ministries has reserved powers which it must exercise effectively. We do not see this as a mere formality. We expect that Providence Ministries will be fully engaged in those matters on which it exercises its reserved powers and that it will have the information and time for discernment needed to make wise decisions. Sponsor, board and management must work together to ensure the integrity of each role is respected in the decision making process.

Experience in other ministries has shown that the role of Sponsor can be viewed in two extreme ways. At one extreme the Sponsor passively receives recommendations and accepts them, but does not participate in identifying issues, placing issues within the context of the role of the ministry, or fashioning potential responses. At the other extreme the Sponsor is actively engaged in all significant matters, but does not distinguish its role as Sponsor from the essential roles of the board or of management. Providence has its roots in community that embraces collegiality, delegation, and respectful distinction of roles allowing each body in governance and management to experience their contribution to the common good. Similarly, we work in communion with the Church to advance the mission of Jesus to the world. We gather with discerning hearts, open to the direction of the Holy Spirit, while honoring those we have entrusted with authority.

We hope Providence Ministries will avoid both extremes and that sponsor, board and management will work collaboratively within their appropriate roles, supporting each other and bringing their special talents and perspectives to the common work. In this way the ministry will be best served, and each body will attract and retain committed and capable people who are willing to serve in the respective roles.

We recognize that organizational structures will evolve in Providence as they have in other ministries that have adopted new forms of sponsorship. We begin our journey as sponsors, both Sisters of Providence and Catholic laity for Providence Ministries. Providence Health & Services will continue to have a board of directors. We do not know whether this initial arrangement will best serve the ministry in the future, or whether some overlapping or more integrated structure would ultimately be preferable. We leave that to the good judgment of those who serve in those roles in the future, and we invite their ongoing assessment of how best to develop structures that will effectively serve the needs of the ministry. We also understand that Catholic ministry is being shaped to more effectively respond to the crying needs of our time. You will be challenged as well to respond to those who call out for our care and the hard choices will be there when our resources are constrained. However, as St. Vincent DePaul commended to us, "Love is inventive to infinity." Compelled by God's providential love, you will be invited to do more than you ever believed possible because of God's goodness and love of all.

CONCLUSION

We know that Providence Health & Services will thrive with the kind of leadership it enjoys today, and we expect that the leadership of Providence Ministries will be equally talented. With people of this caliber and commitment, Providence will continue the Mission for generations to come.

As we express our hopes for the future, we also express our gratitude to all the Sisters of Providence, Little Company of Mary Sisters and the lay women and men who have brought us to this day.

Providence of God, we believe in You.

Providence of God we hope in You.

Providence of God we love You with all our hearts.

Providence of God, we thank you for all.

Dated this 31st day of December, 2009

United Methodist Church
Theological and Historical Statement on Health and Wellness

Health is the ultimate design of God for humanity. Though life often thwarts that design, the health we have is a good gift of God. When God created humankind, God declared it to be very good (Genesis 1:31). Among Jesus' statements on the purpose of his presence is the statement that he came that we might have abundant life (John 10:10). Every account of Jesus' ministry documents how Jesus saw restoration to health as a sign of the Kingdom of Heaven becoming present amongst us. When John the elder wrote to Gaius (3 John 1:2), he wished for him physical health no less than spiritual. The biblical narrative is filled with stories of God's healing presence in the world. This includes spiritual, psychological, emotional, social, as well as physical healing.

For John and Charles Wesley, health was integral to salvation. In the Wesleyan understanding of salvation, Christ's self-giving on the cross not only freed us from the guilt of sin, but restored us to the divine image in which we were created, which includes health. John Wesley not only preached spiritual health, but worked to restore physical health among the impoverished people who heard his call. He wrote Primitive Physick,[1] a primer on health and medicine for those too poor to pay for a doctor. He encouraged his Methodists to support the health-care needs of the poor. Charles Wesley's hymns reflect early Methodism's awareness of spiritual health as a component of salvation.

ACHIEVING HEALTH

Health has, for too long been defined only as the absence of disease or infirmity. The World Health Organization took a more wholistic view when it termed health as "a state of complete physical, mental and social well-being."[2] We who are people of faith add spiritual well being to that list, and find our best definition in the biblical concept of "shalom." Shalom conveys or expresses a comprehensive view of human well being including "a long life of happiness ending in natural death (Gen 15:15)."[3] From the perspective of Shalom, health includes biological well being but necessarily includes health of spirit as well. From the perspective of Shalom, health is social harmony as well as personal well being, and necessarily presumes the elimination of violence. Thus the health that God wants for humanity both presumes and seeks the existence of justice as well as mercy, the absence of violence as well as the absence of disease, the presence of social harmony as well as the presence of physical harmony.

As disciples of the One who came that we might have life and have it abundantly, our first and highest priority regarding health must be the promotion of the circumstances in which health thrives. A leading health expert encourages the study of health not from the perspective of what goes wrong, but of what goes right when health is present. These "leading causes of life" include coherence, connection, agency (action), blessing, and hope.[4] Our lives are healthy when we are linked to a source of meaning, when we live in a web of relationships that sustain and nurture us, when we know we have the capacity to respond to the call God has placed on our lives, when we contribute to the affirmation of another at a deep level, and when we lean into a future that is assured, in this life and forever.

No one portion of the six billion members of God's global family has a monopoly on the expertise of achieving health. Achieving health, therefore, assumes mutual respect among the peoples of this Earth and the sharing of lessons learned in each society among the others.

Physical and emotional health is the health of the bodies in which we live, and we are therefore urged to be careful how we live (Ephesians 5:5).

As spiritual beings, our physical health affects our spiritual health and vice versa. St. Paul has termed our bodies as "temples of the living God (1 Corinthians 3:16; 6:16, 19-20), echoing Jesus himself (John 2:21). We therefore are stewards, custodians, managers of God's property: ourselves, our bodies, minds and spirits. Paul urges us to present to God our bodies as a living sacrifice and this is our spiritual worship (Romans 12:1, 2), and to do everything for the glory of God (1 Corinthians 10:31). When we honor our bodies and those of others, we are honoring God and God's good creation.

The biblical mandate has specific implications for personal care. We must honor our bodies through exercise. We must honor our bodies through proper nutrition, and reducing consumption of food products that we discover add toxins to our bodies, excess weight to our frames, and yet fail to provide nourishment. We must recognize that honoring our bodies is a lifelong process.

The second priority must be the correction of those circumstances in which health is hindered or thwarted. The interconnectedness of life is such that those things that diminish our health are most often things beyond the control of physicians, clinics, or insurers. The Ottawa Charter for Health Promotion identified the basic prerequisites for health as peace, shelter, education, food, income, a stable ecosystem, sustainable resources, social justice, and equity.[5] One estimate of factors influencing health gives medical health delivery only 10 percent of the impact; family genetics account for 20 percent of the variability in health, environment 20 percent, and lifestyle 50 percent.[6] John Wesley recognized the great influence of lifestyle on health and its impact on the ability to perform excellent ministry in his caution against works of supererogation,[7] "voluntary works-besides, over and above God's commandments to do more, for His sake, than bounden duty is required" highlight that faith-influenced lifestyle factors are a factor in health.[8] Thus the achievement of health requires attention to:

- Environmental Factors. Environmental factors include clean air, pure water, effective sanitary systems for the disposal of wastes, nutritious foods, adequate housing, accessible, people-oriented transportation, work for all who want to work, and hazard-free workplaces are essential to health. Environmental factors include not only the natural environment, but the spiritual environment, the social environment, and the political environment, including issues of war and peace, wealth and poverty, oppression and justice, environmental profiling and environmental racism. The best medical system cannot preserve or maintain health when the environment is disease-producing.

- Public Health Factors. Disease prevention, public health programs, and health education including sex education, appropriate to every age level and social setting are needed globally. Services should be provided in a compassionate and skillful manner on the basis of need, without discrimination as to economic status, mental or physical disability, race, color, religion, gender, age, national origin, language, or multiple diagnoses.

- Social Lifestyle Factors. Lifestyle factors detrimental to good health include inadequate education, poverty, unemployment, lack of access to food, stress-producing conditions which include such critical issues as domestic violence and other crimes and social pressures reinforced by marketing and advertising strategies that encourage the abuse of guns, tobacco, alcohol, and other drugs. Other societal pressures that affect health are overachievement, overwork, compulsion for material gain, and lack of balance between family/work responsibilities and personal renewal.[9]

- Spiritual Lifestyle Factors. A relationship with God, learning opportunities throughout life, personal renewal, recreation, green space and natural beauty add essential positive spiritual focus to life which influences health through fulfillment and positives attitudes of hopefulness and possibility.[10]

- Personal Lifestyle Factors. Those factors, which may be choices, habits or addictions destructive to good health include overeating or eating nonnutritious foods, substance abuse, including alcohol, tobacco, barbiturates, sedatives, and so forth. Failure to exercise or to rest and relax adequately is also injurious to health.

- Cultural Factors. Harmful traditional practices such as child marriage can result in serious health problems such as obstetric fistula[11] and the spread of HIV & AIDS. Other practices such as female circumcision can result in pain and the spread of infection.[12] Having multiple partners, a practice in many countries, has significantly increased the spread of AIDS and other diseases.[13]

The biblical view of health integrates the physical and the spiritual, and therefore both are needed in the achievement and restoration of health. In Western Protestant interpretation of health and healing, however, the union of the body and spirit is often dismissed. Cultures that respect and revere that union are often disregarded or looked upon in a condescending manner. Jesus did not make these distinctions, and the early church struggled with it. An illustrative narrative is that of the healing of the woman who suffered from a hemorrhage (Matthew 9:20-22).

She believed that touching his garment would make her well. He told her that her faith had made her whole, which includes physical wellness. We must, if we are to achieve good health, unite the body and spirit in our thinking and actions.

RESTORING HEALTH

The experience of ill health is universal to humankind. When environmental factors have contributed to ill health of body or mind, the restorative powers given to the body and spirit by God, even with the best medical care, will be severely challenged if the environmental factors themselves are not changed.

God challenges our global church, as God has challenged God's servants through the ages, to help create networks of care around the world for those who are sick or wounded. Global networks of care should emphasize:

1. health care as a human right[14];

2. transforming systems that restore health care to its identity as a ministry rather than as a commodity, and reforming those economic, financial and legal incentives to treat health care as a commodity to be advertised, marketed, sold, bought and consumed;

3. citizen leadership from the lowest levels to the highest in each society so that all can have active involvement in the formulation of health-care activities that meet local needs and priorities;

4. public financing mechanisms suited to each society that assures the greatest possible access of each person to basic health services;

5. advocacy care that engages the broader community in what the Ottawa Charter for Health Promotion terms the Five Pillars of Action: building healthy public policy, creating supportive environments that promote health, strengthening community action, developing personal skills, and reorienting health services[15];

6. health promotion and community health education that enables each person to increase control over his or her health and to improve it[16] and then to be a neighbor to another, in the fashion of the Good Samaritan, who took the steps that he could, simply because he was there (Luke 10:29-37);

7. primary care workers who are drawn from the community and are trained to assist with the most common illnesses, as well as educate about the impact that can be achieved by improving environmental factors, such as health and sanitation;

8. basic health services that are accessible and affordable in each geographic and cultural setting;

9. medical care when the degree of illness has gone beyond what can be assisted by primary health workers;

10. hospital care, compassionate and skilled, that provides a safe environment for surgery and healing from illness under professional care; and

11. complete and total transparency to persons (or their designees) under the care of a medical practitioner, of their medical condition, so they can be an active director in their own care.

THE CALL TO UNITED METHODISTS

Therefore, we call upon United Methodists around the world to accept responsibility for modeling health in all its dimensions. Specifically, we call upon our members to:

- continue the redemptive ministry of Christ, including teaching, preaching, and healing. Christ's healing was not peripheral but central in his ministry. As the church, therefore, we understand ourselves to be called by the Lord to the holistic ministry of healing: spiritual, mental emotional, and physical;

- examine the value systems at work in our societies as they impact the health of people and promote the value of shalom in every sphere;

- work for programs and policies that eliminate inequities around the world that keep people from achieving quality health;

- work for policies that enable people to breathe clean air, drink clean water, eat wholesome food, and have access to adequate education and freedom that enable mind and spirit to develop;

- make health concerns a priority in the church, being careful not to neglect the special issues of gender or age, treatment or prevention;

- collaborate as the body of Christ through establishment of networks for information sharing and action suggestions; and

- work toward healthy societies of whole persons.

    o Part of our task is to enable people to care for themselves and to take responsibility for their own health.

    o Another part of our task is to ensure that people who are ill, whether from illness of spirit, mind, or body, are not turned aside or ignored but are given care that allows them to live a full life.

- o A related obligation is to help society welcome the sick and the well as full members, entitled to all the participation of which they are capable.

- o People, who are well, but different from the majority, are not to be treated as sick in order to control them. Being old developmentally disabled, mentally or physically disabled is not the same as being sick. Persons in these circumstances are not to be diminished in social relationships by being presumed to be ill.

- o We see this task as demanding concern for spiritual, political, ethical, economic, social, and medical decisions that maintain the highest concern for the condition of society, the environment, and the total life of each person.

In addition, we call upon specific entities within our United Methodist connection to take steps toward health and wholeness as follows:

CONGREGATIONS

United Methodist congregations are encouraged to:

- organize a Health and Wholeness Team as a key structure in the congregation. Among the team's responsibilities would be to seek each member to develop their spiritual gifts in order that the body of Christ be healthy and effective in the world. The apostle Paul commented that "many are sickly and die among you" (1 Corinthians 11:27-29, NRSV). We suggest that this may have resulted not simply from failing to discern the body of Christ present in the communion bread, but from failing to discern the body of Christ as the congregation. When church members are not allowed to use their spiritual gift, they stagnate or die spiritually and the spiritual affects the physical health of the individual. The spread of health and wholeness should be discerned clearly as a guiding factor in why it is that we make disciples;

- accept responsibility for educating and motivating members to follow a healthy lifestyle reflecting our affirmation of life as God's gift;

- become actively involved at all levels in the development of support systems for health care in the community; and

- become advocates for a healthful environment; accessible, affordable health care; continued public support for health care of persons unable to provide for themselves; continued support for health-related research; and provision of church facilities to enable health-related ministries.

ANNUAL CONFERENCES

We encourage annual conferences to:

- continue their support and provision of direct-health services where needed through hospitals and homes, clinics, and health centers;

- work toward a comprehensive health system which would provide equal access to quality health care for all clergy and lay employees, including retirees;

- undertake specific actions to promote clergy health, physical, mental, emotional and spiritual; and

- support the establishment of Health and Wholeness teams in every congregation.

Seminaries

We call on our United Methodist theological schools to:

- become involved in a search for Christian understanding of health, healing, and wholeness and the dimensions of spiritual healing in our congregations. Include coursework that will train clergy not only in pastoral care, but also in intentional caring of the congregation that promotes the physical and spiritual health of each church member; and

- work toward a comprehensive health system that would provide equal access to quality health care for all clergy and lay employees of seminaries, including retirees.

EDUCATIONAL AND HEALTH CARE INSTITUTIONS

We call on our United Methodist colleges, universities, hospitals, and seminaries to gain an added awareness of health issues and the need for recruitment and education of persons for health-related ministries who would approach such ministries out of a Christian understanding and commitment.

GENERAL AGENCIES

We call on:

- the General Board of Discipleship to develop educational and worship resources supporting a theological understanding of health and stewardship of our bodies;

- the General Board of Church and Society and General Board of Global Ministries to support public policies and programs that will ensure comprehensive health-care services of high quality to all persons on the principle of equal access; and

- the General Board of Pension and Health Benefits to undergird the social teachings of the Church by enacting policies and programs for United Methodist employees that ensure comprehensive health-care services of high quality to all persons on the principle of equal access.

BIBLIOGRAPHY

1. Wesley, John, Primitive Physick: Or, An Easy and Natural Method of Curing Most Diseases. (London: J. Palmar, 1751).

2. World Health Organization. Constitution of the World Health Organization, Geneva, 1946.

3. Richardson, Alan, A Theological Word Book of the Bible, New York: MacMillan,1950, p. 165.

4. Gunderson, Gary and Larry Pray, The Leading Causes of Life, The Center of Excellence in Faith and Health, Methodist Le Bonheur Healthcare, Memphis, TN, 2006.

5. Ottawa Charter for Health Promotion, cited in Dennis Raphael, "Toward the Future: Policy and Community Actions to Promote Population Health, in Richard Hofrichter, Editor, Health and Social Justice: Politics, Ideology, and Inequity in the Distribution of Disease. San Francisco: Jossey-Bass, 2003.

6. Daughters of Charity National Hospital System, 1994.

7. Supererogation is the technical term for the class of actions that go "beyond the call of duty, obligation, or need." Merriam-Webster dictionary (2007 online version). 2004 Book of Discipline ¶ 103, Section 3, Our Doctrinal Standards and General Rules, Article XI, p.62.

8. Wesley, John, Article XI, United Methodist Book of Discipline, Doctrinal Standards and General Rules, 2004.

9. Supererogation is the technical term for the class of actions that go "beyond the call of duty, obligation, or need." Merriam-Webster dictionary (2007 online version). 2004 Book of Discipline ¶ 103, Section 3, Our Doctrinal Standards and General Rules, Article XI, p.62.

10. CAM at the NIH Newsletter, National Center for Complementary and Alternative Medicine, National Institutes of Health (US), Vol. XII, No.1, 2005. Various research and ongoing research; see www.nccam.nih.gov/health.

11. C. Murray and A. Lopez, Health Dimensions of Sex and Reproduction. Geneva: World Health Organization, 1998. Obstetric fistula is a rupturing of the vagina and rectum causing persistent leakage of feces and urine. It is a health risk commonly associated with child marriage because of the mother's physical immaturity at the time of childbirth. (Source: International Center for Research on Women) A majority of women who develop fistulas are abandoned by their husbands and ostracized by their communities because of their inability to have children and their foul smell. It is estimated that 5 perecent of all pregnant women worldwide will experience obstructed labor. In the United States and other affluent countries, emergency obstetric care is readily available. In many developing countries where there are few hospitals, few doctors, and poor transportation systems, and where women are not highly valued, obstructed labor often results in death of the mother. (Source: The Fistula Foundation)

12. Hosken, Fran P., The Hosken Report: Genital and Sexual Mutilation of Females, 4th rev. ed. (Lexington (Mass.): Women's International Network News, 1994.

13. Multiple Partners and AIDS UNAIDS, Practical Guidelines for Intensifying HIV Prevention: Towards Universal Access, March 2007-03-19.

14. UM Social Principle ¶ 162V, Book of Discipline, Nashville: United Methodist Publishing House.

15. Ottawa Charter for Health Promotion, cited in Dennis Raphael, Toward the Future: Policy and Community Actions to Promote Population Health, in Richard Hofrichter, Editor, Health and Social Justice: Politics, Ideology, and Inequity in the Distribution of Disease. San Francisco: Jossey-Bass, 2003.

16. World Health Organization, 1986.

ADOPTED 1984

AMENDED AND READOPTED 2000

AMENDED AND READOPTED 2008

Resolution #3203, 2008 Book of Resolutions

Resolution #109, 2004 Book of Resolutions

Resolution #96, 2000 Book of Resolutions

See Social Principles, ¶¶ 162V and 165C.

From The Book of Resolutions of The United Methodist Church - 2012. Copyright © 2012 by The United Methodist Publishing House. Used by permission.

CPSIA information can be obtained
at www.ICGtesting.com
Printed in the USA
BVOW07s0031270516

449745BV00004B/15/P